# PHARMACOETHICS

## A Problem-Based Approach

DAVID A. GETTMAN, R.Ph., M.B.A., Ph.D.
Wilkes University
Wilkes-Barre, Pennsylvania

DEAN ARNESON, Pharm.D., Ph.D.
Nova Southeastern University
Fort Lauderdale, Florida

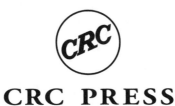

## CRC PRESS

Boca Raton   London   New York   Washington, D.C.

## Library of Congress Cataloging-in-Publication Data

Gettman, David A.
    Pharmacoethics : a problem-based approach / by David A. Gettman and Dean Arneson.
       p. cm. — (CRC pharmacy education series ; 16)
    Includes bibliographical references and index.
    ISBN 1-58716-035-8 (alk. paper)
       1. Pharmacy—Moral and ethical aspects—Problems, exercises, etc. 2. Pharmacy—Moral
and ethical aspects—Case studies. I. Arneson, Dean. II. Title. III. Series.

RS122.5.G48 2003
174′.2—dc21                                                                 2002041505

This book contains information obtained from authentic and highly regarded sources. Reprinted material is quoted with permission, and sources are indicated. A wide variety of references are listed. Reasonable efforts have been made to publish reliable data and information, but the author and the publisher cannot assume responsibility for the validity of all materials or for the consequences of their use.

### Visit the CRC Press Web site at www.crcpress.com

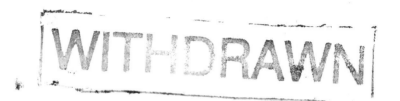
# PHARMACOETHICS

## A Problem-Based Approach

# CRC PRESS
# PHARMACY
# EDUCATION
## SERIES

# Dedication

---

*This book is dedicated to our families and our students, who have helped keep us open-minded and forever young.*

# *Preface*

About 20 years ago, the University of New Mexico School of Medicine (SOM) established a student-centered problem-based learning (PBL) curriculum emphasizing ambulatory care practice competencies. It was designed for small groups of students working together and ran parallel with their more traditional curriculum. The SOM faculty pioneered difficult changes that also paved the way for changes at the SOM's affiliated College of Pharmacy (COP).

Subsequently, other COPs (e.g., at Samford University) have faced the difficult challenge of conversion of their curriculum. Those teachers who have undertaken to embrace this new type of learning usually have done so on the basis of a personal educational philosophy that was in line with student-centered problem-based learning. To many pharmacy professors, their students may have seemed bored and dissatisfied with their professional education and viewed the process as difficult and with irrelevant "hurdles" that have to be overcome to become a registered pharmacist. Students may have had too much emphasis on memorization and seemed to forget readily what was taught them.

The method you are asked to use for learning has a strong influence on how well you will be able to recall and apply what you have learned in the "real world" outside your COP. Problem-based learning can better help you become an independent thinker. It can help you reason through your patient's problems and recall and apply what you have been taught in your COP to care for your patients. Finally, it can help you learn new information, as you need it, and keep your knowledge and skills contemporary.

About the same time that the University of New Mexico Health Science Center was developing its student-centered problem-based learning curricula, it also developed, under the care of Dr. Miriam McIver Gibson, a set of seven clinical ethics competencies for its School of Medicine, College of Nursing, and College of Pharmacy students: (1) professional responsibility, (2) patients' rights, (3) privacy and confidentiality, (4) truth telling, (5) reproductive ethics, (6) distributive justice, and (7) research ethics. In addition to this list of clinical ethics competencies, another list was developed specifically pertaining to research ethics competencies: (1) history; (2) principles, standards, and regulations; (3) integrity in science; (4) research on human subjects; (5) research/testing on animals; and (6) contemporary issues.

Unfortunately, the student-centered problem-based learning cases at the University of New Mexico COP have excluded discussion of these important clinical ethics competencies and research ethics competencies and have instead focused on those competencies specific to the tenets of clinical and basic science.

More recently at the University of New Mexico, there has been the development of the innovative Center for Alcoholism, Substance Abuse, and Addictions (CASAA). It is here that pioneers like Dr. William R. Miller and Dr. Theresa B. Moyers have been able to effectively utilize motivational interviewing in tandem with the transtheoretical model to help vulnerable individuals with destructive behaviors overcome ambivalence and attain more positive outcomes. Again, regrettably, the student-centered problem-based learning cases at the University of New Mexico COP have excluded discussion of these innovative intervention techniques (in addition to the important clinical ethics competencies and research ethics competencies discussed above) and have instead continued to focus on competencies specific to the tenets of clinical and basic science.

All three of these important developments (in student-centered problem-based learning, in clinical ethics competencies and research ethics competencies, and in behavior change using motivational interviewing) at the University of New Mexico have converged here with the development of this innovative book. This book should in no way be construed as an innovation of the authors, but rather as the confluence of the original developments of those professors mentioned above.

Therefore, in summary, the purpose of this book is to have you more effectively focus and learn important clinical ethics competencies and research ethics competencies using student-centered problem-based learning. And, unlike most textbooks on ethics that concentrate on ethical principles and ethical decision making, this textbook goes one step further and tries to help you learn how to utilize motivational interviewing techniques effectively with the people involved to help everyone work through difficult ethical situations to attain more positive clinical, behavioral, and social outcomes.

# Acknowledgments

We are grateful and indebted to five individuals: David B. Brushwood, J.D., University of Florida, who has generated a profound interest among all of his students in pharmacy law and ethics; Paul L. Mann, Ph.D., University of New Mexico, who provided helpful suggestions for those sections of this book involving student-centered problem-based learning; Miriam McIver Gibson, Ph.D., University of New Mexico, who added clarity to both the clinical ethics competencies and the research ethics competencies that are the foundation for this book; and, William R. Miller, Ph.D., and Theresa Moyers, Ph.D., University of New Mexico, who made many important comments involving motivational techniques that have been incorporated into the book.

# About the Authors

**David A. Gettman** received his bachelor of science in pharmacy from the University of Montana, Missoula; his master of business administration from the College of William and Mary, Williamsburg, Virginia; and his doctor of philosophy in pharmacy health care administration from the University of Florida, Gainesville. He has practiced pharmacy for over 20 years in numerous settings: retail, hospital, nursing home, hospice, and military. Dr. Gettman is a military veteran of two wars: he was a naval hospital corpsman stationed with the Marine Corps during the Vietnam War, and he was an Air Force pharmacist in support of the Persian Gulf War. As a lieutenant colonel, Dr. Gettman is presently an Air Force Reserve officer attached to the 45th Space Wing at Patrick Air Force Base, Florida. Dr. Gettman has held academic positions at the University of New Mexico, Nova Southeastern University, and most recently at Wilkes University. He has made over 70 presentations to professional groups at the state, national, and international levels; most of these presentations involved research in pharmacoethics. Dr. Gettman has belonged to more than 20 professional associations, including the American Society for Pharmacy Law and the Association of American Colleges of Pharmacy, for which he recently served as chair of the Ethics Special Interest Group.

**Dean L. Arneson** received his doctor of pharmacy degree, master of science, and doctor of philosophy in pharmacy administration from the University of Nebraska Medical Center. He has been a licensed pharmacist for more than 20 years and has practiced in numerous settings: retail, hospital, and as a consultant. Dr. Arneson has held academic positions at the University of Nebraska, Ferris State University in Big Rapids, Michigan, and Nova Southeastern University in Fort Lauderdale, Florida, where he has served as Assistant Dean for Student Academic Affairs and is currently Associate Professor and Chair of the Department of Pharmacy Administration. He has taught courses in pharmacy law and ethics for more than 10 years and has made many presentations on various topics to professional groups at the state, national, and international levels. Dr. Arneson belongs to various professional associations including the American Society for Pharmacy Law and the Association of American Colleges of Pharmacy, for which he recently served as chair of the Ethics Special Interest Group.

# Introduction

This book represents the answer to a perceived need present in many colleges of pharmacy. Too often, pharmacoethics has been the smaller part of a traditionally taught semester-long pharmacy law course. However, with the advent of problem-based learning, faculties are starting to reexamine their curricula. More specifically, these faculties are starting to understand the ill-structured nature of clinical situations that involve pharmacoethics and/or the use of behavioral interventions. It then becomes easier to understand why student-centered problem-based learning sessions involving the competencies discussed in this book should be conducted in tandem with a more traditional course in pharmacy law.

Most semester-long pharmacy law courses are constrained to a 16-week period. Depending on the college-specific situation, the pharmacy law professor may wish to drop the last two sessions on the list presented in the table of contents, which concern contemporary issues (germline therapy and medical surveillance), and instead devote one session on the shorter list to each week. Alternatively, some sessions with material in common (e.g., research on human subjects and research on animal subjects or unethical experimentation and research principles) may be "doubled up" in a specified week.

Care should also be taken by the law professor to draw associations between the topics discussed in the law course and the problem-based learning sessions. For example, on the week the pharmacy law professor is covering the Omnibus Budget Reconciliation Act of 1990 requirements, it might be prudent for the PBL groups to be working on the professional responsibility PBL session. Or, on the week the pharmacy law professor is covering the dispensing of medications, it might be prudent for the PBL groups to be working on the distributive justice PBL session.

The book begins with four introductory chapters, which discuss the following: (1) the student-centered problem-based learning process, (2) the challenge of our patients' clinical and behavioral problems, (3) the challenge of our patients' ethical issues, and (4) student-centered problem-based learning cases that involve clinical and behavioral problems in the context of ethical issues. The goal of these four introductory chapters is to help "paste together" a framework for conducting the different problem-based learning sessions that revolve around a list of ethical competencies. This framework is displayed next and should be followed by each PBL group member to help optimize personal understanding of each ethical competency. To skip one or more steps in this framework would be unproductive and would "short-circuit" the thoughtful process required to develop the intended educational outcome: a critical set of patient-related skills necessary to practice the profession of pharmacy.

## Framework for Conducting Student-Centered Problem-Based Learning Sessions Involving Ethical Competencies

### Objectives

### Introduction

#### Part one of case narrative

Make a list of the major problems presented in the case.

For the problems in the list, give a cause or a reason for them to happen.

Make a list of learning issues in the form of questions. The goal is to gather the medical, social, and all other relevant facts that might apply to the case.

Look in the local medical library and on the World Wide Web for helpful information.

Identify all relevant values that play a role and determine which values (nonmaleficence, beneficence, respect for persons, loyalty, distributive justice), if any, conflict.

#### Part two of case narrative

List the options open to you. That is, answer the question, "What could you do?"

Choose the best solution from an ethical point of view, justify it, and respond to possible criticisms. That is, answer the question, "What should you do, and why?"

Two group members "role-play": determine the different ways of thinking among people involved and possible techniques for conflict management.

Two group members "role-play": determine how the stages of change and motivational interviewing techniques might help solve the major problem presented in the case.

#### Part three of case narrative

Conclusions: what was learned from the case?

Written or oral feedback to problem-based learning session participants.

# Contents

*chapter one*

# The student-centered problem-based learning process

## The purpose of the problem-based learning cases

The problem-based learning (PBL) case sessions articulated in the appendices to this book have their roots in cases found in the literature for the past 30 years. These PBL cases have been put together to extend your learning experience to ethical problems that might not become available to you during your clinical rotations. Each PBL case contains a real legal case that will be disclosed to you in three staggered fragments. At the end of each of these fragments you will be asked to decide which questions you might ask the other person involved and which tasks you should perform.

The intent of the student-centered PBL discussion in this chapter is to challenge you to understand how to deal effectively with the ethical and behavioral problems that you will have to face in your future pharmacy practice. Most of the information in this chapter is based on the pioneering work of Barrows (see Barrows, 1994, 2000; Barrows and Tamblyn, 1980) and the practical experience of the faculty at the School of Medicine at the University of New Mexico (UNM) (see Mennin et al., 1996). The problems presented also revolve in an innovative way around concepts and principles relevant to pharmacoethics, motivational interviewing, ways of thinking, and conflict management.

Unfortunately, the term *problem* can be narrow in its implications for your learning; it wrongly suggests that it is problems of individuals that are exclusively used. It should be kept in mind that these are not the only problems you must face in your work as you also must understand and work with the more "macrolevel" problems of the community of individuals your pharmacy serves.

Before tackling the PBL cases in this book, it is essential to know what your objectives are or what you hope to accomplish so you can achieve your expectations. The primary objective of the 18 competency-related problem-based learning cases is to make you a more competent pharmacist who can solve ethical and behavioral problems. Therefore, as you consider such an undertaking, you will have to consider carefully the kind of pharmacist you want to become. The methods used in these cases emphasize the development of those abilities, skills, and attitudes you will need during your future pharmaceutical health care practice. The rationale for student-centered problem-based learning as an educational method will become apparent when your educational goals are carefully considered.

Our deeply beloved democratic society has two fundamental expectations of you — a future pharmacist. These are:

1.  Monitoring the medication-associated clinical and behavioral health care problems of your patients in an effective, efficient, and ethical manner. *Effective* monitoring means that your problem-solving skills must be sufficiently developed to facilitate the choice of an appropriate pharmaceutical health care plan. The pharmaceutical health care plan you choose must be designed to provide the most effective care possible, to improve the patient's outcome, and to meet the expectations and needs of the patient with the least risk and cost. *Efficient* means that the care of your patient must be cost effective. This aspect of pharmaceutical health care becomes even more important in our nation's trend toward controlling health care costs. *Ethical* means that you must have cultivated certain observable communication skills that will invoke confidence, trust, and satisfaction. Your care needs to be sensitive to the patient's particular concerns, values, cultural needs, and finances.
2.  Lifelong pharmaceutical health care learning to meet the often unique and changing needs of patients and the problems they present, to face the changing problems and demands of health care systems, and to keep up to date in the practice of the pharmacy profession. The increasingly complex use of drug entities, the ever-changing knowledge of disease processes, the increasingly complex ethical issues related to these advances, and the dramatic changes in information management and health care delivery systems make the task of self-education essential. It is not helpful to have your mind full of facts if you cannot apply them to the care of your patient. A requirement that you must have a rich and extensive knowledge foundation does not address the primary concern that the knowledge must be tailored to your particular patient's circumstances to make a real difference.

## The fundamentals of student-centered learning

You must cultivate the ability to continue learning throughout your entire professional life to meet the often unique and changing needs of patients and the problems they present, to face the changing problems and demands of the health care system, and to keep contemporary in the practice of the profession of pharmacy. Unfortunately, many practicing pharmacists may not have kept up with the developments in their profession, and their skills may have become outdated and potentially dangerous. This may lead to pharmacists losing their licenses or undergoing civil or criminal litigation.

## Self-monitoring

You should be able to monitor your progress with a patient's problem continuously and should note points at which you may be puzzled or lack sufficient knowledge or skills. This requires deliberate awareness of how well you are handling different aspects of each patient's problem or the appropriateness of the pharmaceutical health care plan you have undertaken.

## Self-assessment

In addition to monitoring your performance, you should be able to determine if your functioning is appropriate for your level of training and experience and for the type of patient problems you are encountering. It might become too easy for you later in your practice to just ignore a patient's problem or to refer the patient to the patient's physician and then serve your next patient without considering whether the care of the first patient was sufficient. Of greater concern might be that you might not even be aware of the inadequacies in your work with your patients and that you do not ask for help when it is warranted.

## Defining learning needs

Once inadequacies are recognized in your abilities, these weaknesses should be translated into defined learning needs so that the appropriate learning resource can be identified. What specific areas of information or skills do you need to augment?

## Determining the appropriate learning resource

You should determine which available learning resource would be the most effective and practical for your defined learning needs to obtain up-to-date and accurate information (e.g., from textbooks, peer-reviewed journal articles, computerized information resources, videotapes, computer programs, mentor pharmacists, and accredited continuing pharmaceutical education courses).

## Using the resource effectively

It is one thing to select the right resource; it is quite another to use the same resource effectively. This is particularly true with computerized information resources. Even the effective and efficient use of a library or a reference book requires you to develop certain skills.

### Evaluating the accuracy and value of resource information

It is important for you to question the findings or opinions of your patient's physician. You should evaluate the validity of any conclusions drawn. You should be knowledgeable about the methods used to generate findings or opinions in a printed article. This is increasingly important with the availability of computer databases that, unlike those in the library, are often not peer reviewed.

### Recording or filing the information for future reference

Once information has been obtained, you should have a systematic way to file it for future reference so it can be conveniently found when you need it again.

### Applying what has been learned to the present patient problem and future problems

You have to apply what has been learned to the care of your patients. You must assume responsibility for your future learning. To do this, these unique skills need to be developed and practiced under your instructor's guidance and assistance while in pharmacy school. Student-centered problem-based learning that is self-directed should become a habit so you remain contemporary in your practice and meet the changing problems presented by patients.

The skills required to overcome ethical and behavioral problems and the skills required for student-centered problem-based learning will need to be practiced and feedback given so you achieve the competencies expected of a registered pharmacist. Knowledge acquired in pharmacy school will have to be recalled and applied to the care of your patients.

## The five-step student-centered problem-based learning process

The use of the 18 patient problem cases later in this book will help you utilize specific reasoning processes to achieve your clinical ethics and research ethics competencies. This is the most defining characteristic of student-centered problem-based learning. There have been many studies of this reasoning process (see Norman and Schmidt, 1992; Vernon and Blake, 1993). Most have shown that, when encountering an unfamiliar, difficult, complex, and ill-structured problem, the expert will use a hypothetico-deductive reasoning process. The significance of terms like *unfamiliar*, *difficult*, or *complex* is important here because experts who work repeatedly with the usual and straightforward problems in their fields might tend to take certain shortcuts with these problems. This happens only after working through problems many times before using the hypothetico-deductive process. Undoubtedly, you might have taken shortcuts with repetitive problems and do not think through all possibilities. Instead, you might plunge into what you believe to be the heart of the matter. However, this forward thinking can lead you to err if the problem encountered has unusual features not detected in your shortcut.

The following steps are identifiable in the hypothetico-deductive process: generation of multiple hypotheses, inquiry strategy, data analysis, data synthesis, and preliminary development of a pharmaceutical health care plan. The manner in which you use each stage to meet the challenge of your patient's problems will be stressed with each stage. The emphasis here will be on acquiring this complex skill in pharmacy school to ensure that you can provide effective, efficient, and ethical pharmaceutical health care to your patients.

Most ethical and behavioral reasoning activity occurs quickly and almost unconsciously for experienced pharmacists. However, on reflection, most pharmacists will recognize the presence of these steps.

## *Step 1: The generation of multiple hypotheses*

As soon as you listen to your patient during an encounter and ask a few questions to clarify a problem, you will almost automatically generate hypotheses. These hypotheses are brought to mind by associations with the patient's complaint and a number of other observations, such as the patient's sex, age, and behavior. These hypotheses could be explanations of the patient's problem. The hypotheses have also been called hunches or ideas. Whatever they are called, each represents a label for a collection of facts assembled in your mind. Usually, two or more hypotheses are generated. Among these is the worst-case scenario possible with the patient's complaint; even if remote, it cannot be overlooked. The other hypotheses usually represent the most likely hypotheses, especially conditions that are treatable with medications.

These hypotheses, generated in your head at the outset of the encounter, set the boundaries for your search for more information. Since there is not enough information initially for you to develop a pharmaceutical health care plan for the patient, a guide is needed to determine what additional information is needed. The potential boundaries for information about a patient problem are enormous, and hours could be spent asking all questions possible of your patient. This would be very impractical and tiresome. Hypotheses provide you with guidelines to the kinds of information on a pharmaceutical health care record that would be of most benefit in establishing care decisions.

Hypothesis generation is the creative aspect of patient problem solving. It is an inductive thinking activity used by the experienced pharmacist to think of the possible conditions that might be suggested by the patient's problem.

## Step 2: Inquiry strategy

Using the hypotheses generated as a guide, you need to carry out an inquiry to obtain more data from the patient that will support or weaken these hypotheses. The energy of this inquiry is fueled by taking the patient's medication history. Inquire about the observations that would be expected with the hypotheses considered as well as observations that would tend to separate alternative hypotheses. This is disciplined, logical, deductive, problem-oriented reasoning. An efficient inquiry strategy is of paramount importance when time is limited, as it often is in the real world of pharmacy practice, and there is no time to ask all possible questions.

Mixed together with this problem-oriented inquiry is a more menu-oriented inquiry used when obtaining information about the patient's prior health and family history and to uncover other bits of data that could suggest problems other than those suspected. This inquiry does not require careful reasoning and is mostly a matter of memorizing lists of questions. To provide time to think further about the patient's problem and consider other hypotheses, you also need to use this menu-driven inquiry.

As described, with the ill-structured problems that a patient presents, more information needs to be obtained to understand the patient's problem, and there is no one right way to obtain that information. Hypotheses serve as suggestions to what might actually be responsible for your patient's problem. Therefore, they are a guide to the kinds of clinical and behavioral information needed and the use of a logical deductive inquiry to get the information that will identify the most likely hypotheses. If this is done correctly, the ill-structured problem is efficiently and effectively tackled.

## Step 3: Data analysis

As your patient provides answers to questions and information is obtained for the pharmaceutical health care record, new information beyond that initially present becomes available. As new information is obtained, you have to analyze it against the hypotheses considered. Does it strengthen or weaken any of the hypotheses being considered, or does it suggest a new or unsuspected hypothesis?

## Step 4: Data synthesis

When this ongoing analysis of newly obtained information suggests that the information is significant in terms of understanding or caring for your patient's problem, it is added to the information you are accumulating in your mind about the patient's problem. This growing mental representation of the patient's problem is more than a collection of the important facts learned about the patient during the patient encounter. You organize these facts in a cause-and-effect relationship that suggests the chain of events that led to the patient's present problem and the clinical and behavioral issues responsible. This synthesis records the present and changing shape of the structure of the patient's problem. It is a vehicle for communication between you and other health care practitioners.

In describing a patient's problem to another health care professional for consultation or new ideas, you might present this synthesis in a concise way. The physician with whom you are consulting might incorporate that synthesis and will generate hypotheses based on different experiences or expertise. The physician might say, "Have you thought of so and so?" (hypothesis), or "Did you ask such and such a question or perform such a test?" (inquiry strategy) based on hypotheses generated as a listener. The lack of a synthesis to organize the oral presentation of your patient's case is a frustrating experience because it might make the presentation sound like an immeasurable jumble of facts.

These are the elements of clinical and behavioral reasoning with which you must struggle concerning the patient's ill-structured problem: inductive reasoning, followed by deductive reasoning (hypotheses/inquiry), analysis, and synthesis. This is not necessarily a linear process, as might be suggested by the description above. Inquiry might lead to a blind alley, and new hypotheses need to be generated. An unsuspected finding might suggest new hypotheses. Menu-driven inquiry might need to be employed to find new clues about the problem when problem-based inquiry fails to substantiate the hypotheses considered. The initial hypotheses might be too broad to initiate any care plan, and more refined hypotheses might need to carry the inquiry further.

## Step 5: Preliminary development of a pharmaceutical health care plan

You will have to come to a decision about developing the patient's pharmaceutical health care plan. The time in the encounter it takes to do this relates to the time you have available and the urgency of your patient's situation. Many activities can be sacrificed with time pressure, such as chatting with your patient to get to know the patient as a person, checking into family and personal sociodemographics, reviewing your patient's symptoms again to be sure they are understood, and beginning to carefully develop a pharmaceutical health care plan. The decision to end the encounter is also determined by the impression that no additional helpful data can be obtained from your patient or the patient's caregiver during the present session, or that enough data of sufficient specificity have been obtained to develop your patient's pharmaceutical health care plan. Despite all the ambiguities that might be present and the need for more data for certainty, you will have to make a decision and act. Your patient cannot be told that her or his problem is not well enough understood at this time and to come back later.

This process is well adapted to the challenge of the ill-structured problem-based learning cases in which you cannot be sure that a particular patient's pharmaceutical health care plan is the most perfect one. You have to face ambiguities and insufficiency of data and make decisions on the basis of prevalence, probability, treatment of the treatable, and awareness of the worst possibilities that could be present.

## Metacognitive skills

The term *metacognitive skills* refers to thinking about your own thinking. It is deliberation or pondering and is the direct opposite of impulsivity. Metacognition is the hallmark of the expert pharmacist: "Do I have the right ideas?" "What questions should I ask next?" "Can this pharmaceutical health care problem be put together differently." "Is there something I need to learn to understand my patient's medication-related problem better?" "What would be the correct laboratory tests to order?" These are metacognitive thoughts.

Metacognition is the hallmark of the expert pharmacist when a patient problem is difficult or unusual. It is a skill you must develop in guiding your reasoning process. As mentioned, this reasoning process is often not apparent to you because it is performed almost below awareness and is often executed quickly and nearly automatically. Only when you are confronted by a patient problem that is unusual, difficult, or confusing are you aware of contemplating the problem. This can occur only by actually considering alternative hypotheses, questions that should be asked, laboratory tests that should be ordered (inquiry strategy), reviewing the findings obtained (analysis), or puzzling about what may be going on with the patient (synthesis).

In fact, as mentioned, experienced pharmacists may be so familiar with certain common, recurrent patient problems that they may take quick short-cuts to establish and care for their patient's problem. This has been called using heuristics, rules of thumb, or forward reasoning (the hypothetico-deductive method is considered backward reasoning). However, put an unfamiliar or troublesome problem in front of the experienced pharmacist and you will see metacognition and the hypothetico-deductive process.

The presence of the hypothetico-deductive process may also be unapparent to those watching you perform because they do not know what is actually going on in your mind. The observer can only guess as to the hypotheses being entertained by the questions you ask of your patient. You may jump back and forth from a problem-oriented inquiry to a menu-driven inquiry as you are thinking, and the observer never knows which questions are hypothesis related. The observer also does not know how the data you obtain are being analyzed. Techniques such as asking you to talk aloud during the patient encounter or interviewing you about your thinking immediately after the patient encounter can be helpful in analysis of your reasoning.

## Objectives of student-centered problem-based learning

The 18 problem-based learning cases later in this book ask you to learn by working in the context of an individual patient's medication-related problems. The problems are presented to you in formats that allow you to apply the clinical and behavioral reasoning skills required in the practice of pharmacy. In doing these cases, you will discover which information needs to be learned to understand fully the delicate issues that may surround a patient's problem and the communication skills responsible for helping solve potential patient medication-related problems. In student-centered problem-based learning, you also learn to become responsible for your learning, defining what needs to be learned and the appropriate resources to use (faculty, consultants, books, monographs, peer-reviewed journal articles, computerized information sources, etc.). You will apply what you have learned to the problem at hand and to future problems.

# Requirements of student-centered problem-based learning

This section describes eight things required to prepare for student-centered problem-based learning.

## Student facilitators

Student facilitators have the responsibility of smoothing the progress of student learning in the small group. The role of the student facilitator is like that of a dance instructor who encourages excellence in performance through active guidance from the sidelines. These facilitators should be elected by the members of each PBL group.

Student facilitators must receive training. The success or failure of student-centered problem-based learning could easily rest on the preparation and training of student facilitators since their skills are central to the delivery of the material. The universal experience of all PBL curricula is that the skill of the facilitator is essential to success. This role is central to the students' abilities to achieve the educational goals and outcomes possible with problem-based learning. The skillful facilitator will assist fellow students in developing effective clinical and behavioral reasoning skills, acquire a solid clinical and behavioral knowledge base, become effective student-centered self-directed learners, take control of their own learning, and enjoy the whole process. Skillful student facilitators will also be able eventually to decrease their presence and allow the other members of the group to carry on the process.

The ideal group size is five to seven students. Fewer than that and the amount of pooled knowledge the group can bring to the problem and the value of different points of view and approaches to a problem are seriously reduced. If the group is larger than seven students, it becomes difficult for the student facilitator to keep track of all students and for all students to have a chance to express their particular point of view at all stages of work with the problem. Also, the group's working sessions become longer to allow for each student's ideas and comments in all discussions.

## Faculty consultants

Faculty consultants are pharmacy professors who have agreed to be available to students during their student-centered study as a source for references and for information from their particular area of expertise (e.g., basic science, pharmacy practice, pharmacy administration). Discussions with consultants can be with you, with you and other students, or with the entire PBL group.

Sometimes, PBL groups will ask a faculty consultant to provide needed information in the form of a lecture to. Such a student-requested lecture is perfectly appropriate as it represents student-centered learning. In any discussions with a consultant, it is expected that you will have already carried out your own preliminary study in the areas of your questions. The consultant should question you and others about what you have researched prior to the consultation and ask you enough questions about the topic to see what you already know so that the information given can be tailored to your needs. If the consultants find that you have not done enough prior study, they can suggest references that you ought to read before talking to them.

The consultants indicate the times during the week that they are available to consult with you and how they can be contacted. It is best if they plan to do interruptible work during their scheduled hours so that they get work done if you do not show up. Sometimes, consultants find that they are constantly being contacted about the same subject by different groups of students. This can be alleviated if the consultant puts together a learning resource that covers the subject for student referral. Then, you can come to the consultant if there are still unanswered questions.

### Problem-based learning cases

In problem-based learning cases, the problems present themselves to you in the same way and with the same information that would be available in a real situation. All case formats are designed to allow you to ask the patient any question you feel appropriate in any order — just as in a real situation. In any case simulation, you are never told that a question is inappropriate or would never be asked in a real situation or that no information is available.

The 18 cases in this textbook make use of knowledge about patients and their disease processes. The issues involved need to be discussed by your group members to create answers that would be obtained during development of a pharmaceutical health care plan. Therefore, as in a real situation, you are able to ask inappropriate questions and obtain the responses that would occur with an actual patient. This ensures that the simulations offer the ill-structured problems that your real patients offer and provide the same challenge to clinical and behavioral reasoning.

### Standardized patients

Standardized patients are actors trained to present an actual patient's problem in a manner so convincing that you cannot differentiate the actors from actual patients. Standardized patients can also be members of your problem-based learning group who take the part of the patient during role playing. Each of these people should be interviewed as an actual patient.

The standardized patient allows you to learn and practice developing the pharmaceutical health care plan and communication and interpersonal skills as you work through the problem.

Standardized patients may or may not be actual patients, but they are trained always to present a patient problem in a very real and consistent manner. The so-called time-in, time-out technique allows the standardized patient to be used for clinical and behavioral teaching in the PBL group format. One student takes on the role of the pharmacist and begins the patient interview. Whenever other students or the student facilitator wish to discuss what is going on in the patient problem and to analyze their thinking about the problem at the moment, a time-out is declared. At this time, the standardized patient remains in the role as far as appearances go, but will not respond to any questions while the PBL group discusses what they are thinking about the case. The standardized patient's subsequent performance will continue unchanged or unaffected by any comments made as if the time-out period and discussion had never occurred, continuing when time-in is declared as if no time had passed since the time-out.

## Sequential patient cases

The sequential patient case format, in one variation or another, is used in all 18 of the problem-based learning cases. The patient problems are unfolded in staggered segments. Following each segment, and before going to the next, you will have to discuss what you feel is going on with the patient, generate hypotheses, and decide which questions you would like to ask the patient to substantiate the correct hypothesis if possible. The initial segment usually provides more information than would have been provided when the patient was first encountered in the pharmacy. You then advance to the next segment and read more information about your patient.

You might never learn from the case what you would have discovered with the conduct of your own investigation of your patient. Instead, you passively follow the unfolding of the case as written later in this book, done by the authors of the PBL cases. As you work through your sequential patient case, the new information obtained can be analyzed in the light of the hypotheses that have been generated, and new ones can be generated if appropriate.

Each of the 18 sequential patient cases will not present the same challenge to the clinical and behavioral reasoning skills that would be provided by a real patient. Each case cannot be expected to be an appropriate vehicle for encouraging effective and efficient clinical and behavioral reasoning skills as an objective in problem-based learning. However, the sequential patient case is easier to produce and requires less time to work through in the PBL group. This is probably the main reason for the case format's popularity. It does provide more of a challenge to reasoning than a complete printed case vignette or history.

## Room assignments

Each PBL group should have its assigned room for the group meetings and study. This room provides you with a meeting place for your work. It is where you can bring personal belongings, books, notes, charts, and work materials. The rooms should have a table large enough for you and other PBL members and the student facilitator because it serves as a meeting place for the PBL group and student facilitator to work through the cases and for you to work and study. There should be a large chalkboard, computer access (with informatics capability and connection to the World Wide Web or health science library, if possible).

## Learning resources

In problem-based learning, you determine what you will need to learn as you work through the patient's problems. The challenge of the problems coupled with your awareness of your knowledge deficiencies help you decide what you need to learn. A health sciences library and the pharmacy faculty are major resources. As no textbooks are prescribed in problem-based learning, you are free to use whichever texts you find most helpful. Extra copies of texts that might commonly be used can be put on reserve in the library. The printed resources of the library are enhanced by computer-based information sources (such as Medline and International Pharmaceutical Abstracts) and computer-aided materials (e.g., Epocrates® on your personal digital assistant). Librarians should be alerted and prepared to assist you with information searches so that you can learn the most effective and efficient ways to obtain up-to-date and accurate information from the library.

## Schedules

There should be no schedules in problem-based learning except for the time of the initial orientation for students and student facilitators and weekly unit meetings of students and student facilitators to pass on announcements and to deal with concerns and complaints. All other scheduling should be left to each PBL group to work out because of the following six considerations:

1. The challenge of each problem varies with the background knowledge of students in the PBL group and their particular interests. A problem in a particular case may require more hours to complete (e.g., the problems in the first case). Later, other problems may require fewer hours as knowledge accumulates in the discipline of pharmacoethics.
2. The problem-based learning sessions may vary in length, depending on the discussions, background, and interests of the PBL group members and the issues developed in the group.
3. The type and number of learning issues that each PBL group identifies can vary widely.

4.  It may take a day or two for you and your other PBL group members to obtain and use all the learning resources required for one problem; for another PBL group, this might take only a few hours.
5.  Some learning issues may require more time to accomplish, depending on the availability of faculty or distance involved in obtaining information.
6.  Most important, flexibility in the group's schedule allows each student facilitator to schedule PBL group meetings. PBL groups can meet in the early morning, evenings, or whenever works best for all the members of the group. Each group must be able to schedule its own time for PBL group meetings throughout each week.

# Activities of student-centered problem-based learning

There are 13 activities that the PBL group and student facilitator will have to go through with each problem-based learning case.

## When the small group first meets

At the start, you should be randomly assigned to a PBL group. It is therefore likely that you will not have worked with the other PBL group members before and will not know one another very well. These initial activities are designed to let the members of the group get to know each other, to become comfortable talking with each other, and to set the stage for the PBL group to work as a team.

You are asked to introduce yourselves to the others in the group, covering such areas as college or university attended prior to pharmacy school, majors or studies undertaken, other activities that would be of interest, reasons for going to pharmacy school, anticipated career in pharmacy after graduation, hobbies, and interests. The others in the group are invited to ask questions of each student or comment on anything the student might have said.

This accomplishes a number of important things for the group. It gives each member the opportunity to be recognized as an individual with an interesting and unique background and future expectations. This obviates the need for members in the group to let the others know about themselves through comments and behaviors that can be disruptive during the PBL group process. It also lets group members find areas of common background and interests, facilitating communication and teamwork in the group. It allows each member of the group to recognize the talents and interests of the others and whose particular experiences or expertise might be valuable as a resource.

## Climate and roles

The active learning climate in student-centered problem-based learning is quite different from that in conventional pharmacy curricula. In conventional pharmacy curricula, if you do not know the answer, you should be passively quiet and hope you are not chosen to comment. This is counterproductive if you are to become an effective self-directed learner.

In problem-based learning, you have to admit when you do not know something or are unsure. This is basic to the realization that you need to learn and what you need to learn. In problem-based learning, you are encouraged to say freely whatever is on your mind. In this way, you can find out if what you think or believe is correct. If you hold back from speaking because you are not sure you are right, you may avoid providing a valuable insight or contribution. The student facilitator has to set the stage and make it clear that you and the other members of the group should say whatever is in your minds and freely admit when you do not know something.

There also needs to be a climate of free and open exchange of points of view. The student facilitator stresses the need for each member of your group to speak up when there is disagreement with what is being said by someone else in the group; this includes disagreement with whatever the student facilitator might be saying. The rule must be established that if someone remains silent after a contribution by a member of the group it means that the individual does not have a different opinion or information and agrees with what is being said. It is one thing to say these things and another to be sure they are carried out in your group. The student facilitator must be certain that all comments are respected. The student facilitator must also be sure that all points of view are heard, and that no one dominates your group's ideas.

The student facilitator should review the role of the facilitator with your group. The members of your group should understand that the student facilitator is there to guide them through the problem-solving process and to challenge your group's thinking by asking the members to explain their ideas. The student facilitator must challenge students by asking "Why?" again and again regardless of whether the student facilitator personally feels that a particular student is right or wrong; this is to probe the ability of the student to support or define what the student is saying. The student facilitator should do everything possible to keep the members of your group from knowing his or her opinion. The student facilitator will not provide knowledge to the group about any aspect of the problem even though the facilitator might know the answer to the problem under discussion. As the members of your PBL group gain confidence about how to reason through a problem, the student facilitator will play a smaller and smaller role.

The members of your PBL group must understand that, although the student facilitator should help guide them through the group's problem-based learning cases and student-centered self-directed learning process, the student facilitator also has the responsibility of managing the group's process. The members of your group must challenge each other when they feel statements made by others are not correct, when they feel that the group process is going in wrong directions, or when there are interpersonal problems developing in your PBL group. The student facilitator should eventually become unnecessary.

In the first session with a problem in the problem-based learning case, you and your PBL group take on the problem without prior preparation. This may be difficult for you to accept. You may feel that you do not have sufficient knowledge to begin solving patient problems. You may feel you would do far better if you first gathered some clinical or behavioral information concerning pharmacoethics. There may be a tendency for you to want to have lectures and assigned readings for a period of time before work with the PBL cases begins.

However, as reassuring as such prior preparation might be, there are a number of reasons why it is inappropriate and ineffective in problem-based learning. Taking on the problem as an unknown allows you to discover what you already know or understand about the problem. You have information in your head that may only be recalled in certain contexts and by certain associations. You may have little appreciation of what you already know in your long-term memory from your prior education or prior experiences. The stimulus of a patient problem will often bring to mind information that may actually be a surprise to you.

This ability of the problem to bring forth prior knowledge has two advantages for learning. It indicates areas of information that may not need to be pursued in self-directed study related to the PBL case. More important, the knowledge pulled forth from memory provides a springboard for new knowledge acquired during study, ensuring better recall. Also, the activated knowledge already in long-term memory can enhance the understanding of the related new knowledge that will be acquired by you in self-study.

Most important, taking on the problem as an unknown also allows you to realize what you need to learn to understand and resolve the problem. This is a motivating stimulus in problem-based learning. You become puzzled and challenged by the problem and want to obtain the information needed to understand it. Motivation is further enhanced by the realization that this is the kind of problem you will have to face in the near future as a pharmacist.

The last, and perhaps most compelling reason, for encountering the problem first without prior information is that this is the way you will have to function as a pharmacist for your entire professional life. The patient's problem always comes as an unknown, and you will have to work as far as possible with the problem on the basis of knowledge already possessed.

## Problem-based learning group objectives

When your PBL group sits down to work on one of the 18 problem-based learning cases, it will be essential that you and your PBL group members all agree on the tasks that are to be undertaken. A discussion of PBL group objectives is a way to focus your PBL group's tasks on your work with your patient problems. Any patient problem could raise a wide range of learning issues, from clinical issues to the possible behavioral issues involved. One problem could consume the entire semester.

Therefore, it is important that your PBL group focus on the specific objectives you would like to accomplish with the problem. This is important because it is all too easy for you to become engrossed in the clinical aspects of the problem and forget the behavioral issues that might surround it. A criticism that could be leveled at problem-based learning is that it allows you to play the expert prematurely, and therefore you do not acquire a solid foundation in pharmacoethics. However, it is also appropriate for your PBL group to extend or modify your objectives based on areas of learning about which they are concerned.

A printed set of objectives helps your PBL group agree on the appropriate objectives. The student facilitator must get your group to recognize what the group expects to accomplish in your learning experience and agree on your objectives because this sets the focus for the discussions in your PBL group. If you agree on learning in a certain area, then the problem solving, the hypotheses raised, the understanding of the problem that is developed, the learning issues agreed on, and your group's self-evaluation will be guided by those agreed-on objectives. In accepting problem-based learning, your group should understand that it means going deeper than the "black box" level and going to the roots of the problem as appropriate in your learning issues and study.

When your PBL group becomes immersed in a problem, you often become carried away by the many interesting things that develop, and interests and concerns surface that are peripheral to the agreed-on goals. When this happens, and it is recognized by the student facilitator or one of the members of the PBL group, the agreed-on objectives can be used as a reference point for rethinking the direction of your discussions and learning. Sometimes, it is quite appropriate for your PBL group to revise your goals when you get into the problem and realize that other objectives might be productively pursued in your learning. Setting objectives may seem awkward to your PBL group initially, but it becomes routine when your group realizes it is essential for keeping your work focused and efficient.

## *Mechanics*

When the problem-based learning case is used by your group, there needs to be a large chalkboard next to your PBL group. The chalkboard should be divided into four areas, the last smaller than the rest. One large division entitled "ideas" is where the hypotheses generated by your group about the problem are listed. The next large division is entitled "facts," and it is where information generated from the case and which seems important and relevant to the hypotheses are listed (problem synthesis). The last large division, entitled "learning issues," is where the questions, confusions, and areas of ignorance that emerge during work with the problem and that need to be clarified or learned are listed. The small division is entitled "future actions," and it is where actions that your PBL group wants to carry out in the future are listed as a reminder.

One member of your PBL group (not the student facilitator) should be picked to be the scribe for your group. Your scribe's task is to keep track of your PBL group's process using the board. The scribe lists hypotheses in the idea column as members of your group generate them. The scribe also records the salient facts about the patient that relate to the hypotheses in the facts column and lists the learning issues identified by your group as you work with the problem in the learning issues column. Your scribe is encouraged to abbreviate. Your scribe is also cautioned not to interject personal ideas by altering the way your group's ideas are translated to the board.

It is a difficult job to be the scribe and at the same time be a member of your group. The task should be rotated, and the others in your group should be certain that your scribe's ideas are expressed in all discussions. Until your group is used to each other, it is wise to avoid giving your scribe tasks that would potentially make the scribe the dominant member of your group because the board and chalk can provide great power over any PBL group.

The book will offer some specific questions and answers that may or may not come up during this process. These questions and answers are not meant to exhaust the topics discussed after each segment of each PBL case.

Your PBL group should recognize the limitations of the problem simulations that are used and work around them. Any simulation sacrifices some aspect of reality, and this should be understood. For example, the case describes the patient verbally. There are no visual, auditory, body movement, speech, or nonverbal personality cues available, and you will need to visualize the patient as much as possible. Also, it is impossible to ask a series of questions as easily as it would be with the person involved. Instead, each question has to be requested individually. Although frustrating at times, it can be thought of as an asset for learning because you have to justify each action in light of the hypotheses and not take actions just because they are part of a menu.

When your group has a standardized patient and you utilize the time-in, time-out procedure, your group should agree that during the time-in segment you will act professionally, as if you are working in a real situation with an actual patient. Using the standardized patient in this way not only allows you to develop your clinical and behavioral skills, but also allows you to assess your interpersonal skills. Later, after the encounter, the standardized patient can provide feedback on your interpersonal skills from the patient's point of view.

When the standardized patient is used, it would be better not to use the chalkboard as described above. Here, the actual patient is in front of you. You should keep your own notes concerning ideas, learning issues, and accumulated facts. This again puts you in a professional situation and works toward skills in note taking during a real patient encounter.

## Working through the patient's clinical and behavioral problems

For each PBL case, the problems are reviewed. The student facilitator, communicating at the metacognitive level, may say something such as, "What could be going on with this person?" (hypothesis generation). Often, you may not be ready to come up with ideas until you ask some questions to clarify the patient's problem further. Sometimes, you will answer the challenge for ideas by wanting to ask the patient a question, such as, "I wonder if the patient is taking aspirin?" The student facilitator should then ask, "Why do you want to know if the patient is taking aspirin?" You may answer to the effect that, by taking aspirin, there may be an interaction with the anticoagulant she is taking. The student facilitator can then point out that you actually did have an idea about the drug–drug interaction as a possible cause for the patient's problem that should be put up on the board under the ideas category. The student facilitator sometimes has to nudge you for broader or alternative ideas by making comments such as, "Do you think the patient's adverse drug reaction is caused by an interaction between the anticoagulant and the food the patient is eating?"

Once there are some ideas on the board, the student facilitator can stimulate you to come up with questions. Later, discussion items may be revealed that will help determine which of the ideas listed are more likely or which questions might rule out some of the ideas expressed (inquiry strategy). When you suggest a question for the patient or suggest a laboratory test, the student facilitator should ask why those actions are being taken; this challenges your deductive logic in picking actions related to the ideas (hypotheses) entertained.

After working through a number of patient problems, you may become impatient with such a team approach to asking questions, and you might like to ask a series of questions or perform an inquiry on your own to get to the heart of the problem. One technique that can help is to read the patient's initial problems, then ask each member of your group to write a series of questions they would like to ask the patient and why. The members of your group can then compare questions and the justifications for them. Your list, or a combined list, can be chosen to obtain more information from the patient.

As the patient's responses to questions and the results of items in the pharmaceutical health care report are obtained, your PBL group analyzes the new information against the ideas on the chalkboard and records under the "facts" heading the information that is felt to be significant (analysis). As in the clinical and behavioral reasoning process, hypotheses are generated, an inquiry strategy developed, new data analyzed, and the significant data added to a growing synthesis of the problem on the chalkboard. The student facilitator stimulates the students' knowledge and thinking, guiding them through these steps in the clinical and behavioral reasoning processes as needed. One advantage of the chalkboard is that all entries can be changed, eliminated, reorganized, or expanded as your PBL group progresses in understanding the problem.

As your PBL group becomes more experienced in this process, the student facilitator progressively withdraws from the discussions and enters only when guidance may seem indicated. Occasionally during this process, especially when you seem to be getting off the track or confused about the next step, the student facilitator can ask someone in your group to summarize what has been learned about the patient problem without looking at the facts column on the board (problem synthesis). The rest of the group members are asked to add any important data that was left out of the presentation or to eliminate information felt to be unimportant. This stimulates consideration of the problem synthesis by all of the members of your group and makes sure that all members of your group are seeing the problem in the same way, and that no significant data have been ignored in thinking about the problem.

As time passes and your PBL group becomes more experienced with the process, its presentation of this synthesis should become more concise and organized. A description of the synthesis will often get your PBL group back on the track and present it with an opportunity to review the ideas on the chalkboard to see if something should be changed.

Frequently, you will express the need to do a more complete workup in addition to the development of a plan for your patient. This could become very time consuming in your PBL group problem-solving process, and this ritual requires little cognitive effort and usually provides a small payoff in understanding your patient's problem.

This can be avoided if the student facilitator explains that it is always assumed that you will do a complete workup on patients in future clinical and behavioral work. However, the challenge here is to practice higher-order problem-solving skills to see if you can ask those questions and perform those items that are necessary or that have the greatest payoff in either supporting or eliminating the ideas (hypotheses) considered. It helps to point out that these are the skills you will need as pharmacists when there is no time or luxury to ask all questions.

As the problem-solving process for your patient's problem progresses, the student facilitator must note when you are unsure of facts, seem confused, disagree with other members of your group, or express the need to understand something better. When this occurs, the student facilitator should ask if there is a learning issue that should be put on the chalkboard. If so, it should be listed in the space provided for learning issues. Initially, it may not be easy for your group to be aware of learning issues as they arise in your work with the patient's problem. After the student facilitator does this nudging, it becomes almost automatic for your PBL group to recognize learning issues and to put them on the chalkboard. This conditions you to recognize when you need to learn in your future real pharmacy practice.

An important task for your student facilitator is to make sure that your PBL group reveals the extent of the knowledge and understanding you already have during your problem-solving activities and discussions and, most important, recognizes the knowledge needed. All terminology and concepts mentioned in discussions should be defined. All explanations should be probed to the appropriate level of understanding by the liberal use of "Why?" or "Please explain." If the objective of your group is to acquire clinical or behavioral information in the problem-based learning activity, then the questioning should make sure that you carry explanations and discussions to the appropriate level of inquiry. You soon take up these student facilitator challenges to each member of your PBL group in their discussions. As mentioned, the student facilitator can usually begin to be less noticeable in this process, only interjecting a question now and then as appropriate.

This process continues until your PBL group has carried the analysis of the case as far as it can with its own knowledge and skills. Consistent with pharmacy practice, the results of inquiries are usually not discovered right away, but will be reviewed when your group returns to the problem after student-centered self-directed study.

## Commitment

After you have considered the most probable ideas about your patient's problem, asked all of the questions necessary, and narrowed down your ideas as to the causes of your patient's problem as far as you are able with the knowledge you have, you will come to an important point. Here, your student facilitator will ask each member of your PBL group to commit, on the chalkboard, to what is probably going on with your patient.

Although you will feel that you certainly do not have enough knowledge to make such a decision and would like to look up some things, the student facilitator must insist, in spite of everything, that you must now make your best guess. This commitment provides a strong motivation for student-centered problem-based learning as you will want to find out if your best guesses were correct. It prepares you for the real world of practice, in which decisions often have to be made when data are lacking.

## Reviewing learning issues

When you have reasoned your way through the problem as far as possible with the knowledge and skills possessed by your group and have each made a commitment as to what you feel is the explanation for the problem, your group needs to review the learning issues that have accumulated on the chalkboard and decide how they are to be tackled. The learning issues can be reviewed in the light of the objectives agreed on in the beginning of the session. If your group is learning a specific clinical or behavioral issue and the identification of the issues responsible for the patient's dilemma were agreed-on objectives, then the learning issues can be reviewed and adjusted, if necessary, to emphasize clinical or behavioral learning. Your scribe during the problem-solving process often hastily puts up the learning issues on the chalkboard with only an abbreviation or two to indicate them.

At this point, you should see how each issue should be expressed to best define the area and depth of study required. Some may seem trivial or unrelated to their objectives at this point and can be eliminated. Also, in retrospect, your group may now realize that there are other issues that need to be listed for study relative to the problem at hand. Your group has to make a decision about breadth and depth of learning and how far beyond immediate relevance to the problem the learning should be. Those learning issues that are directly related to analyzing and understanding the problem are the most important. However, the problem may make you realize that there are larger topics or important subject areas raised by the problem that you do not understand or understand fully. These could profitably be reviewed at this time.

Next, your group should decide on how to divide the learning issues. Although there is a tendency for you to want to research and study all the learning issues on your own, there are a number of good reasons not to do this. Usually, there are a large number of learning issues, and if each member of your group takes them all, learning is bound to be superficial. The resources you are accustomed to using are textbooks; it will be hard to get you to use more primary sources of information when each of you feels there is so much to learn. Textbooks, at best, can only give an overview. It would be far more valuable for you to go after resource faculty, other faculty experts, review articles, original articles, computerized information resources, and the like as necessary in your self-directed study. With these resources, you can pursue one or two learning issues in depth using careful searches.

Second, members of your PBL group have a few assigned learning issues, then have the task of transferring this information effectively to the other members in your group in ways in which you will understand it and apply it to the problem at hand. This is a challenge to your communication and educational skills. Of course, the last thing you would want your group to do is to lecture each other, violating the whole point behind problem-based learning. You need to present the information you have acquired in the context of the problem. The appropriate level of detail is important because it makes available to members of your group the proper copies of notes or outlines, diagrams, references, or pictures that you put in your own files for later review.

Sometimes, it is valuable for you to arrange for a resource faculty member or other expert in the area of study to visit your group, comment on the way you have put the problem together, and answer questions from your group. There are usually some learning issues that may be of such central interest to your group that your group members may all want to research them and then compare what they have learned. It is a general observation by most resource faculty that, even though group members have all agreed on their own particular learning issues, they also tend to do a little, perhaps superficial, reading in the area of all the other members.

It is very important that you do not take on learning issues in areas in which you have considerable prior knowledge and experience. For example, if you have worked previously in a large nursing home with a pharmacist, you may repeatedly take on clinical and behavioral problems related to geriatric patient care. It is far more important for you to take on learning issues in your areas of ignorance to achieve a balanced background in your knowledge for pharmacy practice. This allows problem-based learning to be tailor-made for you.

Once the learning issues have been identified and assigned, you should describe the resources you intend to use in your study. This is another important commitment that has to be made. You should eventually be able to decide on the most appropriate and efficient resource for every learning need. This commitment sets the stage for the beginning of the second session, when you return to continue with the problem and are asked to critique the resources you set out to use. As a last step in this first session, your PBL group members then look at their calendars and decide how long you should give yourselves, considering the extent and complexity of the learning issues decided on and the kinds of resources that you plan to use, and when you will meet to continue with the problem, armed with your new knowledge.

## Student-centered learning

The period of student-centered learning that follows the first session is at the heart of problem-based learning. You are learning what you have determined is important for you to learn and what you want to learn. You seek out the information on your own. You go to a variety of resource books in your personal collection, to the faculty, and to the library with unresolved questions about a problem with which you are working and have tried to analyze on your own. You realize the information you are seeking is something you definitely did not know and should know because it relates to being a successful pharmacist.

In contrast to assigned readings in more conventional instructor-directed learning, for which maintaining the attention and interest needed to assimilate information is often a difficult labor for you, this information that you seek on your own initiative to answer your questions literally seems to jump out of the pages. What the resource faculty you consult might tell you, in answer to your questions, makes sense and is eagerly received because you want the information and your own study has not resolved your questions. The resource faculty will often be quite pleasantly surprised to find you act more like a graduate student in the quality, depth, and detail of your questions. Conversations with you can be very stimulating.

Your health science librarians may describe to you their complete surprise at your remarkable increase in library use, at all hours. The members of your PBL group collaborate in their study. You work in pairs and larger groups as you pool resources and your understanding of the information to be learned relative to the problems. In these collaborative discussions, you teach and learn from each other.

## The second session with the problem resource critique

When you return following your self-directed study to continue your work with the problem, you are asked to describe the learning resources you ultimately used to satisfy your learning needs. You are also asked to critique the resources you intended to use, why you went to other resources, and the problems you had with all the resources used. You are asked to comment on whether you would use them again for future learning needs and in what way your approach would change. Early in your attempts at student-centered self-directed learning, you may run into many difficulties. Sometimes, references are difficult to find, some references are superficial and have too little information, and others are too detailed and have too much information. Some resource faculty are hard to contact; you cannot find a satisfactory reference to answer your question. Each member of your PBL group who had problems with resources should describe how he or she would attack a similar learning issue differently in the future.

## Reanalysis of the patient's problem in the light of new information

Having just completed your student-centered self-directed study, you are often excited about what you have learned and the insights you now have achieved about the problem, and you may be eager to tell each member of your PBL group what you have learned. This is less of a problem if there has been a lot of collaborative learning carried out during student-centered self-directed learning.

Nevertheless, there has often been considerable individual learning or work in groups of two or three, and these subgroups may be eager to discuss what they have learned with the whole group. This would, in essence, now put lecturing into the hands of your PBL group, and a number of minilectures by each member of the PBL group would not only be boring, but also would be counterproductive in problem-based learning. Members of your group may not be as interested in displaying the information learned, and there is a need to want to apply it to the problem to enhance understanding and later recall it in real pharmacy practice.

In revisiting your patient's problems, the relevant information obtained from the student-centered self-directed study by each member of your PBL group is brought to bear on those areas that generated the learning issues in the previous session. At these opportunities, you can briefly elaborate on what you learned and hand out summary materials, xerographic copies, notes, and the like that you may have prepared for the members of your PBL group. There may often be a fine line when a brief presentation actually becomes a lecture, and it is something that all in the group need to monitor and discuss.

Any learning issue that was researched by a member of your PBL group but not brought up in the patient-oriented discussion needs to be discussed before the group decides what you have learned from the problem and what your next step will be. This problem usually presents with a learning issue that is a review of a topic or subject area related to the patient's problem. If you have to give a formal presentation, it is a chance to evaluate your ability to get your group's members involved in an interactive discussion with questions and input from the members.

## Summarizing what has been learned

The great advantage to problem-based learning is that the information you acquired in the problem-solving process will be recalled, by association, and applied to similar problems in the future. To capitalize on this advantage, several activities need to be carried out in your PBL group. Without this important step in the problem-based learning process, the recall of information may not be a verbal recollection of the facts learned as much as a recall of which hypotheses should be considered with a new problem and the actions that should be taken. This is seen in experienced practicing pharmacists, who can come up with the right questions and tests that ought to be undertaken and the medication regimen needed. Yet, if you ask yourself why you performed these things, you may not be able to give yourself any kind of a self-discussion of the clinical or ethical principles and concepts involved and, if pushed, may just indicate that the actions just seemed right. Sometimes, you might recall a similar patient problem for which these actions were used.

Knowledge acquired in the context of active learning around a problem is stored in memory as "procedural knowledge," in contrast to the knowledge acquired from readings and lectures, which were memorized for later factual recall, stored as "declarative knowledge," and verbalized in response to questions. The former can be applied to problems but cannot be verbalized, abstracted, and intellectually manipulated for adaptation to new problems; the latter cannot be recalled in work with problems, but can be verbalized in response to questions.

This is one reason for this important stage in the problem-based teaching sequence. When you are encouraged to verbalize what you have learned, you have the best of both methods. You are able to recall and apply the information you acquired to patient problems and also are able to describe the principles and concepts behind your reasoning and pharmaceutical health care plan decisions. You can be challenged to produce definitions, draw diagrams, and make lists.

A second reason for this stage in problem-based learning is to enhance transfer of the information learned and the experience gained from one problem to new problems for which the information and experience are relevant. You need to discuss how your new learning and experience with the present problem relate to the previous problems you have encountered and how it may help you when you encounter similar patient problems in the future.

A third phase of this important stage is for you to develop abstractions as you see how similar facts, structures, principles, or processes from clinical and behavioral pharmacoethics apply in different settings and with different problems and how common features among different problems suggest over-arching principles. You develop your own "big pictures" that your pharmacy professors often try to provide in their lectures during traditional teaching, but to little avail, as you do not have the experiences and personalized frames of reference needed to own them. These concepts have to be developed, as for the expert, through experience with many different instances and problems; with reflection, these produce a personally constructed, and therefore owned, big picture.

## Self-evaluation and peer evaluation

In this last stage of the problem-based learning process, you will be asked to assess your own performance during your PBL group's process in three areas: (1) ability as a problem-solver, (2) ability as a self-directed learner, and (3) ability as a member of the group.

You will be asked to make an evaluation of your reasoning for the problem. As your PBL group worked on the problem together, the challenge is for you to separate your thinking and its adequacy. You should attempt to recall and comment on the adequacy of the ideas you generated about the problem (hypotheses), the questions and actions you suggested with the patient (inquiry), the way you put it together in your own mind (synthesis), and the decisions you made about the underlying processes involved and how these might have been managed. Furthermore, you should address the appropriateness of learning issues undertaken and whether appropriate references were used. Finally, you should evaluate your support of your PBL group in its task with the problem at hand.

After you present your self-assessment, the other members in your group are then asked to comment on their self-assessments and to add their comments, good or bad, about your performance. The ability to provide honest, accurate, and constructive feedback to a peer may be even more difficult for you. In the beginning, you may all be very civil to each other.

If, for example, during a self-assessment one member of your group should express concern that you did not get enough information to your group about the learning issue you were assigned, the other members will invariably reassure that member that it was a difficult topic or that there were no good resources available to you. The student facilitator must then interject. If, indeed, a poor job was done, the student facilitator needs to openly comment on this. More important, if there was a poor performance by you or a member of your PBL group that was not mentioned during self-assessment, the student facilitator must comment on this poor performance. Once any group has been together for a week or so, they will get beyond the usual initial civilities and become open in their criticism or support of other members of the PBL group.

Self-assessment requires you to monitor your performance and to judge its adequacy. The development and practice of this ability is central to lifelong, self-learning skills. The practicing pharmacist must be aware of inadequacies in daily work to be able to recognize the need for more learning and to update knowledge and skills to keep contemporary and meet the new challenges faced in practice. The ability to provide constructive feedback to others is an essential skill for working effectively in health care or research teams.

## Moving toward individual learning

In the above sequences, you work in a PBL group to take advantage of the peer support and accumulated knowledge that occurs in collaborative learning. You learn to work effectively in team settings and to increase the personal and individual contact between members of your PBL group and faculty. However, once you have become proficient in this learning process and have developed experience with a sufficient number of patient problems in the 18 cases in this textbook, you can and should begin to work individually with patient problems. You will use the same sequence of activities; afterward, as part of a group, you will confer and compare your individual approach and learning just before the step at which you summarize what has been learned.

## References

Barrows, H.S., *Practice-Based Learning: Problem-Based Learning Applied to Medical Education*, Southern Illinois University School of Medicine, Springfield, 1994.

Barrows, H.S., *Problem-Based Learning Applied to Medical Education*, Southern Illinois University School of Medicine, Springfield, 2000.

Barrows, H.S. and Tamblyn, R.M., *Problem-Based Learning: An Approach to Medical Education*, Springer, New York, 1980.

Mennin, S.P., Kalishman, S., Friedman, M., Pathak, D., and Snyder, J., A survey of graduates in practice from the University of New Mexico's conventional and community-oriented, problem-based tracks, *Acad. Med.*, 71, 1079–1089, 1996.

Norman, G.R. and Schmidt, H.G., The psychology basis of problem-based learning: a review of the evidence, *Acad. Med.*, 67, 557–565, 1992.

Vernon, D.T. and Blake, R.L., Does problem-based learning work? A meta-analysis of evaluative research, *Acad. Med.*, 68, 550–563, 1993.

*chapter two*

---

# The challenge of the patient's clinical and behavioral problem

Many of pharmacists' difficulties in intervening to modify a patient's clinical and behavioral problem may be the result of assuming that patients are ready to act on their inappropriate practices. Trying to persuade patients who are not yet ready to change may push them into a defensive position that may result in the pharmacist experiencing a decreased sense of self-efficacy and in the patient being put off by the pharmacist's attitude (Rollnick et al., 1992).

If the patient is not ready to change, it is more effective for the pharmacist to assist with the decision-making process rather than to provide advice on how to change. If pharmacists used the concept of readiness-to-change to match patients to different forms of intervention, their commitment to pharmacy (Prochaska and DiClemente, 1986) may provide the conceptual framework through which patient-based interventions would be enhanced because they would experience a greater sense of self-efficacy in dealing with all types of patients.

## The stages-of-change model

The stages-of-change model proposes that those who need to change could be optimally allocated to different types of interventions depending on their level of readiness to change. Prochaska and DiClemente (1986) proposed the existence of five stages that reflect a process of change. The model conceptualizes change as a process, not an event, a linear continuum with individuals going through a state of being unaware or unwilling to act on the problem (precontemplation stage), to a state of considering the possibility of change (contemplation stage), then to becoming determined and prepared to make the change (preparation stage), and finally to taking action (action stage) and maintaining the change over time (maintenance stage).

Precontemplation describes the stage at which a person is not considering change. Precontemplators are mostly aware of the positive aspects and are less inclined to process information on the negative aspects of the behavior or to reevaluate themselves; they do not put much effort into overcoming their problem. Usually, precontemplators do not consider that there may be adverse effects associated with their behavior or that change is possible.

Contemplation is the stage at which a person is considering change. Contemplators are usually of two minds about changing; they will often convey that part of them wants to change and part does not.

Preparation describes the stage at which the individual has made the decision to change and is now choosing strategies. The impetus to move into this stage occurs when the negative aspects of the behavior outweigh the positive. A person in this stage really wants to change.

Action is the period when the person engages in efforts aimed at modifying the inappropriate behavior. The person usually implements the plan made in the preparation stage. This stage is said to be a stressful one because individuals are not accustomed to the new lifestyle.

Maintenance is the period when the person is working toward maintaining the changes made earlier. As time passes, the person becomes adjusted to the new lifestyle, and the behavior in question is no longer a problem.

## Is the model applicable to pharmacoethics?

It is true that the greatest body of research supporting the stages-of-change model comes from the area of substance addiction, such as smoking and alcohol dependence. Whether the behavior in question is drinking, lack of exercise, smoking, low self-esteem, risky sexual behavior, or other behavior, the structure of change appears to be the same. Individuals go from being unaware or unwilling to do something about the behavior to contemplating change, then to preparing for self-change, taking action, and finally maintaining behavior change. Insofar as the model is concerned with differentiating patients according to their preparedness to change rather than the idiosyncrasy of the behavior, it is reasonable to assume that the model applies to a broad range of high-risk behaviors, including unethical professional practices.

Evidence of the robustness of the model across different types of behavior is provided by the fact that researchers have been able to replicate basic findings from the smoking and alcohol area across a diversity of behaviors, such as weight control, exercise, psychological distress, radon exposure, sun exposure and sunscreen use, mammography screening, high blood pressure risk reduction, and adolescent delinquent behavior (Prochaska et al., 1992).

## Motivational interviewing

If a patient does something that may violate a legal or ethical code and walks into a pharmacy, the individual can be at any point in the process of change.

A style of counseling known as motivational interviewing was developed in the addiction fields by Miller, a clinical psychologist (1983); this interviewing technique facilitates movement from one stage of change to the next. Motivational interviewing recognizes that not all patients who have problems enter a pharmacy in a state of readiness to change their way of doing something. Within a motivational interviewing framework, the role of the pharmacist is to assess the individual's stage of change and then trigger the unfolding of the process of change using techniques that are specific to the patient's stage of change.

An important feature of motivational interviewing is the fact that it is the patient's task to convince the interventionist that a problem exists and not vice versa. Providing strong advice to a patient who is not ready to change will most likely make the patient argue to defend his or her behavior. According to motivational interviewing principles, eliciting opposing arguments from the patient is the worst thing the interventionist can do because it will make behavior change less likely to occur. There is a well-established principle in social psychology: "I learn what I believe as I hear myself talk" (Miller, 1983). This means that having the patient verbalize the reasons why he or she should continue certain inappropriate behavior will make the patient more committed to maintaining the inappropriate behavior (Miller, 1983).

In motivational interviewing, the interventionist raises the patient's awareness about the inappropriate behavior and then assists the patient in the process of weighing the costs and benefits of the behavior in question to facilitate a decision on whether to continue it.

## Intervention methods

This section describes a brief intervention based on the stages-of-change model and motivational interviewing principles. It is based on the assumption that not everybody who performs an inappropriate behavior is ready to change. The appropriate strategy is determined by the patient's level of readiness to change.

### Opening strategy

A good opening strategy would be to raise the subject of the inappropriate behavior with an open question like, "How do you find this behavior?" or "Do you find it does the job?" This is useful for building a certain degree of rapport before talking about the behavior in more detail. It also allows understanding the context in which the behavior is being used, and it helps the pharmacist assess whether the patient is acting inappropriately.

### Assessment of readiness to change

If it is established that the patient is using a behavior inappropriately, the next step is to assess the patient's readiness to change. To identify a patient's stage of change, the pharmacist should ask a very simple question: "How do you feel about . . . ?" (mention drug-related problem, for instance, "How do you feel about this behavior?") The patient's answer should provide the pharmacist with an indication of the patient's readiness to change, allowing the pharmacist to tailor the intervention specifically to that individual.

## Intervention strategies for precontemplators

Those who use inappropriate behaviors and are not even thinking about change (precontemplators) will most likely resist any attempt from the pharmacist to discuss the problem behavior. The question to be asked in this situation is, "How do we as interventionists facilitate progression from a state of not thinking about change to a state of contemplating change?"

One of the strategies that facilitate movement from the stage of precontemplation to that of contemplation is to raise awareness about the behavior, that is, to make the individual more aware of his or her inappropriate behavior. Precontemplators will need to be provided in a nonthreatening manner with more information about their practices and their consequences. The pharmacist should ask for permission to provide the information because this will minimize resistance. When providing information, the pharmacist should talk in the third person, that is, talk about what happens to people rather than to the individual. The pharmacist should encourage the patient to think about the information and make it clear that the pharmacist will be there to help if the patient decides to talk about it at a later stage.

The pharmacist should be mindful that it is not the role of the pharmacist to make patients face up to the inappropriateness of their behavior or to convince them to change. The pharmacist should simply provide patients with insight into the behavior. Remember that strong arguments for change will cause the patient to take up the other side, becoming more committed to the inappropriate behavior (Miller, 1983).

## Intervention for contemplators

When individuals enter the contemplation stage of change, the negative aspects start to outweigh the positive aspects of the behavior, although both are still very important for the individual (Prochaska and DiClemente, 1986). On the one hand is recognition of a problem; on the other is avoidance of change due to what the patient perceives as the benefits of the inappropriate behavior.

Contemplators will need to be helped with the decision-making process so they can work through ambivalence about behavior change. The use of motivational interviewing techniques can accomplish this best. A good strategy is to do a decisional-balance exercise with the patient. Simply ask the patient about the good things related to the inappropriate behavior, for instance, "What are the good things about the behavior?"

The pharmacist should always start by asking about the positive aspect of the behavior to minimize resistance and to motivate the patient subsequently to talk about the negative aspect of the behavior. Talking about the positive aspect of the inappropriate behavior also helps the pharmacist demonstrate empathy by recognizing that there is also a good side to the inappropriate behavior.

Once the patient finishes talking about the positive aspect of the inappropriate behavior, the pharmacist should briefly summarize it and then get the patient to talk about the negative aspects of the inappropriate behavior by asking, "What are the not-so-good things about the inappropriate behavior?" The pharmacist should prompt the patient to elaborate on the not-so-good things about the inappropriate behavior by asking such questions as "How does it affect you?" "What else?" or "What don't you like about it?" If patients verbalize the need to change often enough, they will experience greater propensity to act. Remember the social psychological principle: "I learn what I believe as I hear myself talk." Simply by allowing the patient to talk about the willingness and the need to change, the pharmacist facilitates behavior change.

Another important aspect of this exercise is to generate in the individual's mind a state of psychological discomfort known as "cognitive dissonance," which is created when an individual's behavior is discrepant with personal beliefs, attitudes, or feelings (in this case, "I need to change my behavior").

One of the interventionist's roles will be to heighten the psychological discomfort experienced by the patient by highlighting the inconsistency between the behavior and the patient's concerns about it. This can be done by succinctly summarizing the good things and the less-good things.

## Intervention for those in the preparation stage of change

If an individual is ready for change, the limited time available to the pharmacist may be better spent providing practical advice on how to go about making the change rather than on further boosting the patient's motivation. The pharmacist's task will be to help the patient determine the best course of action to change the inappropriate practices. A good way of starting is to set a date for behavior change to occur. If the misbehavior is being caused by misinformation, the patient may commit to change on being provided with information on how to behave appropriately. However, in the case of chronic misbehaviors, the individual will most likely need a few days to prepare for changing behavior.

Patients will need to learn a new set of skills that will enable them to cope with the change. The cognitive–behavioral approach advocates the replacement of the inappropriate behavior with more adaptive ways of satisfying the needs that it fulfilled. Patients should be encouraged to think about alternative behaviors. If appropriate, the pharmacist should also provide the patient with self-help materials.

### Intervention for patients in the action stage

In the action stage, patients put into practice the skills acquired in the preparation stage. Support from the pharmacist is crucial in this stage; it is important for patients to have someone with whom to discuss the progress and difficulties encountered in making the change.

Reinforcement, finding and playing back to the patient the efficacious behavior, will help increase the patient's self-esteem and sense of mastery of the changing process. The pharmacist should arrange follow-up visits of 3 to 5 minutes to assess the patient's progress and reinforce success.

## Rollnick, Mason, and Butler: seven-step process for behavior change

If we want a pharmacist to be able to handle a patient's pharmaceutical care problems effectively, efficiently, and humanely, the challenge that the patient problem presents to a pharmacist's reasoning needs to be well understood. Rollnick, Mason, and Butler, in their groundbreaking book, *Health Behavior Change: A Guide for Practitioners* (2000), outlined a seven-step process to elicit change in patients.

Patient problems can be characterized as follows:

1.  When the patient is first encountered, there is always insufficient information available for the pharmacist to decide immediately what may be going on with the patient and to determine an appropriate plan of care. More information is needed for the pharmacist to understand what is probably responsible for the patient's problem and to decide which actions may be required to provide relief or resolution. Most patients present with only a prescription, and it is quite obvious that more information will have to be obtained by the pharmacist through a pharmaceutical care history form and maybe one or more laboratory tests to derive a care plan. In fact, no matter how much information may be present when the pharmacist first encounters the patient (pharmaceutical care history form, laboratory results), the pharmacist will always want more to decide on a care plan. Presenting students with patient problems that contain most of the information needed is inconsistent with what they will face.

    Pharmacists have to obtain the necessary additional information needed for patient care through a deductive inquiry process. The pharmacist needs to fill out the patient's medication history with more information to create a pattern that can be compared with those of the pharmacist's knowledge and verify or eliminate possibilities. A second important point is that the real challenge to the practicing pharmacist is the patient problem that does not fit into any common pattern. Experience with real patient problems, as students learn from the very beginning of pharmacy school, provides them with the best opportunity to develop the flexible thinking necessary to accommodate these challenges of practice.

2. There is no one right way for the pharmacist to obtain the additional information needed. If different pharmacists are given the same patient problem, each will go about getting more information for that same patient problem in different ways. Although there may be some common questions shared by all, each will ask different questions in a different order, order different laboratory tests, and counsel a patient in a different way. Despite these differences, they will often come up with similar pharmaceutical care plans. Each pharmacist has different patient and educational experiences in long-term memory. These produce unique configurations of data and different experiences of what works to make and care for a particular patient. As a consequence, each requires different information to support or deny the ideas considered. This means that each pharmacist has to inquire, explore, and probe based on personal past experiences and education to obtain the data needed to fill out a more complete picture of the patient's situation and establish ideas on how best to care for the patient.

3. As new information is obtained, the patient's problem may change and result in something quite different from what was initially suspected. The way the patient presents information to the pharmacist is not unlike the tip of the iceberg. As the pharmacist begins to inquire and new data are added to the patient's picture, it may become more complex or serious than suspected and may possibly involve significant unsuspected behavioral complications.

4. Despite the most careful and complete investigation of the patient's problem, and even with the most straightforward patient problems, the pharmacist can never be sure that the care plan decided on is correct and represents the right decision. Important data that a pharmacist might like to have to make a pharmaceutical care plan decision may not be available from the patient for a variety of reasons. Data obtained from the patient on a pharmaceutical care history form may be conflicting or ambiguous, and communication with the patient may be difficult. Even in straightforward cases, there can be an unsuspected complication to care management.

   Despite all of this, the pharmacist has to make decisions and take actions. The patient's problem cannot be set aside for another day when it might be more clear-cut or until medical science can provide better-defined treatment guidelines. Unlike problem solving in other professions or in scientific investigations, the pharmacist has to provide care for the patient then and there, taking action despite the fact that there is a chance of being wrong.

5. The patient is a necessary and important partner in the treatment process. The value of data obtained by the pharmacist from a pharmaceutical care history form depends on the patient's ability to un-

derstand, communicate, and cooperate. The effectiveness of the care plan depends on the patient's understanding, cooperation, emotional state, and ability to communicate. Cooperation and communication can be affected by a multitude of factors that may be beyond the control of the pharmacist and can tax the pharmacist's communication skills, such as the patient's level of consciousness, mental aberrations, or ability to speak English.

However, many of the factors that do affect cooperation and communication are within the pharmacist's control and therefore depend on clinical and humanistic skills. The patient expects to receive professional service from the pharmacist and expects care and understanding. A frightened, hostile, unhappy, or confused patient will not communicate, cooperate, or comply with the care plan as well as a reassured patient who understands the care being offered and is satisfied with it. It is not sufficient for the pharmacist to have good technical and problem-solving skills to care for patients. Interpersonal, communication, and patient education skills are equally essential.

With these characteristics of patient problems in mind, we now need to look at how the effective, efficient, and ethical pharmacist can effectively deal with the challenges patient problems offer. It is also important to have faculty from different disciplines and content areas periodically review the specific problems in each PBL case to see if the seven-step method discussed below produces the necessary behavior change.

## Step 1: Establish rapport

Sometimes, it is difficult to get started on a discussion about behavior change with a simulated patient. Good rapport is essential for an honest discussion and for constructive understanding of a patient's behavior and openness to change. Rapport is sometimes quickly established, and the agenda is often obvious. In a community pharmacy, there may already be an existing relationship between the pharmacist and patient, and this will provide a setting for the current counseling session. It is not difficult to get things off to a good start. Three items, discussed below, are essential for establishing rapport: physical setting, thoughts and feelings about the counseling session, and a typical day.

### Physical setting

The physical setting for the counseling session may either promote or obstruct the development of rapport. An equal power relationship is essential for successful negotiation.

### Thoughts and feelings about the counseling session

The patient's expectations will affect rapport. The patient will expect to be handled by the pharmacist in a certain way. Check these expectations and clarify any misunderstandings. The patient may also have immediate concerns that will need to be addressed before the patient will be comfortable about addressing other matters like behavior change. It is important to identify these and respond appropriately. It is also worth acknowledging the context of the consultation for the patient. It may be necessary to switch focus from the patient's medications to negotiating behavior change. If the patient feels respected and cared for from the beginning, any subsequent discussion will be easier.

### A typical day

One useful strategy for establishing rapport is to use a strategy called "a typical day," highlighting its benefit to information exchange. Here, the patient describes a typical day and usually says where the behavior under discussion fits into this context. The pharmacist's role is to practice restraint and develop an interest in the layers of personal detail provided. It is useful to employ this strategy near the beginning of a counseling session, even if the subject of behavior change has not been raised. If one has time to spare, it can be a most worthwhile experience for both parties. One can follow the account of a typical day in general without reference to any behavior. If this is carried out skillfully, rapport will be considerably strengthened.

## Step 2: Set agenda

Sometimes, there are so many things contributing to a person's poor health that it is hard to know where to begin. Of all the judgments made in a behavior change counseling session, the poorest often arise from a premature leap into specific discussion of a change when the patient is more concerned about something else.

Sometimes, it can be a relatively routine matter that prevents a focus on behavior change: a patient who arrives at a counseling session upset about a minor accident might not be able to concentrate on anything the pharmacist says. Sometimes, it is a personal matter that concerns the patient and that he or she might want to talk about; someone who has recently had a heart attack might be preoccupied with matters of life and death. It would be poor timing, even insensitive, to talk about getting more exercise or changing diet under these circumstances. A critical early task, therefore, is to agree on the agenda.

Even when behavior change is a possible topic for discussion, one is often faced with multiple interrelated health behaviors. For example, many excessive drinkers also smoke. Thus, health behaviors deemed risky often coexist in individual patients. Those who suffer from diabetes, heart disease, and other chronic conditions frequently face the challenge of changing more than one behavior. Deciding what to talk about is thus a crucial first step.

A clear distinction should be made in the pharmacist's mind between single and multiple behavior change discussions when setting an agenda. Pharmacists will need to make a clear and conscious choice between using either a strategy for multiple behaviors or a strategy for a single behavior.

This is because so many health care practitioners, when faced with a range of possible behaviors, prematurely compel a patient to discuss one particular behavior at the expense of others. At this stage of the counseling session, the patient should be given control of its direction.

### Multiple behaviors

Negotiating behavior change is a specific process. It is applicable to a range of behaviors, but can only be used with regard to one specific behavior at a time. It is not possible to negotiate a "healthier lifestyle" in general. Everyone is at a different stage of readiness to change due to different issues. Even within one topic, such as diet, a patient may be ready to make one change (e.g., eat more fruit), but not ready to make another (e.g., eat less fat). Sometimes, changing one behavior will also begin change of another, but it is important to keep the process to one behavior at a time. When there is a range of behaviors that could be discussed, it is essential to prioritize and focus on one clear objective. This makes the whole process more manageable.

The aim here is to be open and honest about the agenda the pharmacist may have, to understand the agenda the patient may have, and to help the patient select a behavior, if appropriate. The patient, however, might prefer to talk about a pressing personal matter. The pharmacist's behavior and tone of voice should reflect an attitude of curiosity about what the patient really wants to discuss. This agenda setting can be done informally by asking a series of open questions.

Consider talking about the importance of change and the building of confidence. If time is running out, you might consider asking the patient to keep a diary of the behavior or simply to think about it.

Many behavior change discussions have stress as an underlying theme. Rather than leave this topic to one side, it can be helpful to bring it out into the open and consider which behavior changes, if any, might help. The aim here is to help the person take an initially very broad view of stress, its causes, and its consequences. Having done this, if you sit back and are prepared to tolerate a period of uncertainty with the patient, the patient will often lead you to talk about a change. A genuinely curious tone needs to be adopted; the practitioner sits back and tries to understand how the patient sees things.

Everyone has different causes or reasons why stress builds up. Some causes can be changed; others cannot. Some come in a downpour, others in a slow stream. Symptoms are the things that happen to the patient as the level rises. They affect the body (e.g., heart rate, development of aches and pains, dizziness), the mind (e.g., poor concentration and memory, feeling tired, worrying too much), and behavior (e.g., difficulty sleeping, smoking, drinking, eating habits). Solutions are the things that lower the level of stress in the patient (e.g., talking to someone about worries, relaxation, exercise, altering one of the causes).

This kind of discussion often leads to talk about change. If this happens, be careful not to close the discussion prematurely. Patients can sometimes seem confused, and silences can follow as they talk about the possibilities. The only guideline is to stay with them and retain a genuinely curious tone that reflects the underlying spirit of the exercise. It is not essential to make decisions now. The aim is just to have a look at the situation.

### Single behavior

In some circumstances, the pharmacist may clearly identify one particular behavior to discuss. In the pharmacy, a patient may present with a particular symptom, and the pharmacist may identify a probable or certain link with a particular behavior. Alternatively, there may be a single behavior that is clearly compromising the patient's best health according to the patient's physician.

Pharmacists may believe that it is their professional duty to raise a concern about risky health behavior, and not raising the issue would be to shirk this responsibility. This can make some patients uncomfortable when a problem raised by the pharmacist "hits them in the face." But, if the pharmacist has good rapport with the patient, the patient can talk about any subject. Therefore, the pharmacist should consider this the first priority. Remember that both the pharmacist and the patient are on the same side: they both have an interest in improving or maintaining the patient's health. Be honest about your agenda and invite the patient to express personal views on the subject.

There are some occasions when raising the subject can be difficult. There is no better formula than taking time to establish good rapport. Raising the subject of heavy smoking is a good example. A proud person who feels concerned about being stigmatized as a smoker can make things difficult for the pharmacist concerned about his or her health. The mere mention of the word "smoker" produces immediate resistance. Put bluntly, undermine someone's self-esteem, and the person will resist any efforts. Under these circumstances, it seems easier to say what one should not do. Obviously, no reference should be made to words like "smoker," "problem," or even "concern." It should be left up to the patient to reach this kind of conclusion. "Use of tobacco" is the safest phrase. If one encounters immediate resistance, this is a signal to change strategy. In truth, there is no easy route through this problem, no simple strategy that will unlock a patient's willingness to talk, apart from conveying a genuine concern for the person. A productive way of building this kind of rapport is to use the typical day strategy.

If the pharmacist raises the subject and gets the impression that the patient is feeling threatened, it can be useful to give the patient time to think. This is fairly easy in a pharmacy, where continuity of care is a possibility. The patient can come back and see the pharmacist again. Back off in a nonthreatening way, and come back to it later.

## Step 3: Assess importance and confidence (and readiness)

It seems that some patients cannot change, and others do not want to change. Having agreed to talk about a particular behavior, the assessment of importance and confidence is a useful next step. Put simply, it will help the pharmacist understand exactly what the patient feels about change. This task need not be carried out in every counseling session. A pharmacist might, for example, know how a patient feels about change or at least have a strong intuition.

A patient's readiness to change is influenced by personal perceptions of the importance of the change and confidence that the change can be made. A patient might be convinced of the personal value of change (importance), but not feel confident about mastering the skills necessary to achieve it (confidence). This applies to many smokers. Heavy drinkers, on the other hand, can be quite different: they often have mixed feelings about the value of change (importance), but say that they could achieve this fairly easily (confidence) if they really wanted. When it comes to changes in eating patterns, people often have relatively low levels in both dimensions.

A pharmacist can assess readiness in addition to importance and confidence. Particular emphasis, however, will be placed on importance and confidence given the subtle interaction between them. The assessment can be done informally by simply asking the patient to clarify how he or she feels about importance and confidence. It can also be done more formally using a standard set of questions. In either case, the assessment can take as little as 2 to 3 minutes, but the patient must be actively involved.

There is no single way of doing this. The most direct questioning would be something like this: "How do you feel at the moment about [change]?" "How important is it to you personally to [change]?" "If 0 was 'not important' and 10 was 'very important,' what number would you give yourself?" Sometimes a patient will simply respond by saying, "Very important." In this case, the pharmacist can move directly into the process of exploring importance. In this particular assessment, though, the pharmacist is interested in penetrating the patients' feelings and views about the costs and benefits of change — its personal value or whether it will lead to an improvement in their lives.

In keeping with the meaning of the term self-efficacy, here confidence is about mastering the various situations in which behavior change will be challenged. The most direct questions are: "If you decided right now to [change], how confident do you feel about succeeding with this?" "If 0 was 'not confident' and 10 was 'very confident,' what number would you give yourself?"

The outcome of this assessment is sometimes clear. The patient has little concern about one dimension, and the obvious difficulty lies with the other one. It is then a matter of deciding which strategy will help this person to either explore importance or build confidence.

Sometimes, the outcome of this assessment is not clear, or both dimensions appear salient. Under circumstances like this, a pharmacist will need to lower his or her sights if the contact time is brief. Being too ambitious is probably the biggest mistake to make, often taking the form of a premature recommendation. Resistance is a likely outcome. One possibility is that the discussion returns to agenda setting and moves on to another issue. If behavior change is to be talked about, a period of uncertainty is likely to prevail in which the pharmacist should ultimately use the patient as the guide for deciding whether to focus on importance or confidence.

There can be situations for which it is useful to assess readiness, either instead of or in addition to importance and confidence. It can be a useful platform for taking a counseling session a step further. This more global dimension is often viewed as something to be aware of throughout the session, not necessarily something to be assessed. It often provides an explanation for resistance if you overestimate the patient's general readiness to change. The assessment of readiness is a process, not an event, involving conversation and reflection. A pharmacist can use a numerical scaling method here, too. For example, the pharmacist asks, "If 0 was 'not ready' and 10 was 'ready,' what score would you give yourself?" The pharmacist can follow the response with a series of follow-up questions, such as, "You gave yourself a score of x. Why are you at x and not [a lower number]?" or "You gave yourself a score of x. What would have to happen for you to move up to [a higher number]?"

Having assessed the importance of change for a patient and the patient's confidence to put plans to change into action, the pharmacist reaches a critical junction. The pharmacist needs to decide the next step and which of these two dimensions receives focus. Here, the pharmacist has a selection of strategies for working within either dimension. Which to use depends very much on the circumstances, the pharmacist's goals, and the patient's needs.

In moving both within and between these dimensions, the pharmacist will require considerable skill to lead a partner through a sequence of movements, simultaneously leading and being led, keenly alert to subtle threats to the synchrony of the partnership. Resistance from the partner is not met by force, but by transforming the movement in a constructive direction if at all possible. No amount of dedicated adherence to the strategies described below will be effective if this state of mind is absent. A certain degree of relaxation is required to maintain this spirit in the counseling session. It is useful to develop a committed but curious state of mind when talking about behavior change. The pharmacist cannot be expected to have all the answers. Indeed, the pharmacist must believe that these lie mostly within the patient.

## Step 4: Exploring importance

Some of the strategies for working on importance are best used at fairly high levels of this dimension (i.e., with scores above 5 of 10 on the formal assessment). Use of words to describe different degrees of concern about a behavior can be critical. If the pharmacist gives people a chance to talk, they will use a variety of words about change. The pharmacist should watch for these and match them as much as possible. Many of the strategies below start with a leading question that implies knowledge of how concerned the patient is about a behavior. Sometimes, however, one does not get a lead from the patient, and one has to take a deep breath and see what happens.

If one imagines a continuum of importance, from 0 to 10, different words are suitable at different points along this continuum. In ascending order, the following terms are appropriate as the level of importance increases: dislikes or less-good things (2 or 3 of 10), concerns (6 of 10), difficulty or problem (7 or 8 of 10). If you use one of the last terms with low levels of importance, the damaged rapport will be the pharmacist's responsibility to repair.

The range of strategies for exploring importance is best viewed as a menu. Care should be taken not to view these strategies as techniques applied to patients. If this happens, it is an indication of detachment that will damage rapport. The strategies are simply ways of structuring a purposeful conversation. Creative adaptation, not mindless adoption, should be the goal.

### Do little more

If a patient's level of perceived importance is markedly low, particularly if accompanied by a low level of confidence, it might be advisable to close the discussion of behavior change and turn to a more important issue or end the counseling session. How this is done is important. The pharmacist could leave the patient feeling downhearted or even reluctant to come back.

Acknowledge the uncertainty; do not just leave the patient hanging. If the pharmacist is unsure what to do, then ask the patient. For example, the patient might want to talk about it again in another encounter. Many health care practitioners faced with this situation are tempted to take a deep breath and simply provide information, seeing it as their professional responsibility at least to inform the patient of existing or potential risks. If this does not damage rapport, the approach seems understandable and justified.

### Scaling questions

Scaling questions involves using a set of questions designed to understand the patient and to encourage the patient to explore personal value or the importance of change in more detail. Typically, having elicited a numerical judgment of importance, the six recommendations listed below can open a very productive discussion in which the patient does most of the talking and thinks hard about change.

1.  Ensure that the pace of the discussion is slow and develop a genuine curiosity to know how this person really feels. You should listen to the answers to your questions, using techniques like reflection and other simple open questions to help patients express themselves as fully as possible. Your attention should not be on your thought processes (e.g., "What should I ask next?"), but as much as possible on the meaning of what the person is saying. Trust the process and the patient.

2. Watch carefully for resistance because this is a signal that you are going too far.
3. A first method for scaling questions moves down from the number given by the person. You can then follow these questions with other open questions or reflective listening statements. This method of scaling questions should not be used if the patient's rating of perceived importance is too low (i.e., around 1 or 2 of 10). Ask why he or she scored a given number and not a lower number.
4. The patient's answers amount to positive reasons for change or, in the jargon of motivational interviewing, a series of self-motivational statements.
5. Your task is now to elicit the range of reasons why the person wants to change. The pace should be slow, and simple open questions can be very useful here. If the answers are obvious, then elicit them and move on. If the answers are more complex, then take your time trying to understand all the ramifications.
6. A second method for scaling questions moves in the opposite direction, up the scale from the number given by the person. Note that one can ask about either the score or just the person. The second method often feels like the better one.

### Examine the pros and cons

The pharmacist's role is to provide structure, listen carefully, and then summarize at the end. The patient's role is to explain how he or she really feels. Start with the positive, which will help with rapport building and place the behavior in a normal context. This can be a shock in some situations, particularly when the patient believes that the behavior is a problem. Try to deal with this in a straightforward way by explaining that there must be benefits from the activity or behavior, otherwise the person would not be doing it.

### Explore concerns about the behavior

Exploration of concerns about the behavior focuses solely on the costs of the current behavior. One can only use it if the patient appears concerned. Misjudgment of this will result in resistance. Otherwise, it is ideal for helping the patient take time to express exactly what the issues are. Two principles guide the use of this strategy. First, the patient expresses the concerns; second, once the patient has reached the end, the pharmacist asks some key questions about the possibility of change.

Then, simply follow the patient's description, attempting to understand exactly why the patient feels this way, under which circumstances, and so on. Take your time. Go through any other concerns the patient might have. Exchange information if appropriate, but try not to wander off task. The pharmacist's role is to help the patient paint a picture of exactly why he or she is concerned. Then, summarize these concerns for the patient.

Ask the patient about the next step. Do this in a gentle and nonconfrontational way. This kind of question is deliberately phrased in neutral terms. The patient can either move toward or away from a decision to change. A question that explicitly asks about change can be useful, but carries the risk of the patient feeling pushed too far.

## *Step 5: Build confidence*

A patient was recently heard to say something that seemed like an echo from many other discussions: "I need to lose weight. I understand why. I know what to do, and why I should do it." Some patients really want to change. It is important to them to do so. However, they feel pessimistic about the success of such a venture. This section describes strategies for building confidence to succeed. These strategies provide a framework for something that is pervasive in counseling sessions: helping people find practical solutions to their difficulties.

The strategies described below are not meant to be counseling strategies for dealing directly with low self-esteem and helplessness. Rather, they deal with more specific changes in self-efficacy about behavior change. Sometimes, however, the pharmacist will find that if someone can be encouraged to look at small changes and succeeds with these changes, they often have a bearing on gradually improving self-esteem. If not, simply acknowledging the way a person feels can start a process of reversal of low self-esteem, particularly if you can offer further support.

There are different terms to describe people's efforts to change behavior. Goals, strategies, and targets are among the most widely used. It can be useful to note the way in which the use of terms like these varies from the general to the specific. They can be likened to signposts on a journey. The start might be with talk about a general goal. Usually, this refers to behavior change, although the goal of losing weight provides an interesting exception: losing weight is an outcome of behavior change rather than a behavior. The journey often continues with talk about strategies and, becoming more specific, about targets. Thus, numerous strategies might be considered in pursuit of a single goal; in turn, numerous targets might be considered in pursuit of a single strategy.

A menu of strategies was constructed for exploring importance. Choose a strategy that fits the way the patient describes his or her lack of confidence. These strategies are not completely separate from each other. They are overlapping, different ways to approach the subject of confidence building.

### *Do little more*

Most decisions to change do not take place during a single discussion. The patient does not necessarily need to set specific targets in conversation with you. It might be enough simply to raise the issue, mention the possibility of taking action, and leave it at that. If you plan to see the patient again, this is often a very good starting point, much better, for example, than pushing too hard for change.

### Scaling questions

The scaling questions strategy is linked to the numerical assessment of confidence. It is simply a way of opening the door to talk about strategies and targets. The patient does most of the thinking and talking, while your role is to ask questions and help clarify the stumbling blocks to change. Having conducted an assessment of how confident the person feels to make a particular change, you have been given a rating on a 10-point continuum. You now have a platform for understanding exactly how the patient feels and what might lead to successful change. Keep the pace of the discussion slow and adopt a curious attitude. Your hope is that the answers lie within the patient.

### Brainstorm solutions

Some patients, in some situations, apparently want to be told what to do. Certainly, if someone has an acute life-threatening condition, the person will probably take your advice. In most behavior change counseling sessions, however, patients probably prefer greater autonomy of decision making. If clinical judgment tells you that a patient really wants you to tell him or her what to do, then you should respond accordingly. However, most will react against simple advice giving.

The alternative to simple advice giving is a single strategy that can be learned quite quickly. In essence, rather than advising patients what to do, you encourage them to select targets and strategies for achieving the targets. Your expertise is used to enrich this process, not to overwhelm it. You construct a range of options with the patient and then encourage the patient to choose the most appropriate one. You can suggest any number of options as long as you help the patient choose the most suitable one.

### Past efforts — successes and failures

Our expectations for ourselves are frequently related to past experiences. We can learn what we are good at and what we find most difficult by looking at previous attempts to change. This can be a good way of learning, a slightly more sophisticated form of trial and error. However, sometimes people allow their confidence to be undermined by what they see as repeated failures.

Helping someone to see the past as a valuable piece of information to help plan a more successful future is a skill. Patients with low self-esteem may be particularly likely to recount stories of their "relapses" as evidence of their general worthlessness.

Affirm the person's hard work and persistence in trying more than once. Courage and perseverance are important. Patients can be encouraged to give themselves credit for applying these qualities to the issue under discussion. Encourage them to see themselves as competent, determined people who are potentially able to make changes, but have not yet hit on a successful plan for doing so.

Look for even transient evidence that change is possible. If someone feels it would be impossible to go half an hour or more without a cigarette, check if the person has ever succeeded, even if coerced rather than choosing such an action. Perhaps the person went on holiday by air or was in a social situation that made escaping for a cigarette impossible for an hour or so. If someone finds it hard to imagine refusing a drink offered by a friend, inquire if the person has ever done so (e.g., when driving or on medication).

Keep the discussion of past experiences focused as much as possible on things that are, and are seen by the patient as, within the patient's control. If a previous attempt failed because of unforeseen circumstances, acknowledge that there were real difficulties and move on to look at things for which the patient could plan and take control over another time.

## Step 6: Exchange information

A large part of the pharmacist's job is giving information to the patient. A large part of the patient's job is giving information to the practitioner. Done badly, this task will make the patient a passive recipient of expert knowledge, disconnected from personal context and concerns. Done well, it is a vehicle for true understanding and, it appears, a better outcome. For the pharmacist, information exchange will be linked to specific medical or behavioral matters. For the patient, it often also includes broader personal concerns. To deal with the former at the expense of the latter could be a serious mistake. Improving various aspects of the information exchange process can enhance compliance. This is not only a "technical matter," but also something that involves the use of skillful listening, careful questioning, and well-timed intervention. There is little of this part of the counseling session that does not involve eliciting or providing information.

Given its obvious importance, it is something of a surprise to notice that information exchange is seldom taught as a specific topic in its own right. It is difficult to find clear and teachable strategies that help pharmacists carry out this task. Rather, they are left to find their own ways of doing this. The purpose of this section is to bring together what is the most effective and satisfying way to exchange information in a form that can be learned and practiced.

Information exchange is an art as much as a technique or procedure. It is as much about maintaining rapport and having a conversation as it is about the exchange of facts. The two strategies outlined below are designed to help pharmacists achieve these goals.

### General information exchange
The following principles are important:

- Does the patient want or need information? About what? How much does the patient already know? There is no point in providing irrelevant information or information the patient does not want to receive. The best time to provide information is when the patient asks for it.

- Make a distinction, if at all possible, between factual information and the personal interpretation of it. You present the information and encourage the patient to interpret its meaning.
- When presenting information, present it in a neutral tone of voice and avoid too much use of the word "you."

### Gathering information — a typical day

The strategy of gathering information about a typical day emerged in the development of brief motivational interviewing when looking for a way of conducting assessment by a conversation led by the patient. The strategy is easily learned, provides the pharmacist with a profusion of hard facts, and gives a clear idea about the relevant personal context of health behavior. Its usefulness extends beyond information exchange. It is ideal for establishing rapport. If focused on a particular behavior and its place in the person's life, it can also help to establish readiness to change.

This strategy involves simply asking the patient to take you through a typical day in his or her life. It is described here with reference to a particular behavior or problem, although this is obviously not essential. Having agreed to talk about a particular behavior or problem (e.g., diabetes), you can launch straight into this strategy. It can take as little as 3 to 5 minutes to use; the ideal time is about 6 to 8 minutes. Much longer can be tiresome for both parties. Of course, the strategy does not have to focus on a typical day. One can ask about a typical drinking or eating binge, a typical afternoon, or anything else.

The spirit of this strategy is the most important: it is like asking the patient to paint a picture. Your role is simply to try to understand the picture that is painted. You might ask for a bit more detail here or there, but your task is simply to understand. The interviewing style shows curiosity rather than being investigatory. This strategy is easy to practice with patients.

### Review and summarize

Sometimes, it is not necessary to review and summarize, and the pharmacist can move on to another topic. If a pause is made to take stock, a useful question is: "Is there anything else at all about this picture you have painted that you would like to tell me?" This is also a good opportunity to be honest with the patient about your reaction and to provide affirmation whenever you can. Having listened so carefully to the patient, you will now be able to change the topic quite easily.

## Step 7: Reduce resistance

Some patients seem to resist your best efforts to help them. You think you are making good progress, and then it all becomes difficult again. The three practical strategies that follow are ways by which pharmacists can respond to resistance. The forms of resistance that emerge will vary across discussions and contexts. Sometimes, it takes the form of a patient's quiet reluctance; at other times, it is outright denial. Although there appears to be less outright conflict, pharmacists may sometimes have to tread a skillful path to avoid conflict with a patient.

Resistance can arise when the patient brings conflict into the discussion, when the pharmacist elicits it, or as a result of a combination of the two. The patient can be in a state of internal conflict about change in which different internal voices are pressing for different outcomes. The stronger and more conflicting the voices, the more likely it is that resistance will arise. If the person is in conflict with others as well, it can be even more pronounced. Sometimes, the person might not be in a state of conflict, but in a state of learned helplessness about lifestyle change. Whatever the personal source of resistance for the patient, the patient will be particularly sensitive to the way you speak to them.

It is unrealistic to view resistance as a sign of failure in the counseling session, something that is abnormal and should be eliminated from the discussion at all costs. Some health care practitioners even say that, with good rapport, resistance provides the kind of energy that generates change. However, in most time-limited discussions, it is a nuisance. Hence, on an ongoing basis, pharmacists should look out for resistance and move toward reducing it. This is not just a matter of what you say or which strategy you use, but how you say it and having a sufficiently flexible state of mind to roll with the resistance and avoid argument.

Awareness of strategies for dealing with resistance should not over-shadow the most important guideline: listen and watch. If you meet resis-tance, change tack. Resistance is often a signal to you to change gears and to repair damaged rapport, usually by coming alongside patients and talking in a way more in sympathy with their feelings and attitudes. Be watchful for the patient who is in verbal accord with you, but whose body language demonstrates obvious resistance.

### Emphasize personal choice and control

If a person is struggling to maintain some sense of control over life, it does not take much to threaten this sense of stability. All one needs is a confrontation, and resistance to change will emerge. It does not take much to fall into the trap of undermining the personal autonomy of the patient. Health care practitioners, even when giving advice, appear to be well aware of these subtleties and apparently adjust their message accordingly. Hence, it has been discovered that they make their advice ambiguous to avoid becoming too personal: they present their advice in neutral terms, as if it is information. Another viable option to avoid threatening auton-omy is to make this explicit. A simple phrase added to a piece of advice can make all the difference: "I think that you should stop smoking now, but it's really up to you." This might well avoid eliciting resistance. Leave out the second half, and you could be in trouble.

It is also not merely a matter of what is being said, but how it is being said. The pharmacist's attitude and the atmosphere of the counseling session will contribute to the patient's reaction. The same words used in two different atmospheres will have quite different effects.

### Reassess readiness, importance, or confidence

A common cause of resistance is when the pharmacist falls into the trap of overestimating or misjudging readiness, importance, or confidence. Most often, this results in premature action talk. If readiness is seen as a continuum and the patient is at the not-ready end, a pharmacist who assumes that the patient either is or should be at the ready end will elicit resistance. Seen in this light, resistance is a measure of the extent to which the pharmacist has jumped ahead of the patient. The obvious practical implication is that a shift in the pharmacist's strategy is necessary to ensure congruence with the patient's state of readiness. The same overestimation mistake can be made when the talk is about either the importance of change or the confidence to achieve it.

For example, a pharmacist establishes that a smoker would very much like to give up smoking (i.e., importance is high), but the smoker is concerned about achieving cessation (confidence is low). The pharmacist makes the mistake of assuming that this confidence should be higher and more amenable to shifting than it really is, and that a few bits of simple advice will suffice. Some suggestions are offered. The outcome is resistance.

This discussion has assumed that the patient would like to talk about behavior change. However, a more dramatic, yet very common, example of overestimation is to focus on behavior change when the patient is more concerned about something else. Thus, the pharmacist might talk about exercise when a patient in cardiac rehabilitation is feeling depressed and fearful about having another episode of myocardial ischemia.

A pharmacist can also misjudge a patient's feelings by focusing on confidence instead of importance or vice versa. People often come into action-orientated clinics and slip into talk about practical measures to improve confidence to change. Health care practitioners are trained to do things to people and to solve problems.

If you have made the mistake of either overestimating one of these qualities or focusing on the wrong one, the most obvious response to the resistance that can arise is to reevaluate the direction you are taking. This can be done explicitly by asking the patient to tell you how he or she really feels, particularly about the distinction between importance and confidence. This can be achieved in a few minutes.

This reassessment does not necessarily have to be done in an explicit manner, but can be achieved simply by sharing with the patient your confusion about exactly what the patient's concerns are.

### Back off and come alongside the patient

The strategy of backing off and coming alongside the patient is designed to counter the trap of meeting force with force. It captures the heart of motivational interviewing, that is, responding to resistance by keeping in a state of mind in which one does not "take the bait" or meet force with force, but comes alongside the patient. The technique of making reflective listening statements is a direct way of achieving this.

Avoiding argument is not just a passive process in which one sits back in a defensive posture and uses reflective listening until the fire dies down, but one in which the pharmacist tries to come alongside the patient and understand how the patient is feeling. If successful, resistance usually subsides, and the discussion can move in a different direction.

Reflective listening involves making statements designed to show that you understand the meaning of what the person is saying. The effect of using such statements, as opposed to questions, is to encourage the patient to continue talking and expressing personal views and feelings. The reflective statements can take a variety of forms: repeating exactly what the person has said, rephrasing what is said in different words, or adding new meaning to that expressed by the patient.

## References

Miller, W.R., Motivational interviewing with problem drinkers, *Behav. Psychother.*, 11, 147–172, 1983.

Prochaska, J.O. and DiClemente, C.C., Towards a comprehensive model of change, in Miller, W.R. and Heather, N., Eds., *Treating Addictive Behaviors*, Plenum, New York, 1986, pp. 3–27.

Prochaska, J.O., Di Clemente, C.C., Velicer, W.F., and Rossi, J.S., Comments on Davidson's "Prochaska and DiClemente model of change: a case study?" *Br. J. Addict.*, 87, 825–828, 1992.

Rollnick, S., Heather, N., and Bell, A., Negotiating behaviour change in medical settings: the development of brief motivational interviewing, *J. Ment. Health*, 1, 25–37, 1992.

Rollnick, S., Mason, P., and Butler, C., *Health Behavior Change: A Guide for Practitioners*, Churchill-Livingstone, Edinburgh, 2000.

# chapter three

# The challenge of the patient's ethical problem

Pharmacists have a professional commitment to the care of their patients. Pharmacoethics is thus central to the understanding of pharmacy practice as a profession. In this chapter, five ethical principles are identified in the tradition of pharmacy practice: nonmaleficence, beneficence, respect for persons, loyalty, and distributive justice. These ethical principles establish ethical duties, obligations, and rights and provide a standard for rationalization of ethical decisions.

Pharmacists may meet head-on ethical conflict in their practices. Ethical dilemmas arise when two or more of these ethical principles appear to be in conflict and may be resolved through closer scrutiny of the situation or thoughts concerning other courses of action. Ethical dilemmas occur in pharmacy practice when two principles conflict and signal that a pharmacist may be unable to act fully on responsibilities and duties.

A fundamental task of pharmacoethics is to probe the meaning of these ethical principles through important examples of ethical conflicts, to examine the implications of the principles for professional integrity, and to recognize priorities when principles conflict. Nonmaleficence, which requires avoiding harm, also provides a framework for trust in the pharmacist–patient relationship. The ethical tradition of pharmacy historically has been expressed in an ethic of beneficence and patient benefit. However, especially in cases of paternalism, a commitment to beneficence may conflict with patient autonomy and dignity, including a patient's right to have health care professionals respect her or his informed and voluntary decisions. Loyalty and fidelity engage the conscientious pharmacist in an ongoing process of negotiation and a thoughtful deliberation about personal and professional roles. Justice demands that pharmacy professionals seek a fair allocation of benefits and burdens in pharmacy practice.

Depending on interpretations of the meaning and priority of these ethical principles, a pharmacist may affirm a professional self-understanding of technician, parent, advocate, or partner. Such models also have ramifications for the conception of the "patient" in pharmacy practice.

The principles of pharmacy practice are most appropriately understood as presumptions or *prima facie* obligations rather than ethical absolutes or ethical maxims. This method permits flexibility to the particularities of a clinical situation without compromising the obligatory force of ethical principles. Deliberation and discernment among conflicting principles can enable better patient care and a pharmacy practice that embodies professional ideals.

## The ethical realities of pharmacy

Buerki and Vottero, in their insightful book, *Ethical Responsibility in Pharmacy Practice* (1994), have outlined the reasons for the transformation of the practice of the profession of pharmacy from a product-orientation to a more patient-orientation. Furthermore, they laid the foundation for most of the contemporary discussion on ethical pharmacy practice and how ethical principles must be considered when the pharmacist must make a decision involving a clash of these principles.

However, an individual pharmacist might find that many decisions central to the health of a patient are largely out of the pharmacist's hands. The pharmacist sometimes is perceived as an "extension" of the physician, and the pharmacist's exercise of moral agency can be severely circumscribed not only by the directives of physicians, but also by the regulations of government and the marketing methods of the pharmaceutical industry. Someone else, in short, has often already made the ethical choices a pharmacist might make about patient care, and the role of pharmacist may thereby seem largely restricted to the activities of "filling and following orders."

However, pharmacists are much more than technicians of transfer for health-related products. They instead have undertaken a professional commitment to the health care and interests of persons who present themselves as patients. An ethical choice about providing benefits to fellow human beings is central to the self-understanding of pharmacy. As articulated in the 1994 revision of the American Pharmaceutical Association's (APhA's) Code of Ethics, "a pharmacist promises to help individuals achieve optimum benefit from their medications, to be committed to their welfare, and to maintain their trust." The ethical tradition embedded in pharmacy has been formalized since the 1850s through various codes of ethics that express a collective "profession" of moral self-identity.

It also is not the case that pharmacists are mere passive puppets of physicians, regulators, or entrepreneurs. The discrete encounters and ongoing relationships between pharmacists and patients continually confront practitioners with perplexing ethical choices that require the exercise of personal and professional autonomy.

# Ethical perplexity and justification

The process of ethical justification can be conceived in terms of an ascending and descending relation of judgments regarding particular choices or actions, ethical rules, and ethical principles.

In an encounter with a patient, a pharmacist might make a judgment to fill a prescription based on a professional rule to promote patient health care, which in turn is rooted in the principle of beneficence, or respect for persons. The pharmacist might also inform the patient of the nature of the medication, its prescribed dosage, any side effects, and the like, also based on a principle of beneficence. The process involves moving back and forth between decisions in other situations and the general direction offered by the ethical principles. The decisions might be modified by competing ethical principles in multifaceted circumstances.

The nature of ethical rationalization in pharmacy practice will reflect different kinds of ethical situations. In many instances, a person's ethical responsibility is clearly evident, and the person's performance is justified by appeal to one (or more) ethical principle. Alternatively, we may know what our responsibility is and fail to do it. Imagine that a pharmacy student is eagerly anticipating an arranged discussion with the professor of a student-centered problem-based case in pharmacoethics, but the professor fails to attend. It turns out that the professor found the idea of a day at the park overpowering and headed for the local park. We can correctly conclude the professor failed to meet ethical and professional responsibilities set by the ethical principles of justice and respect for persons.

Genuine ethical dilemmas occur for pharmacists in their personal lives generally and in their pharmacy practices because it is unclear what the right or good thing might be after considering everything. It may turn out, for example, that the professor did not meet with the student for a quite different reason: While preparing for the discussion, his wife became ill and required attention. The professor has an ethical responsibility to meet with the student because of his previous promise, but he also has a moral responsibility to obtain necessary care for his wife. There may be alternatives to avoid the ethical dilemma, such as contacting the student to reschedule the meeting, but this option might be difficult if the pharmacy student cannot be reached.

The language of "ethical dilemma" signals that the person will be unable to act fully on personal responsibilities because of a conflict of ethical principles. Our professor, for example, cannot aid his wife and carry out the teaching commitment. Thus, in an ethical dilemma, ethical considerations could be offered for alternative and seemingly incompatible courses of action, and careful deliberation is necessary to determine which principle, that of beneficence or that of promise keeping, should have priority. The nature of ethical justification in a dilemma involves discerning which of the conflicting actions has greater ethical weight and offering persuasive reasons to various stakeholders for the decision. While some ethical dilemmas are only obvious because satisfactory alternatives can be investigated, a real ethical dilemma cannot be resolved solely by more investigation of the facts of the situation. It necessitates a value choice that expresses the ethical character of the person.

## *The principle of nonmaleficence*

A fundamental duty in patient care and in social life generally consists of not inflicting harm, injury, or death to other persons. This duty is expressed in the ethical principle of nonmaleficence. This principle is implicit in the Hippocratic maxim "first of all, or at least, do no harm." We also acknowledge this ethical duty in our legal and philosophical traditions, which allow a broad scope to personal freedom but permit the imposition of ethical and legal restrictions when individual actions pose risks of harm or injury to others. The principle of nonmaleficence is the bedrock of social life, and it is difficult to conceive of a society or a profession functioning without a commitment to it.

A commitment to nonmaleficence, in contrast, provides a context for the expression of trust in human relationships, and this capacity for trust is especially significant in health care because of the vulnerability of patients. Patients give professional caregivers privileged access to their bodies and selves in the trusting expectation that they will not be harmed unnecessarily. Trust is so vital to the encounters of caregivers and patients that we commonly perceive their relationships as "fiduciary" in character. The cultivation of reliance and confidence is especially relevant to pharmacist–patient relationships. In marked contrast with the levels of trust expressed in other health care professions, pharmacists are considered to possess high levels of integrity; they are afforded a social trust generally given to friends, neighbors, and relatives.

While the principle of nonmaleficence is clearly essential to ethical research and testing for safe and effective drugs, it plays an equally significant role in the activities of the practicing pharmacist. To avoid harming patients, even unintentionally, the pharmacist must be technically competent and knowledgeable about new product developments, the interactive qualities of various medications, and the characteristics of the particular patient, who may suffer an allergic reaction to a medication that is entirely safe for most others. The principle of nonmaleficence thereby provides justification for specific professional duties delineated in the 1994 APhA Code of Ethics, including the duty "to maintain knowledge and abilities as new medications, devices, and technologies become available and as health information advances." The principle of nonmaleficence, as well as respect for persons, supports the professional duties of honesty and integrity.

A pharmacist has a duty to tell the truth and to act with conviction of conscience. A pharmacist avoids discriminatory practices, behavior or work conditions that impair professional judgment, and actions that compromise dedication to the best interests of patients. If pharmacists fail to observe these duties, patients may be harmed due to dated knowledge or technical skills and can rightly claim that their trust in the fiduciary relationship has been violated.

Of course, such a relationship entails that the expression of trust is mutual, and the pharmacist can be placed in a difficult situation if patients or their proxies seek to exploit the trust.

## The principle of beneficence

Only a very minimalistic morality would claim that our moral responsibilities are exhausted by duties to refrain from harming or injuring others. Our common life requires affirmative efforts to benefit others by promoting their welfare, although disagreement often ensues about who is obligated to assist or provide the benefits. Few persons dispute, for example, that receiving health care is substantially beneficial. However, there is controversy over whether a person's access to health care should be based on need, personal responsibility, or ability to pay, and there is controversy over who should be obligated to provide access.

The principle of beneficence expresses this sense that morality requires more than just staying out of another's way; rather, on occasion we may be obligated to step in and aid others, or we may already be in relationships, such as families, that require mutual assistance for viability. In most instances, duties of positive benefit are accepted as part of the various roles and relationships we assume, such as husband–wife, parent–child, teacher–student, and health care professional–patient. Indeed, what makes the health care professions morally distinctive is the prominence of duties of positive benefit as part of the profession's self-identity. We have already discussed, for example, how patient health and safety are deemed the "first consideration" of the ethical pharmacist, and fulfilling that duty requires both acts of nonmaleficence and the positive concern for patient benefit expressed by beneficence. It is arguable whether a society can survive without beneficence; our society, for example, has largely repudiated legally compelled beneficence expressed in "Good Samaritan" laws, preferring to leave acts of charity and love to personal ideals and discretion. It is clear, however, that a health care profession cannot survive ethically without beneficence: the act of "professing" is just that a person voluntarily assumes certain affirmative responsibilities toward a patient's welfare.

Philosophers often have specified a threefold content to beneficence, holding that it encompasses duties to (1) prevent harm, (2) remove harm, and (3) provide benefits. The professional responsibilities of pharmacists can reflect each of these dimensions. One rationale for disclosing the potential effects of a medication to a patient or in monitoring patient compliance is clearly to prevent harm to the patient. Pharmacists do not perform the kinds of invasive procedures that remove harm as a surgeon or dentist might, but a pharmacist might take steps to intervene in medication patterns to alleviate or minimize causes of harm. Finally, the intention and expectation of dispensing drugs and medications is that they will bring benefit to the patient by improving the patient's condition.

While beneficence is central to the profession's sense of ethical identity and integrity, its priority is a source of controversy in pharmacoethics. The dispute is not over whether pharmacists should express commitment to patient health and safety, but rather over who defines "health and safety" — the pharmacist or the patient. The patient's understanding of health or safety is set in relation to the pharmacist's particular way of life and set of values. On that basis, the pharmacist might, for example, be willing to accept certain levels of risks or side effects that are different from the standard professional recommendation. Or, some patients with protracted terminal illness may be willing to trade safety for a chance at health by seeking to use nonvalidated drugs.

The conflict between the perspective of the professional and that of the patient regarding health and safety constitutes the moral conflict of paternalism. The paternalistic medical model depicts the relation of professional and patient in terms of parent and child. The parent/professional makes decisions and provides directive information, based on experience and specialized knowledge, to enhance the best interests of the child/patient as perceived by the parent/professional. The beneficence-based rationale of paternalism is that the professional, like parents, "knows best." The child/patient is excluded from the decision-making process because of lack of education and minimal understanding about the consequences of choices. It becomes clear that, because of significant disparities in power, information, and experience, the potential for paternalistic practice is embedded in all interactions between health care professionals and patients. As an important participant in these relationships, pharmacists can find themselves involved in paternalistic conflicts regarding refusals of patient requests for a particular medication or disclosure and nondisclosure of information.

## The principle of respect for persons/autonomy

The ethical vision of the intrinsic dignity of human beings lies behind the ethical principle of respect for autonomy. This dignity is expressed in our capacities for free action and rational choice; in our political culture generally, and in health care specifically, the possibility of exercising these capacities without interference from others commonly gives rise to the language of "rights." For example, a claim of a right to information about a proposed medication allows the patient to make a rational choice about whether to use the medication and accept its risks or to seek other alternatives. We treat others as rational beings and respect their autonomy by allowing them a zone of personal liberty in which to enact their ways of life and worldviews and by requiring that they offer reasons for their choices and decisions regarding their interests. That is, the necessity of ethical justification is itself a part of what it means to express respect for another person as a rational being.

Conversely, the principle of respect for autonomy prohibits us from treating a person merely as an instrument or means to achieve our ends and purposes or to achieve ends and purposes they do not share with us, even if we think they should. This is what makes paternalistic pharmacy practice ethically problematic.

Current trends in pharmacoethics and practice clearly signal an ascendancy of respect for personal autonomy. A shift in language from "patient" to "client" or "consumer" to describe the recipient of the pharmacist's services reflects this trend: a patient embodies the passivity of "the sick role," in contrast to the more informed and participatory role required of a client or consumer. This emerging ethical vision of the person who requests medication requires a corresponding modification in the understanding of the ethical role of the pharmacist.

## The principle of loyalty

In one of its aspects, loyalty is concerned with the fulfillment of the ethical self. It therefore overlaps with issues of personal autonomy and integrity, although it entails more than self-determination in decision making. Loyalty also requires commitment and deep devotion to the kind of person one aspires to be.

Loyalty also presumes a social and institutional context to our ethical choices. It reveals a relational dimension to the ethical life that an exclusive focus on personal autonomy can conceal. We do not find ourselves to be free-floating, unencumbered atoms in an ethical universe; instead, our ethical responsibilities are interwoven with and mediated by our interrelationships with others, which in the context of pharmacy may include family, patients, physicians, professional colleagues, administrators, employers, and others. We express concern about devotion, fidelity, and "betrayal," the antithesis of loyalty, in these relationships that are core to our sense of self-identity. Loyalty answers our need for unification of the personal and relational dimensions of our lives, a harmony of the private and public ethical worlds.

It would be incorrect, then, to associate the principle of loyalty with the model of pharmacy as a technical, unethical practice. Loyalty instead engages a conscientious ethical agent in an ongoing process of negotiation and accommodation through which commitment and faithfulness are displayed to sometimes converging, sometimes diverging, claims. It requires thoughtful, discriminating deliberation about priorities and the relative importance of responsibilities, whether personal, professional, or institutional. The principle of loyalty is thus ethically richer than a professional model of following and filling orders, and within this model to question an order is itself a form of disloyalty rather than an autonomous expression of devotion and fidelity.

As an ethical principle, loyalty requires that we give the persons to whom we are loyal their ethical due. It is often expressed in interpersonal or interprofessional relationships in the rule of fidelity, including the keeping of promises, while in broader social settings, loyalty overlaps with the ethical principle of justice. That is, the nature of the roles and relationships of the persons conditions the answer to the question of what is "due" another on the principle of loyalty. This requires, in turn, that we give meaningful content to professionalism in pharmacy.

The participation in many relationships can, on occasion, make conflicts of loyalty an unavoidable part of the ethical life of the pharmacist. Resolving the conflict could involve extricating oneself from the relationship, but this obviously does not occur without ethical loss.

## *The principle of distributive justice*

It is not always ethically possible in pharmacy practice to avoid harms (nonmaleficence) and provide benefits (beneficence). In such situations, we need to be concerned with who receives the benefits and who bears the burdens or harm. The question of the allocation of benefits and burdens is the focus of the principle of distributive justice. It is a central principle for pharmacoethics because of the broader social context in which pharmacists practice, one aspect of which is that some persons may be restricted in terms of their ability to have access to the services of a pharmacist. The principle of distributive justice requires the pharmacist to consider whether the resources the pharmacist provides to patients are distributed fairly and equitably.

## *The ethical status of principles*

We identified five ethical principles of pharmacy practice. The meaning and priority of these principles are in part conditioned by prior conceptions of professionalism in pharmacy. It is useful to address the question of priorities among conflicting ethical principles.

One possible interpretation of the ethical status of principles is to understand them as expressions of ethical absolutes. This interpretation can be difficult to sustain when, as in our view of pharmacoethics, an ethical framework offers a plurality of principles. It simply is not always possible to avoid harm, provide benefits, and respect rights without ethical conflict. One method of resolving this sense of incompleteness associated with ethical absolutism is to prioritize one principle and to consider others as reflecting important, but subordinate, responsibilities. The 1981 APhA Code of Ethics was suggestive of this method in its designation of patient health and safety as the "first" consideration of the pharmacist. Yet, prioritizing one principle can neglect some ethical matters, such as patient and professional autonomy, that should be more prominent.

Another alternative is to treat ethical principles as maxims that may illuminate a situation of ethical conflict, but do not themselves give moral direction or prescribe ethical obligations. On this account, the principle of loyalty, for example, would have a moral status analogous to the medical maxim, "Take two aspirin, get plenty of rest, and call me in the morning." An ethical maxim expresses the generalized experience and wisdom of the past, but can be set aside or ignored in the exigencies of any situation.

While the flexibility of this approach is appealing, we believe it is possible to accommodate flexibility and sensitivity to the distinctive setting of an ethical problem without abandoning the ethical or obligatory force of a principle. Perhaps it is that the principles of pharmacoethics are understood as establishing presumptive or *prima facie* duties or obligations. All other things being equal, a pharmacist is obliged to avoid harm, promote welfare, respect autonomy, express loyalty and fidelity, or distribute benefits equitably. However, often things are not equal, and the ethical pharmacist is required to choose one principle that provides definitive ethical direction in the dilemma.

An instructive analogy for presumptive principles can be drawn from the law. A basic principle of our legal system is that a person is presumed innocent until proven guilty. The legal presumption of innocence imposes a burden of proof on those who seek to establish guilt. Similarly, the ethical decision to infringe one principle, such as beneficence, for the sake of another, such as loyalty, imposes an ethical burden of proof on the pharmacist; the burden of proof can be met through the reason-giving process described above as ethical justification. Thus, unlike the absolutist approach, this account accommodates both ethical conflict and flexibility, but unlike the maxim account, it demands conscientious deliberation and public accountability rather than allowing laxity.

## *Ethical decision making*

When faced with an ethical problem, how should the pharmacist proceed? There are many ways of answering this question, but a particularly useful way is to approach the decision-making problem systematically (Weinstein, 1996):

1.   Gather the medical, social, and all other relevant facts of the case.
2.   Identify all relevant values that play a role in the case and determine which values, if any, conflict.
3.   List the options open to you; that is, answer the question, "What could you do?"
4.   Choose the best solution from an ethical point of view, justify it, and respond to possible criticisms; that is, answer the question, "What should you do, and why?"

Good ethical decision making begins with getting the facts straight. Thus, the first step for making ethical decisions, in the clinical setting or anywhere else, is gathering the relevant facts.

Information we may have for a patient in a common scenario is that she has a history of orthostatic hypotension, that this is one of the major side effects of the drug prescribed for her, and that there are other drugs available that do not commonly have this side effect. While not necessarily life threatening, orthostatic hypotension may place the patient and others at great risk of harm since the condition may involve loss of consciousness, and the patient may be operating machinery, descending a staircase, or holding an infant when this occurs. Since legal obligations are ethically relevant, the pharmacist should consider what the law requires of a pharmacist. Although there is a general legal duty to inform physicians and patients of the potential risks of drug therapy, the specific laws in a case such as this vary from state to state.

To resolve an ethical dilemma such as this common one, facts are necessary, but not sufficient. Addressing ethical problems differs from addressing mere technical ones in that the former involves a consideration of values as well as facts. In addition to the relevant facts, an appropriate response to the question, "What should you do?" requires an account of the values that play a role in the case and which ethical guidelines those values suggest. Identifying values is thus the second step of ethical analysis. Certainly, one important value suggested by the case is the welfare of the patient, which gives rise to the ethical rule, "Protect others from harm." The pharmacist has good reason to believe that filling the prescription for the guanethidine will result in harm, not only to the patient, who already has experienced one of the known side effects of the prescribed drug, but also possibly to others who may come into contact with the patient. The ethical commitment to do no harm justifies the feeling the pharmacist has that it would be wrong to fill the prescription.

If avoiding harm to patients were the only important ethical consideration in the case, the pharmacist would not be faced with a dilemma since it would be clear that the pharmacist should not fill the prescription. There are other values, however, that play a role here. One of them is the pharmacist–physician relationship. Pharmacists are rightly obligated to promote a good relationship with the physicians with whom they work, and this obligation includes a responsibility to fill the prescriptions the physicians provide. A third value is respect for patient autonomy or, more specifically, the patient's right to have information that will enable her to make an informed decision about her health care. This value gives rise to the rule requiring both the physician and pharmacist to provide the patient with the relevant facts about the likely consequences of various drugs, as well as of no drug therapy.

The final value that plays a role in this case is respect for the law, which requires the pharmacist to do what is legally required. We now have the makings of a genuine ethical dilemma: the pharmacist is bound to avoid harming patients and others, but is also committed to promoting a professional relationship with the prescribing physician, as well as to counseling the patient. To which ethical rule, and thus to which group of people, does the pharmacist ultimately owe allegiance?

This brings us to the third stage of ethical analysis, generating options. In other words, we might ask, "What could the pharmacist do?" This is the creative step of the process. Among the options open to the pharmacist are to (1) fill the prescription, but counsel the patient about the risks of the medication; (2) refuse to fill the prescription and explain to the patient why; and (3) attempt to persuade the prescribing physician to change the prescription. There are other possible courses of action, but these are the most obvious ones and correspond most closely to the values presented above. Which option is best from an ethical point of view, and why?

To answer these questions, we take the fourth and final step of ethical analysis, choosing an option and justifying it. If it were the case that the pharmacist had to choose between competing loyalties, it would be difficult to hold that the pharmacist's final decision must be to respect the wishes of the physician. After all, the primary commitment to the welfare and rights of patients distinguishes pharmacy as an ethical practice. Still, it might not be necessary for the pharmacist to choose between these apparently conflicting responsibilities. The pharmacist might call the physician back and provide the justification for the belief that alternative antihypertensive medications offer fewer risks to the patient than guanethidine. Sometimes, ethical conflicts can be handled adequately by exercising personal skills rather than by having to make tough choices, and this may be one of those cases. Only if such an attempt is unsuccessful will the pharmacist have to decide whether loyalty to the physician requires placing the patient and others at risk.

One conclusion that may be drawn from this common scenario is that turning to the law will not always help us resolve ethical quandaries. Even if it is legally permissible for a pharmacist to dispense the medication, the pharmacist still may ask, "What is the right thing for me to do?" The analysis also suggests that some approaches to ethical problems in the clinical setting are more ethically defensible than others, and that through ethical analysis one is able to distinguish better from worse approaches. It is sometimes the case that any option will have unfortunate consequences, but this is not the same as saying that there are no answers to ethical problems. Indeed, the circumstances of pharmacists often require some kind of decision or action; thus, in many instances it is impossible to avoid making ethical choices. Through ethical analysis and reflection, as well as discussion of the problem in a systematic way with others, one is more likely to achieve a reasoned and justifiable decision.

One might think that the process of ethical decision making is too time consuming and complex to use in the clinical setting. Obviously, in emergency situations, the ethical mandate of the pharmacist is to save the patient's life or prevent irreversible harm. For troubling ethical problems, it is both prudent and ethically appropriate to take some time to reflect on one's options and consider the best reasons for choosing some rather than others.

## References

Buerki, A. and Vottero, L.D., *Ethical Responsibility in Pharmacy Practice*, American Institute of the History of Pharmacy, Madison, WI, 1994.

Weinstein, B., *Ethical Issues in Pharmacy*, Applied Therapeutics, Vancouver, WA, 1996.

*chapter four*

---

# Creating a framework for student-centered problem-based learning sessions involving pharmacoethics

Using what we discussed in the first three chapters, we now turn to ways of thinking, conflict management, and feedback. These features are incorporated into the new framework for conducting PBL sessions involving pharmacoethics. We then turn to a discussion of the list of clinical ethics and research ethics competencies.

## Ways of thinking

At the heart of every discourse is the question of perspective. Different people make different assumptions about reality and the nature of information. How one sees the world affects the kind of questions asked and what can be accepted as explanations. Of the hundreds of questions about pharmacy that can be asked, each presupposes a "normative perspective" for that particular question. Some questions will be more productive than others for obtaining answers, especially those for which the questioner correctly assumes the perspective of the respondent.

Due to selective perception and conditioning, people analyze problems differently. Everyone has sources of knowledge that range from untested opinion to highly systematic styles of thinking. As we go about our daily lives, we rarely think about how we "know" something or where this knowledge originated. From ancient times to the present, we have pursued the discovery of how we know. In the process of this discovery, we have depended on an ability to discriminate among information sources. Pharmacists must therefore identify those sources of high quality and high value that will produce the best results for a given situation or decision. The philosophy of science provides six of the styles of thinking: (1) untested opinion, (2) self-evident truth, (3) persons of authority, (4) literary, (5) scientific, and (6) postulational. Each of these styles of thinking is discussed in turn (Mitroff and Mason, 1982).

There is a way of thinking that is often called *untested opinion*. People cling to untested opinion despite contrary evidence. In the indoctrination programs of less-enlightened organizations, it is not unusual for new employees to hear remarks that confuse entrenchment and habit with efficiency. Most families have an aging relative who holds steadfastly to a conspiracy theory for a memorable world event despite overwhelming contrary evidence. Historically, myth, superstition, and hunch have been serious competitors for scientific thinking. One writer notes that, before an event occurs — an event that one is trying to predict or control — myth, superstition, and hunch offer "the reassuring feel of certainty" (Hoover, 1991), although seldom does that feeling of certainty persist after the event is over. Pharmacists will find little to improve their patient's understanding of reality from untested opinion, even though human nature indicates they should be prepared to cope with its use by contemporaries when searching for solutions to ethical dilemmas.

There is another way of thinking that is often called the method of *self-evident truth*. It may be self-evident to a person that people will die no matter what precautions are taken by a conscientious pharmacist. If citizens do not die because of a drug-related problem, then they will die as a result of something else. Death is inevitable; it can be deduced from known laws of nature. But, what about propositions that appear reasonable to one person or even to many at any time, but are not true? For example, "Everyone drives on the right side of the road." This "truth" is self-evident only to some of the world's drivers. Other propositions once considered reasonable include: "Women make inferior pharmacists"; "Men of noble birth are natural leaders"; and "Japanese quality practices are universally applicable to U.S. productivity problems." We now dismiss these once self-evident propositions.

Since not all propositions or assumptions are self-evident, we rely on *persons of authority* to improve our confidence in our knowledge. Authorities serve as important sources of knowledge, but should be judged by their integrity, the quality of the evidence they present, and their willingness to present an open and balanced case. Too often, authority may depend on status or position rather than true expertise. Such celebrity authorities, when acting outside their area of expertise, are often wrong. You would be wise to accept the views of such sources cautiously. Even authorities who do meet the standards of integrity, quality evidence, and balance may find their knowledge misapplied.

The *literary style* of thinking is used in many classic case studies in the social sciences. Case studies play a prominent role in the development of knowledge; our nation's best graduate programs use case studies extensively. Portions of anthropology, psychiatry, and clinical sociology also trace their roots to this origin. Abraham Maslow's theory of motivation is one example from psychology that is well known (Maslow, 1987). The literary perspective is one in which "a person, a movement, or a whole culture is interpreted, but largely in terms of the specific purposes and perspectives of the actors, rather than in terms of the abstract and general categories of the scientist's own explanatory scheme" (Kaplan, 1964). Because it is difficult to generalize from individual case studies, the literary style of thought restricts our ability to derive generally applicable knowledge or truths.

There is a way of thinking referred to as the *scientific method*. The essential tenets of science are: (1) direct observation of phenomena; (2) clearly defined variables, methods, and procedures; (3) empirically testable hypotheses; (4) the ability to rule out rival hypotheses; (5) statistical rather than linguistic justification of conclusions; and (6) the self-correcting process. "Current scientific methods merge the best aspects of the logic of the rational approach with the observational aspects of the empirical orientation into a cohesive, systematic perspective" (Howard, 1985, p. 7).

Finally, there is a way of thinking referred to as the *postulational style*. Competing styles of thinking influence research directions throughout the social and behavioral sciences. Many firms run computer simulations of their new medication before a product rollout. These might examine different pricing levels or manufacturing output levels designed to optimize profitability. One goal of this perspective is to reduce the object of study to mathematical, formal terms. These terms, called postulates, are used to devise theorems that represent logical proofs. The objective is to deduce a mathematical model that may account for any phenomenon having similar form.

There is no single best perspective, only preferred perspectives, from which to view reality or to practice pharmacy. The range of available styles of thinking offers many frameworks to confront the diverse problems of practicing pharmacy. Useful knowledge abounds; one should simply be aware of the vantage point selected to find information and the strengths and weaknesses of that position.

## Conflict management

By recognizing the innate differences in styles of thinking, it will become easier for you to gain entrée into other innate differences between you and your patients before you can truly understand the basic tenets of conflict management. Any type of problem solving requires effort and sensitivity to other causes of conflict.

Conflict almost always arises because one person believes that the achievement of personal goals is being threatened. Conflict can arise when people are competing for limited resources, whether tangible (a promotion) or intangible (respect, power, trust).

Maybe most important, conflict can also arise over differences in values. Because of the way values are learned in childhood, people often see values as absolute "rights and wrongs." When opposing values or beliefs are encountered, conflict occurs. Opposing values, beliefs, or ideas call our beliefs into question. This unsettles us because the possibility then exists that we have spent a substantial portion of our life believing something that may not be true. Unfortunately, most people do not see this as an opportunity to question their thinking. Many people see conflict as a chance to defend their beliefs — even if their beliefs are incorrect.

The best strategy for managing conflict can be described as problem solving. There are five steps to the problem-solving process (Daft and Steers, 1986):

1.  It is important to identify the exact problem and its nature and who "owns" the problem. Keep in mind that we are not responsible for solving other people's problems.
2.  By brainstorming with others, multiple solutions to a problem are sought; parties understand that important decisions/solutions may take time; and all possible ideas must be expressed. People are striving for quantity at this point, not quality, and are free to seek combinations or improvements of ideas.
3.  Decide which solution is best. After all the solutions have been identified, choose the one that is best for the problem at hand.
4.  Determine how to implement the solution. After choosing the best solution, decide on a plan of action for carrying it out.
5.  Assess the outcome of the solution. Were both parties satisfied with the outcome? Could this problem have been prevented?

Through problem solving, the persons involved may negotiate to accept and approve a desired change (Filley, 1990). When we avoid a conflict or a problem, three things happen: (1) we still have the original problem; (2) we create a new problem when we deny the existence of the problem so we do not feel defeated by it, therefore distorting reality; (3) we undermine ourselves because we know we have avoided a problem, it does not feel good, and we have impeded our growth. Often, problem solving entails one or more of the following:

1.  Educating others helps to provide information they may be lacking, which can clear up inaccurate perceptions and help to effect change. Counseling patients about the proper use of their medications may avoid misconceptions and improper use. The language of problem solving focuses on attacking the problem, not the person. It expresses a desire for a mutually acceptable solution that achieves both parties' goals. Open, honest feelings, facts, and opinions are expressed by both parties. There is a shared responsibility to ask questions and to seek clarification of the issues. An important part of clarifying and accurately defining the problem is through feedback.

2.  Those adjusting to change need encouragement. Active listening and empathy will offer the needed support for people having difficulty accepting change. Patients having a hard time accepting a chronic illness need this kind of support. People in conflict typically engage in a specific type of communication that attacks the other person. They make statements such as, "You make me angry!" "You're too sensitive!" "If it weren't for you . . . " "You always do that!" Then, both people are off and running into an argument that is separate from the original issue. The problem does not get solved, and a new one is created. Both people feel hurt or angry.
3.  The change process is easier when those involved are included in the decision making. The patient should be actively involved in decisions that affect personal health and life.

## *Framework for conducting student-centered problem-based learning sessions involving ethical competencies*

Although the problem-based learning process is an important vehicle for applying the pharmacist's clinical knowledge to the patient's problem in a logical way, it would be of limited value without extensive knowledge of ethical issues that might surround the patient's problem and ways to communicate with the patient or physician effectively about these possible issues. It is impossible for any pharmacist to have all the knowledge that will be needed for all ethical issues surrounding the patient problems that will be encountered. In fact, it is not uncommon that a particular patient problem will be one for which the pharmacist does not have sufficient knowledge of its ethical issues, but careful reasoning with the knowledge available about the patient's situation can carry the pharmacist quite far with the patient at the moment. After obtaining even more information about the patient's situation, the pharmacist can skillfully approach the patient or physician to work through the issues together.

The knowledge pharmacists bring to bear on the patient's problem is integrated from all the health disciplines basic to pharmacy practice through a rich network of associations. This integrated information is almost automatically recalled to mind with the cues presented by the patient's problem. More can be recalled through thoughtful metacognition. The recalled information is structured through associations with information from a variety of disciplines and applied to the understanding of the patient problem as it unfolds. As an example, the understanding in the workup of a patient with a suspected socially transmitted disease depends on recall of anatomical, physiological, pathological, biochemical, and pharmacological information associated with the evolving information on history and laboratory tests.

The pharmaceutical care of the patient may require considerable legal and ethical knowledge. Often, the experienced pharmacist is unaware of the knowledge itself, but its presence is clear in the care decisions made for the unique picture a particular patient presents. Importantly, this rich, integrated, and structured information base is enmeshed with the pharmacist's clinical and ethical reasoning processes. Furthermore, it is responsible for the hypotheses generated through association with the cues in the patient's problem as well as the pharmacist's skill with inquiry, analysis, synthesis, and decision making. The ethical reasoning process, like the clinical reasoning process, employs recalled information for application in work with the patient and is not apparent to most practicing pharmacists because it is recalled and applied almost automatically and below consciousness. Only when deliberation or puzzlement intervenes and there is an active attempt to recall relevant information are pharmacists aware of their thinking and the information in memory.

The pharmacist has information integrated from ethical knowledge and ethical decision making to structure around the cues and information coming from the patient's clinical problem, and it is enmeshed with the stages of the clinical reasoning process. Most information will be acquired during clerkship, internship, and practice because much of the information acquired during conventionally taught courses is forgotten.

In contrast with the integrated, patient-structured information that the pharmacist has enmeshed with the clinical reasoning process, pharmacy students in the traditional preclinical years are asked to learn information from ethics in isolated subject contexts. Even the so-called integrated curricula still present information from ethics in isolation from each other, but coordinated in the teaching schedule. Integration occurs in the schedule, not in the minds of the students. Information from each ethical competency is learned in the context of that discipline and not in the context of patient problems. Concepts are learned within hierarchies of a particular discipline.

The students learn definitions and concepts in ways that will help them pass written examinations in subject contexts. The important cues for the recall of information acquired are the questions that will be on the examination, not cues that will appear in later clinical work, when the information will be needed for the care of patients. The principal cognitive skill students employ is rote memorization to recall the information given in the course when cued by examination questions aimed at the recall of content for its own sake. Student performance on an examination at the end of an ethics course does not measure long-term recall or what the student actually learned because students will always cram to tune their long-term memory using rote memorization and mnemonics.

Even if some ethical knowledge were to be remembered by the time of the clinical years, it would not be associated with clinical phenomena (cues from the patient's history, laboratory tests) or the clinical reasoning process employed. This severely reduces the odds that it will be recalled in subsequent clinical work. Context is important in the recall of information.

To manage the health problems of patients in an effective, efficient, and humane manner, the pharmacist has to acquire an expert clinical reasoning process enmeshed with rich associated ethical information structures that are recalled in the context of patient problems. Conventional ethics courses do not stress the development of clinical reasoning skills in the context of learning ethics. The students are involved in passive learning in which their heads are force-fed with "inert" knowledge as they try to absorb and memorize the many facts thrown at them in lectures and reading assignments. The term *inert knowledge* is defined as knowledge that can be recalled to answer questions, but cannot be applied even though it is relevant to the task at hand. Students' knowledge is acquired in the context of individual subjects and not integrated in the mind of the student around the pathophysiological, psychobiological, or ethical problems of patients.

The design of problems for practice-based learning has already been discussed. The design of problem formats that present the patient problem as it is actually presented clinically and that permit the student to carry out a free inquiry (asking any questions on history, performing any laboratory tests in any sequence) is essential to allow the students to develop an effective and efficient clinical reasoning process. Commonly used formats to accomplish this in practice-based learning are the PBLM (problem-based learning method) and standardized patient. These problem simulations should be based on actual patient cases, ensuring the students that such a problem really existed and allowing the problem designers to use the actual patient's problems.

## Criteria for problem-based learning session participant feedback

Feedback is a way of helping a student consider changing personal behavior in order to become a better pharmacist. Feedback is communication to a person that gives information about how effective the person's work or actions are during the PBL session. Feedback helps an individual keep behavior "on target"; thus, it helps a person better achieve personal goals. The University of New Mexico School of Medicine developed the following criteria for oral or written PBL session participant feedback:

1. *Feedback is descriptive rather than judgmental.* Describing one's reaction to another person's work leaves the other person free to use the feedback or not use it as the person sees fit. Avoiding judgmental language reduces the other's need to respond defensively.
2. *Feedback is both positive and negative.* A balanced description of a person's behavior or actions takes both the strong and weak points into account. Both points give the other information for change.
3. *Feedback is scientific rather than general.* To make a general statement about another person's work as a whole does not tell a person which parts of that performance or those actions need changing and which might serve as models.

4.  *Feedback takes into account the needs of both the receiver and the giver.* What you say to a person about that person's performance not only reflects his or her work or actions, but also reflects how you think or feel about the person at the moment.
5.  *Feedback is directed at behavior that the receiver can do something about.* When a person is reminded of some shortcoming for which the person has no control, the major change is in terms of an increased frustration level.
6.  *Feedback is solicited rather than imposed.* Feedback is most useful when the receiver has formulated the kind of question for which he or she most wants an answer.
7.  *Feedback is checked to ensure clear communication.* What the giver intends to say is not always synonymous with the impact it has on the other person. Asking about the meaning of doubtful feedback can clear up the discrepancy.
8.  Feedback is directed primarily at a person's performance or behavior rather than at the person.
9.  Feedback is most useful when given immediately after work has been completed or behavior has been exhibited.

## Clinical ethics competencies and research ethics competencies

Choosing the patient problems is the essential ingredient in providing a curriculum of study. Any patient problem will require the students to apply a certain body of facts and concepts to assess the problem, determine the basic mechanisms involved, and attempt resolution. If the students are ignorant, unsure, or confused about the facts and concepts required in their problem-solving activity, they will recognize the need to put them on the board as learning issues and tackle them during self-directed study. In this way, practice-based learning will cause them to learn and apply the facts and concepts important to their medical education.

There are two ways to approach the selection of problems for a practice-based curriculum. The first is based on the professor's knowledge or belief regarding what students ought to learn from their disciplines. This approach allows the professor to be more comfortable in the conversion from the teacher-centered, didactic learning approaches always used to the student-centered practice-based learning. They can be reassured through problem selection that a curriculum is still intact, and they are able to determine what the students should learn. However, the question can always be asked: "How does the pharmacist know what a pharmacy student should learn?" In the clinical realm, the clinical faculty have assembled lists. In the pharmacoethics realm, lists of clinical ethical competencies such as the one given next are extremely useful for problem-based learning.

UNM's Health Sciences Center has developed the following list of clinical ethics competencies for its School of Medicine, College of Nursing, and College of Pharmacy students. UNM's Health Sciences Center expects these clinical ethics competencies to apply throughout its programs. The competencies were developed by the Perspectives in Medicine (PIM) program at the UNM School of Medicine, the Professional Attitudes and Values group, and the Task Force on Ethics and Humanities.

## *Clinical ethics competencies: University of New Mexico Health Sciences Ethics Program*

### *1. Professional responsibility*
Assume responsibility for profession as a whole.
Understand emergency treatment duties.
Do no harm.
Do not abandon patients.
Understand own biases.
Provide for continuity of care.
Keep abreast of important research and changing practice standards.
Understand rights and duties of both patients and professionals.
Understand own limitations.

### *2. Patients' rights*
Understand autonomy and informed consent.
Obtain valid consent or refusal of treatment.
Understand medical and legal dimensions of decisional capacity.
Know how to proceed if treatment is refused.
Understand appropriate use of ethics committees and consultants.

### *3. Privacy and confidentiality*
Understand how to protect patients' privacy as well as the duty to
     inform.
Inform patients of limits of confidentiality.
Understand legal requirements of reporting.

### *4. Truth telling*
Tell the truth.
Understand those specific circumstances when it might be morally justified to withhold or delay information.

### *5. Reproductive ethics*
Understand ethical and legal issues of reproductive decision making:
     abortion, birth control, sterilization, sexually transmitted diseases,
     and appropriate referrals; reproductive research; genetic screening
     and counseling; treatment decisions for seriously ill neonates.

### 6. *Distributive justice*

Understand issues of access and barriers to health care: alternative models of equitable delivery; individual rights and the public good; impact of technology, managed care.

### 7. *Research ethics*

Understand the ethics and law of research on humans as well as animals: informed consent; patient care/comfort vs. research imperatives; access to new therapeutic research treatments; use of placebos; conflicts of interest; duty to share research results.

## Research ethics competencies: University of New Mexico Health Sciences Ethics Program

The responsible researcher:

### History

Is familiar with sentinel events in 20th century research ethics (e.g., research in Nazi Germany, the Tuskegee syphilis study, the Willowbrook studies, the human radiation studies)

### Principles, standards, and regulations

Is familiar with the major codes, statements of ethical principles, and laws/regulations that prescribe responsible conduct in research (e.g., the Nuremberg Code, the World Medical Association Declaration of Helsinki, the Belmont Report, applicable government and institutional regulations)

### Integrity in science

Understands the meaning of scientific misconduct (fabrication, falsification, plagiarism) and knows how to respond
Understands the duty to report research errors due to mistake or negligence
Keeps good records and manages, stores, and retains data responsibly
Claims authorship, performs peer review, and allocates credit for research responsibly
Understands the legal, regulatory, and professional definitions of conflicts of interest and avoids exploiting his or her position for personal or financial gain
Mentors or supervises students/trainees in a responsible manner (i.e., assumes responsibility for their academic, technical, and ethical development)

### Research on human subjects

Understands the elements of and can secure a legally and ethically valid informed consent

Understands ethical issues around selection of subjects and research on
   special populations (e.g., minorities, patients, persons with developmental disabilities, prisoners, infants and children, fetuses)
Understands the function, structure, and requirements of institutional
   review boards (IRBs)

### Research/testing on animals

Is familiar with and respects professional and institutional regulations
   and guidelines concerning responsible research on animals
Understands and can apply assessment criteria for conducting responsible research on animals (e.g., the nature and measurement of pain
   and suffering in animals, the purpose of the experiment, policies on
   pain and death, alternatives to the use of animals)

### Contemporary issues

Keeps abreast of current and emerging important national and interna-
   tional research ethics issues, such as:
   Ownership of data, intellectual property, and the right to patent
   Genetic research (gene therapy, genetic testing, cloning, uses of ge-
      netic information, banking of genetic material)
   International research standards and practices (international ac-
      quired immunodeficiency syndrome [AIDS] research, indus-
      try-sponsored research in developing countries, subject selection
      and subject consent outside the United States)
   Research versus medical surveillance in the work setting

## *Framework for conducting student-centered problem-based learning sessions involving ethical competencies*

The goal of the four introductory chapters has been to help "paste together"
a framework for conducting each different problem-based learning session
that revolves around a list of ethical competencies. This framework is displayed on the next page and should be followed by each PBL group member
to help the person optimize his or her understanding of each ethical competency. To skip one or more steps in this framework would be unproductive
and would "short-circuit" the thoughtful process required to develop the
intended educational outcome: a critical set of patient-related skills necessary
to practice the profession of pharmacy.

### *Objectives*

### *Introduction*

   *Read first part of case narrative, then work through the following:*
   Make a list of the major problems presented in the case.

For each problem in the list generated above, give a cause or a reason for it to happen.

From your two lists above (problems and causes/reasons), make a list of learning issues — medical, social, legal, ethical, and so on.

Look in the local medical library and on the World Wide Web for helpful information.

Identify all relevant values that play a role and determine which values (nonmaleficence, beneficence, respect for persons, loyalty, distributive justice), if any, conflict.

*Read second part of case narrative, then work through the following:*

List the options open to you. That is, answer the question, "What could you do?"

Choose the best solution from an ethical point of view, justify it, and respond to possible criticisms. That is, answer the question, "What should you do, and why?"

Two group members role-play: determine the different ways of thinking among people involved and possible techniques for conflict management.

Two group members role-play: determine how the transtheoretical model/stages of change may help you understand why some people involved are not changing and what motivational interviewing techniques might be brought to bear on the situation.

*Read third part of case narrative, then work through the following:*

Conclusions: what was learned from the case?

Written or oral feedback to PBL session participants.

## References

Daft, R.L. and Steers, R.M., *Organizations: a Micro/Macro Approach*, Scott Foresman, Glenview, IL, 1986, pp. 575–580.

Filley, A.C., *Interpersonal Conflict Resolution*, Scott Foresman, Glenview, IL, 1990, pp. 41–43.

Hoover, K.R., *The Elements of Social Scientific Thinking*, 5th ed., St. Martin's Press, New York, 1991, p. 5.

Howard, G.S., *Methods in the Social Sciences*, Scott Foresman, Glenview, IL, 1985.

Kaplan, A., *The Conduct of Inquiry*, Chandler, San Francisco, 1964, pp. 259–262.

Maslow, A.H., *Motivation and Personality*, 3rd ed., Harper & Row, New York, 1987.

Mitroff, I.I. and Mason, R.O., Business policy and metaphysics: some philosophical considerations, *Acad. Manage. Rev.*, 7, 361–371, 1982.

*case one*

# Professional responsibility

This problem-based learning session is based on the following: *Wright v. Abbott Laboratories*, 97-1333-JTM, U.S. District Court for the District of Kansas, 62 F. Supp. 2d 1186; 1999 U.S. Dist. Lexis 13531. August 16, 1999, Decided. August 16, 1999, Filed. It is reprinted with permission of LexisNexis.

## Objectives

To investigate the roles and responsibilities of pharmacists to create a professional atmosphere. These responsibilities include:

- A responsibility to the patient
- A responsibility to self and society
- A responsibility to the profession as a whole

Professional responsibility in the field of pharmacy is a very emotional issue. Many court decisions often involve pharmacists and their patients. Pharmacists have a responsibility to a patient to prevent negative outcomes of drug therapy as it relates to the pharmacist's professional knowledge. As a result, states have mandated specific guidelines for pharmacists to follow. The role of the pharmacist includes responsibility to the patient, themselves, to society, and to their profession as a whole.

## Part one

Eric Wright was born at Wesley Hospital in Wichita, Kansas, on November 10, 1992, at 6:51 P.M. At birth, he had good color and respiratory effort, but shortly afterward he went limp and required resuscitation. Because of his low blood sugar levels, Wright was started on intravenous fluids and was transferred to the neonatal special care unit (NSCU) for blood pressure monitoring, thermoregulation, and continued intravenous fluids.

Wright arrived at the NSCU at 9:45 P.M. with low blood pressure after resuscitation. Prior to transfer, his treating physician, Dr. Barry Bloom, had given an order to monitor blood sugar every hour. Nurse Donna Benjamin put Wright on a machine that read his blood pressure automatically every 15 min. Shortly after the third reading, Nurse Benjamin had Dr. Bloom paged due to the infant's low blood pressure reading.

At approximately 10:50 p.m., Nurse Rhonda Martin took the following telephone order from Dr. Bloom for Eric Wright: "Piggyback normal saline, 20 cc over 30 min." Dr. Bloom prescribed normal saline (0.9% sodium chloride) to raise the infant's blood pressure levels. Eric Wright was not hyponatremic (that is, suffering from a low sodium condition) at the time and did not have an electrolyte imbalance.

Nurse Karen Diltz overheard Nurse Martin repeating Dr. Bloom's order and asked if she could help. Nurse Martin said, "Yes, if you could draw it up."

Wesley Hospital's Department of Nursing "Medication Administration Policy" provided in pertinent part:

> the registered nurse and/or licensed practical nurse is legally accountable to know the medications, the action, adverse reactions, and implications of nursing care for each medication administered.

The policy required the following checks prior to administering any medication:

> The name of the patient (if able, a patient should be asked to verbally state their name), the patient's identification band and specialty bands (if applicable), drug, dosage, route, and time on the medication label three times.

In both nursing school and again at Wesley, nurses were taught to check and double-check the "five R's" — whether they have the right patient, the right drug, the right route of administration, the right dose, and the right time for administration. The plaintiff's nursing expert, Emily Jansen, R.N., testified that when a nurse administers a drug, the nurse must follow the five R's. According to Jansen, learning the five R's is one of "the basics" in nursing school and in hospital practice.

Nurse Diltz did not read Dr. Bloom's order. Relying on what she had overheard, Diltz believed Dr. Bloom wanted normal saline to be given. In her deposition, she admitted her action was a departure from hospital policy.

At approximately 11:00 p.m., Nurse Diltz removed a vial from the medication cart in the workroom of the NSCU. The medicine cart contained, in drawers on different levels, 0.9% sodium chloride and 14.6% sodium chloride. Although it was Nurse Diltz's practice to read a drug label three times before administering a drug, she did not read the label on the vial to determine the concentration of sodium chloride she had retrieved.

She knew at the time that normal saline solution and 14.6% sodium chloride were stocked in the same medication cart, but in different drawers. The drawer of the medication cart containing 14.6% sodium chloride had a label identifying its contents.

Nurse Diltz knew before she took the vial from the cart that Eric Wright was not hyponatremic, and that none of the indications for using concentrated sodium chloride was present. She also knew the difference between normal saline and 14.6% sodium chloride. She knew that normal saline (0.9% sodium chloride) was used as a volume expander for hypotensive patients, whereas 14.6% sodium chloride was used to replace electrolytes for hyponatremic patients. Before November 10, 1992, she had administered 14.6% sodium chloride more than 10 but less than 100 times. Nurse Diltz knew that a medication error involving 14.6% sodium chloride could result in serious injuries. She knew that if too much sodium was injected into a patient, sodium levels would increase, resulting in a possible imbalance of the fluid distribution in the body. She also knew that such a condition could result in an intraventricular bleed, causing permanent brain damage.

Nurse Diltz knew that the order left by Dr. Bloom was for normal saline "because you would never add . . . 20 cc of sodium chloride to an i.v. solution, it would be too large an amount to add to an i.v." Moreover, she knew that the order was for a volume expander and testified: "We do not give 14.6% sodium chloride as a volume expander."

Still, Nurse Diltz drew 25 cc of 14.6% sodium chloride from the vial and gave the syringe to Nurse Benjamin. Nurse Benjamin injected the sodium chloride into a porthole in Wright's intravenous tubing.

Less than an hour later, Dr. Bloom ordered another 20 cc of normal saline. Again, Nurse Diltz went to the medicine cart, took a vial of 14.6% sodium chloride from the drawer, and drew 25 cc with a syringe. She again handed the syringe to Nurse Benjamin, who, at around 11:50 p.m., injected the sodium chloride into Eric Wright's intravenous tubing.

Nurse Diltz testified that she knew the normal saline vial only held 10 cc, and that when she went for the vial with the larger amount in it, she looked only "at a portion of the label and did not look at the percentage." She testified that, in both instances, she failed to follow nursing policies, failed to read the concentration on the vial, and handed the syringe to a nurse who was not authorized to administer the solution.

Nurse Diltz also testified that, as soon as she retrieved the empty vial from the trash, she knew "it was the wrong vial . . . it was the vial that I used, but I should not have used it . . . because I knew it wasn't normal saline. . . . It was the wrong concentration." She knew it was wrong because "it's on the label." Diltz testified, "I made a mistake," and that her "thought process did not continue on where it should."

As a result of this injection of concentrated saline into the intravenous tubing, plaintiff Eric Wright has incurred substantial, severe, and permanent physical injuries.

Wesley Medical Center is a 760-bed tertiary care hospital located in Wichita, Kansas. According to their brochure, Wesley provides sophisticated health care services to residents of Wichita, Sedgwick County, the State of Kansas, and out-of-state patients. It is a major teaching hospital and provides clinical services, medical research, and outreach care programs. It was one of four incorporating hospitals that formed Health Frontiers, a network of 30 midwestern hospitals seeking to provide joint purchasing power, expertise and office sharing, and economies of scale.

Throughout the relevant period, Wesley had three levels of neonatal units: (1) receiving nursery or "well baby" nursery, (2) neonatal special care nursery or neonatal special care unit (NSCU), and (3) neonatal intensive care unit (NICU). The NICU mainly treated children needing alternative feeding approaches, those with mechanical ventilation, children with cardiovascular instability, and children recovering from surgery. The NSCU cared for newborn infants between well baby status and newborn intensive care candidates. The NICU and NSCU are in the same building, but on different floors of the hospital.

- At all relevant times, Michael Hurst was the director of Pharmacy Services at Wesley, a position he has held since 1987 and still holds. Hurst obtained a degree in pharmacy from the University of Kansas in 1966 and a master of business administration from Wichita State University in 1978. He joined Wesley as a staff pharmacist in 1966 and was later promoted to senior staff pharmacist and then assistant director of Pharmacy Services. Hurst has memberships in the American Society of Hospital Pharmacists and the Wichita Academy of Pharmacists. As the director of Pharmacy Services, Hurst reports to the Vice President, Administration for Professional Services, and is responsible for the complete operation of the pharmacy department, including proper policies and procedures.
- Ella Hamilton obtained a pharmacy degree from the University of Kansas School of Pharmacy in 1974. Shortly after graduation, she worked for Wesley for approximately 7 months. In 1979, she returned to Wesley and has been a staff pharmacist ever since. Hamilton was responsible for and performed monthly inspections of the drug storage areas on the NSCU.
- Barry Bloom is a medical doctor specializing in neonatology who has practiced at Wesley since 1986. In 1992, Dr. Bloom was the medical director of the NICU and NSCU, and he was Eric Wright's treating physician. Dr. Bloom is currently medical director of Wesley's NICU.
- Delaine Bartsch is a registered nurse who graduated from the Medical University of South Carolina in 1982. She began working in the NSCU at Wesley in 1988. In October 1991, she became the department director of Special Care Nurseries and held that position when Wright was admitted to the NSCU.

- Karen Diltz is a registered nurse who obtained her degree from William Jewell College in 1985. She began work in the NSCU at Wesley in 1987 and has worked in that unit, as well as in the NICU, until today.
- Donna Benjamin is a licensed practical nurse who was employed by Wesley during the relevant period. She received her diploma from nursing school in 1981, and in November 1991, Wesley sent her to a 10-week class for intravenous administration.
- Cynthia Harmon is a registered nurse who has been employed by Wesley since 1974. She has been the nurse manager of Wesley's NICU since 1978 and is in charge of the other nurses working in the NICU.

## Make a list of the major problems presented in this case

- 
- 
- 
- 

## Hypothesis and mechanism

For the problems in your list above, give a cause or a reason for each to happen:

- 
- 
- 
- 

## Learning issues

Make a list of learning issues in the form of questions. Remember, your goal is to gather the medical, social, and all other relevant facts that may apply to the case.

- 
- 
- 
- 

### Responsibility to the patient

1. All health care providers have a responsibility to their patients to do no harm. What sorts of actions would fall within the meaning of "do no harm"?

- Unintentional harm by mistakenly filling a prescription for the wrong drug for the wrong person
- Deliberately harming the patient by dispensing expired medications knowing it may harm the patient

2. Health care providers must understand their own biases. Can you give an example of some common examples of personal biases?
   - An individual pharmacist might state that floor stock is an inherently flawed method of drug distribution, and that all drugs and drug admixtures should be obtained from a pharmacist.
3. Define unprofessional or dishonorable conduct.
   - In defining unprofessional conduct, the definition of professional conduct and duty should be considered: failure of the health care provider to conduct herself or himself professionally in conformity with all applicable federal, state, and municipal laws and regulations.

*Responsibility to self and society*

1. What is meant by providing for continuity of care through continuing education?
   - Keeping abreast of current developments in the field
   - Being aware of future investigations that will improve the quality of care to patients
   - Attending continuing education classes for continued licensure
   - Completing a law review
2. One or more of the health care providers in the case could have been under the influence of alcohol or some other mind-altering drug. What is the prevalence of drug abuse among pharmacists and the concurrent need for counseling?
   - 16.4% prevalence of psychiatric substance abuse disorder
   - 13.3% prevalence of alcohol abuse or dependency
   - 5.9% prevalence of other drug abuse or dependency
3. If the circumstances in the case had been slightly different, the pharmacist may have been asked to help with emergency treatment for Eric Wright. What examples of emergency treatment duties should a pharmacist understand?
   - Inappropriate drug therapy may require emergency treatment.
   - Adverse drug reaction, drug interaction, and the like.
   - Prevention of inappropriate medication use.
   - Importance of indications, contraindications, and warnings.
   - Drug utilization review intervention.
   - Pharmacists' role in teaching emergency action for poisoning. Expertise in using antidotes to treat various poisonings.
   - Poison centers are staffed with pharmacists.
   - Advising mothers to keep a bottle of ipecac syrup at home.
4. What limitations to duty should a pharmacist understand?

- System-related medication errors will occur, but need to be investigated to understand how to avoid them in the future.

*Responsibility for the profession*

What can pharmacists do to assume responsibility for the profession as a whole?

- Risk management programs
- Continuous quality improvement programs
- Expansion of roles
- Initiate, monitor, evaluate, and adjust drug therapy
- Responsibility for outcomes
- Pharmacist prescribing

## Literature review

To help you get ready to answer certain questions you anticipate being asked during the second part of the case, you start to look in the local medical library and on the World Wide Web for helpful information. Please indicate in the spaces below (1) several helpful articles or books you found and (2) several helpful Web sites you found.

- **Helpful articles/books:**

  Baldwin, N.J. et al., ASHP statement on the pharmacist's role in substance abuse prevention, education, and assistance, *Am. J. Health-Syst. Pharm.*, 55, 1721–1724, 1998.

  Belkin, L., *First, Do No Harm*, Simon and Schuster, New York, 1993.

  Buerki, R.A. and Vottero, L.D., *Ethical Responsibility in Pharmacy Practice*, American Institute of the History of Pharmacy, Madison, WI, 1994.

  Flake, J.L., Developing an immunization program, *Am. J. Health-Syst. Pharm.*, 56, 2398, 2403, 2408, 1999.

  Gasbarro, R., Does the Rx look suspicious? *Am. Druggist*, 216, 48–51, 1999.

  Grabenstein, J.D. and Bonasso J., Pharmacists' role in immunizing adults against pneumococcal disease and influenza, *Am. J. Health-Syst. Pharm.*, 56(17 Suppl. 2):S3–S22, quiz S23–S24, 1999.

  Iverson, K.V., Sanders, A.B. and Mathieu, D., *Ethics in Emergency Medicine*, Galen Press, Tucson, AZ, 1986.

  Jonsen, A.R., Siegler, M. & Winslade, W.J., *Clinical Ethics*, 4th ed., McGraw-Hill, New York, 1998.

  Melton, C., Clinical management of poisoning and drug overdose, *Ann. Emerg. Med.*, 34, 304–305, 1999.

  Phipps, J., Educational evolution: perpetual progression of pharmacy, *J. Am. Pharm. Assoc.*, 38, 121, 1998.

  Rutberg, P.M., Medical record confidentiality, *Neurol. Clin.*, 17, 307–311, 1999.

- **Helpful Web sites:**
  The National Center for Public Policy Research: www.national-center.org
  American Pharmaceutical Association: www.aphanet.org
  Drug topics: www.drugtopics.com

*Identify all relevant values that play a role in the case and determine which values, if any, conflict*

Non-maleficence:

Beneficence:

Respect for persons:

Loyalty:

Distributive justice:

*Learning issues for next student-centered problem-based learning session*

- List the options open to you. That is, answer the question, "What could you do?"
- Choose the best solution from an ethical point of view, justify it, and respond to possible criticisms. That is, answer the question, "What should you do, and why?"
- What are the different ways of thinking about the problem? Which conflict management techniques can be used in the situation?

- Could it be that some of the persons involved are in various stages of change about how to solve the problem? How can motivational interviewing be used to help some people change?

## Part two

Wesley's Pharmacy Department was responsible for providing continuing pharmaceutical services to the hospital. Wesley had a central pharmacy that was staffed 24 hours a day and two satellite pharmacies. One satellite pharmacy was located in the area of surgery and labor and delivery; the second was near the NICU. The satellite pharmacies were staffed for the first and second shifts during the week and only the first shift on weekends.

The Pharmacy Department had the responsibility to distribute drugs to the patient care areas in an efficient manner, which will ensure their availability when needed for administration and ensure their safe use. Wesley pharmacists were expected to keep up with the professional literature and maintain a working knowledge of current trends in therapeutics. The Pharmacy Drug Information Center, within the Pharmacy Department, maintained a reference library containing textbooks, journals, commercially published drug information, and reference files categorizing information alphabetically by generic name, disease state, or special topic heading (such as sodium content, teratogenic agents).

The Pharmacy and Therapeutics Committee (P&T Committee) of the Wesley medical staff developed or approved policies and procedures relating to the selection, distribution, handling, use, and administration of drugs and diagnostic testing materials, among other functions. The P&T Committee includes one physician from each of the following areas of specialty: infectious disease, cardiovascular disease, pediatric allergy, anesthesiology, family practice, oncology, pulmonary disease, obstetrics/gynecology, orthopedics, otolaryngology, urology, and pediatrics/neonatology. Each physician member of the committee has one vote. Also participating on the committee, without a vote, are two members of Nursing Services, the Quality Assurance director, the director of Pharmacy Services, the clinic coordinator, the Drug Utilization Evaluation coordinator, a representative from Administration, the pharmacy supervisor, and a recording secretary.

All pharmacy policy implementation and change requests are submitted to the P&T Committee by the director of Pharmacy Services. In addition, all Pharmacy Department policies are reviewed annually by the P&T Committee for the purpose of establishing their consistency with current practices within the hospital.

Because drug storage areas throughout Wesley are under the supervision of the director of Pharmacy Services, the director of Pharmacy Services or one of the director's pharmacists or designees is responsible for monthly inspections of all nursing units or other areas of Wesley where medications are dispensed, administered, or stored.

During Michael Hurst's more than 30 years at Wesley, there has been a continuous quality improvement program. It is uncontroverted that the subject of medication errors has been of great concern at Wesley. As a result, Wesley has a Pharmacy Quality Assessment Program to undertake a continuous analysis of medication dispensing errors. The director of Pharmacy Services prepares monthly reports of medication dispensing errors for the P&T Committee. Wesley policy provided, "Critical errors will be evaluated immediately and the Chairperson of the Pharmacy and Therapeutics Committee will be contacted to determine if policy changes are required to reduce serious errors in the future." In an effort to minimize the risks associated with the use of drugs, the P&T Committee also developed a list of restricted drugs and guidelines for use of those drugs.

In the early 1980s, Wesley developed an intravenous admixture pharmacy to minimize intravenous preparation, storage, and handling outside the pharmacy. With respect to orders for additions to intravenous solutions, the Pharmacy Department's I.V. Admixture Guidelines provided:

> *The pharmacy will not make additions to i.v. solutions once they have been started. If the physician deems it necessary to add medication to a solution that is already being infused, the addition is to be made by the nurse on the unit. The medication to be added may be obtained from the emergency supply on the unit or from the IV Admixture Pharmacy if not available in emergency stock.*

*Floor stock* at Wesley means those "items that nursing has immediate access to for patient use." Floor stock requests, either additions to or deletions from, are within the purview of the P&T Committee.

It is uncontroverted that, when reviewing a floor stock request, the P&T Committee assesses the additional risk of medication errors against the need for nursing to have access to the proposed floor stock item for patient use. Ultimately, however, it is the practice of the P&T Committee "to defer to the judgment of the medical director of the affected nursing area whether there was a medical need to floor stock the medication."

In November 1992, concentrated sodium chloride was a floor stock item for electrolyte therapy in critical care areas. Before that time, Hurst knew that concentrated sodium chloride could cause serious injury if administered improperly or if the nurse selected the wrong concentration. He knew that 14.6% sodium chloride should never be injected without dilution. According to Dr. Keck Hartman, who chaired Wesley's P&T Committee in 1991 and 1992, the committee also appreciated these risks. It knew that injection of concentrated sodium chloride could cause serious injury.

Before 1992, a patient at Wesley had been injured when he received excessive quantities of 3% sodium chloride through an intravenous bag.

That incident prompted Wesley to adopt restrictions for sodium chloride concentrations greater than 3%. Beginning in September 1991, intravenous sodium chloride (3% or greater) was listed as a restricted drug, and there were published guidelines for its use. This policy was created due to the danger of hypernatremia, impairment of renal function, fluid, solulate overload, tachycardia, seizure, and coma.

In 1992, the NSCU was an approved floor stock nursing area. The P&T Committee approved the floor stock of concentrated sodium chloride on the NSCU because of the medical staff's perceived need to have it immediately available if necessary. Dr. Bloom testified that there are times when a patient will need "immediate action" to correct an electrolyte disturbance. P&T Committee chair Hartman concluded that, based on the opinions of Dr. Bloom and Dr. Curtis Dorn, the neonatologist member of the committee, there was a medical need for nursing to have immediate access to concentrated sodium chloride on the unit for patient use. This decision to have concentrated sodium chloride as floor stock on the NSCU took into account the potential additional risk created by dispensing the solution from floor stock on the one hand and the need for immediate access to those drugs on the other hand.

As director of Pharmacy Services, it was Hurst's duty periodically to review the NSCU's medication floor stocking policy. In November 1992, the NSCU stocked concentrated sodium chloride in an immobile medicine cart that was located in a supply room on the unit. The standard floor stock consisted of 2 vials of 14.6% sodium chloride and 25 vials of normal saline (0.9% sodium chloride).

Hurst has testified that, before the Eric Wright incident, he knew dispensing medications from floor stock could increase the risk of medication errors. He also knew that nurses could make mistakes when using sodium chloride. For instance, he knew that nurses could select the wrong concentration, draw up too much or too little of the right concentration, and not dilute a medication properly before administration. They could administer a medication in improper ways, by improper routes, and to the wrong patients.

Hurst knew in 1992 and before that one approach to reducing the risk of medication errors was to reduce floor stock items. It was standard hospital practice for the pharmacy to control the dispensing and administration of drugs to minimize errors, and Hurst stated that he has read literature on the subject. Hurst knew that there were reasons for minimizing or attempting to eliminate floor stocking of drugs that invoked risks if improperly administered.

Hurst has stated that he probably read the package insert for 14.6% sodium chloride. It is uncontroverted that Hurst knew in 1992 and before that there was a risk of serious adverse reaction if an excessive dose of concentrated sodium chloride was administered to a newborn by the intravenous route and if a doctor had prescribed normal saline, but 14.6% sodium chloride was inadvertently administered instead.

To obtain information about a particular drug product, Hurst testified that the Pharmacy Department personnel "would go to the package insert[s] themselves." They could also go to resources such as the American Hospital Formulary and the Micromedex drug information program.

Wright's treating neonatologist and head of the NSCU, Dr. Bloom, testified:

> *I didn't have to have the FDA tell me that there's a risk of [inadvertent administration of concentrated sodium chloride] . . . if you asked me when I was a second year medical student if administering 14% sodium chloride solution would harm someone, I would say absolutely. Direct intravascular administration is harmful.*

Bloom further testified that he knew that medication errors could occur almost anywhere: "If it could occur at the bedside, it could occur in the drug room, it could occur in the pharmacy, it could occur anywhere. So where they restricted this to or where they put it, I don't know that we could prevent the kind of error that occurred in this situation."

Nurse Diltz testified that she knew, in 1992 and before, that a medication error involving 14.6% sodium chloride could result in serious injuries, including an intraventricular bleed that could cause permanent brain damage. Nurse Harmon testified that every nurse's training includes procedures for mixing and calculating dilutions for electrolytes, including concentrated sodium chloride, and the importance of avoiding medication errors. According to Nurse Harmon, that nurses should read medication labels is "more or less drummed into nurses and nursing students."

Ella Hamilton, Wesley's staff pharmacist, testified that she was aware of a risk of inadvertent administration of concentrated sodium chloride created by the floor stocking of concentrated sodium vials in proximity to vials of normal saline.

*List the options open to you. That is, answer the question, "What could you do?"*

- 
- 
- 
-

*Choose the best solution from an ethical point of view, justify it, and respond to possible criticisms. That is, answer the question, "What should you do, and why?"*

- 
- 
- 
- 

*Select one member of your PBL group to role-play as the pharmacy director and have another member of your PBL group role-play the nursing director. How might the two converse about different ways of thinking and techniques for conflict management?*

- 
- 
- 
- 

*Again, please select one member of your PBL group to role-play the pharmacy director and have another member of your PBL group role-play the nursing director. How might the pharmacy director use what is known about stages of change and about motivational interviewing to solve what you consider the major problem presented in the case?*

- 
- 
- 
- 

## Part three

On January 7, 1994, the plaintiff filed a medical malpractice action in the District Court of Sedgwick County, Kansas (Case 94 C 66), against HCA Wesley Medical Center and Dr. Barry Bloom, M.D. On February 10, 1994, the petition was amended to remove Dr. Bloom as a defendant. The plaintiff prayed for damages in the sum of $17,807,317.

On November 14, 1994, the plaintiff entered into a settlement agreement and release with Wesley. The settlement agreement provides for an initial lump sum payment of $3,574,710.62 on November 14, 1994, and smaller lump sum payments on four other occasions. It also requires periodic payments over the plaintiff's lifetime, beginning on December 15, 1994, with

$5,588.12 per month and escalating annually until they reach $81,217.04 per month on November 15, 2022, just after plaintiff reaches the age of 30.

The payments from December 1994 through November 2009 are guaranteed. Payments beginning in December 2009 and continuing for the remainder of plaintiff's life are contingent on his survival.

Eric Wright is 6 years old. The plaintiff's experts project a life expectancy of an additional 57 to 67 years. Plaintiff is thus guaranteed to receive over $7 million (the initial lump sum payment plus the payments certain through 2009). If plaintiff reaches the age predicted by his experts, he will receive between approximately $45 million and $63 million. The plaintiff's damage expert based his opinion, in part, on a third projected life expectancy of an additional 75.64 years.

The plaintiff's life care plan expert proposed three alternatives for the plaintiff's day-to-day care under the two different life expectancy projections: 57 additional years and 67 additional years from November 1998 (or a total of 63 years and 73 years, respectively). Based on these life care plans, as well as a third projected life expectancy of an additional 75.64 years, or a total of 81.64 years, the plaintiff's damages expert, Dr. Harold Goldstein, prepared three reports estimating the plaintiff's loss of earning capabilities and the sums that the plaintiff's conservator will need to cover the plaintiff's future expenses. Dr. Goldstein opinioned that, if the plaintiff reaches 63 years of age, he will lose earning capacity of $2,113,220 and will incur expenses between approximately $11.7 million and $15.7 million. If he reaches 73 years of age, he will lose earning capacity of $2,404,153 and incur expenses between approximately $16.1 million and $20.2 million. If he reaches age 81.64 years, he will lose earning capacity of $2,404,153 and incur expenses between $20.6 million and $24.6 million. Thus, the range of damages under Dr. Goldstein's theory is approximately $13.8 million to $27 million.

## Discussion of case

### Responsibility to the patient

Apply the principle of beneficence.
Do no harm by preventing or removing harm.
Be kind and civil to others.
Promote autonomy when appropriate to avoid patient abandonment.
A pharmacist cannot quit service without a valid reason, and if abandonment becomes necessary, give reasonable notice of termination of care to patient when alternate care exists for patient.

### Justification of biases

The pharmacist should never let personal biases cause a patient to have a negative outcome. This would be unprofessional conduct that would damage the patient–pharmacist relationship and disrupt the patient's optimal drug therapy.

### Responsibility to self and society

Pharmacists should step out from the satellite pharmacy or from behind the counter and counsel all health care providers and patients.

Various pharmacy groups have developed programs to train and certify pharmacists interested in new areas of practice.

Substance abuse among patients and health care providers frequently can cause psychiatric disorders and physical immobility; intervention is key.

### Clinical management of poisoning and drug overdose

Appropriate use of drugs can prevent drug-induced illness, hospitalization, and even death. Pharmacists' role in teaching health care providers and society in general about emergency treatments contributes to overall improved health care.

### Justification of limitations

A pharmacist must exercise his or her professional judgment in any situation as proactively as possible.

### Expanding roles

Interests of pharmacists should not be product driven, but patient driven.

Patient outcomes will fuel future pharmacy-based clinical practice.

We must move to a more professional pharmacy practice with the implementation of continuous quality improvement programs.

We must start to show our value in the management of patient care and play a more integral role in our patients' care.

## Conclusion

Pharmacists are forced to balance three areas of responsibility. They have a medical responsibility to the patient. Pharmacists also have a responsibility to themselves and to society to enhance the level of care provided. Professional responsibilities promote guidelines for pharmacists to ensure consistency. In addition to balancing these responsibilities, the pharmacist must meet the needs of the patient to ensure positive therapeutic outcomes that accompany the emergence of pharmaceutical health care.

# Patients' rights

This problem-based learning session is based on the following: *N.O. v. Callahan*, Civil Action No. 85-0836-Mc, U.S. District Court for the District of Massachusetts, 110 F.R.D. 637; 1986 U.S. Dist. Lexis 23961, June 19, 1986. It is reprinted with permission of LexisNexis.

## Objectives

The objectives of this problem-based learning case are:

- To discuss the responsibilities of health care providers
- To understand the rights of patients

## Introduction

According to the National Association of Boards of Pharmacy (NABP), the patient has a right to expect that his or her pharmacist will be professionally competent, treat him or her with dignity, act in his or her best interest, and serve as his or her advocate when making pharmaceutical care decisions. In addition, the pharmacist must protect the patient's medical records and ensure confidentiality. Provision of counseling and monitoring of drug therapy for safety, efficacy, and compliance and instituting appropriate remedial interventions when necessary are also mandated.

In return, the patient is responsible for providing accurate personal information, a medical history, and payment for services. It is also the patient's responsibility to implement the drug therapy regimen conscientiously and report the clinical response, especially untoward reactions and adverse changes in their health status, to the pharmacist.

The following case illustrates situations a pharmacist may encounter for which the potential for conflict between patient's rights and pharmacist's responsibilities exists, and that the proper course of action may not be obvious. Such scenarios may require action that could deviate from the parameters set forth by the NABP.

## Part one

This is a civil rights action brought by seven plaintiffs who are or were inpatients at mental health facilities operated by the Massachusetts Department of Mental Health (DMH). They claim they have special or chronic medical or nursing care needs that cannot adequately be treated by the DMH medical care system and allege that the defendants' "gross, systematic and continuing failure to provide them adequate medical care and facilities" violates the federal and state constitutions and federal and state law.

Two motions were referred to the court: (1) plaintiffs' motion to compel defendants Murphy and Bennett to permit plaintiffs to inspect, photograph, and videotape designated facilities; and (2) plaintiffs' motion to compel discovery. A hearing was held on these motions on June 4, 1986. The action on the first motion is presented next, and action on the second motion is presented in Part two.

### Motion to compel defendants Murphy and Bennett to permit plaintiffs to inspect, photograph, and videotape designated facilities and for entry of protective order

On June 13, 1985, plaintiffs requested defendants to permit them to enter, inspect, photograph, and videotape eight DMH facilities "for the purpose of observing and determining the manner in which medical care is provided to clients of the facilities," including, but not limited to, the observation of the physical design and conditions of the facilities; the location, number, and types of wards, clinics, and beds; the types, duties, and location while on duty of personnel included in delivery of medical care; the location, type, number, and working condition of medical care equipment and facilities; the location, design, and staffing of laboratories, pharmacies, infirmaries, and other medical care facilities; and the manner of making and maintaining medical records.

On July 1, 1985, defendants responded that they would permit "plaintiffs' counsel to enter and inspect the facilities listed in their motion at a mutually convenient time" and in a manner that would not interfere with the operation of such a facility, but that "photographing or videotaping of the facilities, personnel and patients will not be permitted."

On December 24, 1985, plaintiffs filed a motion to compel defendants to permit the photographing and videotaping. They also moved for a protective order to limit disclosure of any "sensitive photographic material" that contains an "individually identifiable image or recording of any DMH inpatient client" to certain counsel, assistants, and experts.

On January 2, 1986, defendants opposed the motion to compel the "indiscriminate photographing and videotaping of patients at Department of Mental Health facilities." They argued, among other things, that the "proposed Protective Order does not adequately address the privacy interests of these non-party patients." Defendants had no objection to photographing and videotaping the named plaintiffs.

Plaintiffs' motion to compel is allowed because federal law permits the entry on property for the purpose of inspection and photographing "of the property or any designated object or operation thereon." The defendants raised no valid objections to the photographing or videotaping of the various facilities and objects on those facilities as long as such filming does not interfere with the operation of the facility.

Defendants have not articulated any basis for their objection to the photographing or videotaping of the types, numbers, duties, and location of on-duty medical care personnel at the facilities. As long as the filming is limited to the purposes outlined in plaintiffs' request, this request is allowed.

Defendants' objection to the videotaping and photographing of non-party patients, who have not given their consent, has merit. The Court has not yet certified a class, and the proposed protective order does not deal with the valid concern that some mentally ill patients may not consent to being photographed and filmed by persons not designated by the Court to represent them.

According to Fed. R. Civ. P. 26(b)(1), parties are permitted to obtain discovery regarding any matter "not privileged" that is relevant to the subject matter involved in the pending action. Evidentiary privileges in federal courts are governed by Fed. R. Evid. 501. This rule also applies to pretrial discovery disputes. This Court is instructed by Fed. R. Evid. 501 that recognition of a privilege "shall be governed by the principles of the common law as they may be interpreted by the Courts of the United States in light of reason and experience." Rule 501 envisions the flexible development of the federal common law of privilege on a case-by-case basis. In developing a federal common law privilege, this Court must balance the particular federal interest involved against the rationale and comparative strength of the particular state evidentiary interest claimed.

The First Circuit has suggested an analytical framework for balancing state and federal interests to determine whether, and to what extent, the federal common law of privilege would recognize a state privilege:

1. Would the Courts of Massachusetts recognize such a privilege?
2. Is the State's asserted privilege "intrinsically meritorious in our independent judgment"?

This Court will follow that analytic framework in balancing the privacy interests of the non-party patients, asserted by the defendants, and plaintiffs' litigation needs.

The Commonwealth of Massachusetts has recognized the privacy rights of mentally ill patients in state mental hospitals. The state law provides that each patient or resident of DMH facilities is entitled to "privacy during medical treatment or other rendering of care within the capacity of the facility." Videotaping of mentally ill patients, no matter how well intentioned, could well involve an intrusion into the most private aspects of the lives of these patients.

However, under both federal and state law, privacy rights of patients are not absolute. This Court must weigh the merits of the privacy interests against plaintiffs' need for the information in light of their claim of violations of constitutional and statutory rights. Plaintiffs argue that the videotaping and photographing are necessary to enable plaintiffs' counsel and experts to assess the care and treatment provided by state-run institutions and to preserve evidence of present conditions. However, at the hearing, defendants' counsel agreed that plaintiffs' experts could personally tour the facility. Expert assistance and testimony would adequately meet plaintiffs' litigation needs without unduly infringing on the privacy interests of the mentally ill.

Certainly, any competent inpatient could consent to being videotaped and photographed during the inspection of DMH facilities. Under state statutory and common law, even involuntarily committed patients are deemed competent until adjudicated incompetent. However, the procedure for obtaining consent should fully protect the rights of patients. The parties should obtain written consent of the patient in advance of filming; should explain to the patients the purpose of filming and the extent of release of any films; and should ascertain, when possible, if the patient has been adjudicated incompetent.

The parties are instructed to negotiate a practical procedure for obtaining the consent of the patients during the inspections and a protective order like the one proposed by plaintiffs to limit release of any sensitive films. If the parties are unable to work out a mutually agreed procedure and protective order, they should submit their proposed procedures by July 18, 1986.

## Make a list of the major problems presented in this case

- 
- 
- 
- 

## Hypothesis and mechanism

For the problems in your list above, give a cause or a reason for each to happen:

- 
- 
- 
-

## Learning issues

Make a list of learning issues in the form of questions. Remember, your goal is to gather the medical, social, and all other relevant facts that may apply to the case.

- 
- 
- 
- 

What are the responsibilities of health care providers?

- Provide the best quality of care within their power to every patient
- Promote optimal therapy through the practice of beneficence (includes reducing cost to the patient when possible)
- Protect the confidentiality and integrity of patient records and information relating to medical conditions

What are the rights of patients?

- Access to the best quality of care available
- Confidence in the notion that the health care professionals will act in the best interest of the patient
- Protection of confidentiality concerning health and treatment records

## Literature review

To help you get ready to answer certain questions you anticipate being asked during the second part of the case, you look in the local medical library and on the World Wide Web for helpful information. Please indicate in the spaces below (1) several helpful articles or books you found and (2) several helpful Web sites you found.

- **Helpful articles/books:**
  As drug costs rise, health plans shift the burden, *Capitation Manage. Rep.* 4, 153–158, 1997.
  Cardinale, V., Time for bill of rights, *Drug Topics*, 131, 8, 1987.
  Lo, B. and Alpers, A., Uses and abuses of prescription drug information in pharmacy benefits management programs, *JAMA*, 283, 801–806, 2000.
  McPherson, M.L., Pain management and ethical dilemmas in the terminal patient, *ASHP Annu. Meet.*, 55, 1–66, 1998.
  O'Harrow, R., Prescription sales, privacy fears: CVS, giant share customer records with drug marketing firm, *Washington Post*, Feb. 15, 1998, p. A1.

Oliver, W.W., Ethical considerations in pharmacy practice, *Georgia Pharm. J.*, 19, 11–17, 1997.

Simonsmeier, L.M., "Nobody told me it was wrong," the pharmacist's corresponding liability, *Pharm. Times*, Sept. 2000, p. 38.

Tisdale, C. and Woloschuk, D.M., Terminal sedation: is there a role for the pharmacist? *Can. Pharm. J.*, 132, 28–33, 1999.

Ukens, C., Too many prescriptions, too little time for OBRA, *Drug Topics*, 137, 15, 1993.

U.S. Department of Justice (Drug Enforcement Administration, DEA), *Pharmacist's Manual: An Informational Outline of the Controlled Substances Act of 1970*, 1990, p. 368.

Younger, P.J.D. et al., *Pharmacy Law Answer Book*, 1996, p. 321.

- **Helpful Web sites:**

Arizona State Board of Pharmacy: www.pharmacy.state.az.us/link2.html

Fountain of Healthy Living Presents Patient Rights and Responsibilities: www.va.gov/station/501-Albuquerque/fountain/prights.html

American Pharmaceutical Association: www.aphanet.org/lead/committe2.html

*Identify all relevant values that play a role in the case and determine which values, if any, conflict.*

Nonmaleficence:

Beneficence:

Respect for persons:

Loyalty:

Distributive justice:

## *Learning issues for next student-centered problem-based learning session*

- List the options open to you. That is, answer the question, "What could you do?"
- Choose the best solution from an ethical point of view, justify it, and respond to possible criticisms. That is, answer the question, "What should you do, and why?"
- What are the different ways of thinking about the problem? Which conflict management techniques can be used in the situation?

## *Part two*

### *Plaintiffs' motion to compel discovery: medical records concerning non-party patients*

Plaintiffs moved to compel the production of the medical records of the approximately 210 class members who the DMH determined require more intensive or skilled nursing or medical care than is available at DMH facilities.

First, defendants object on the grounds that the medical records are privileged under state law, which provides that medical records are "absolutely exempt from mandatory disclosure." The affidavit of Gerald Morrissey states that the medical records contain "highly personal information regarding the client as the client's past medical and psychiatric history, present medical and psychiatric diagnoses, psychological and family history and present family involvement (family members named), past and current treatment plans, behavioral problems, psychological evaluations and profiles," and so forth.

Plaintiffs argue that there is no absolute privilege associated with the medical records they seek, that the records of medical treatment are essential to any evaluation of the adequacy of medical care provided to DMH clients, and that the proposed protective order adequately protects patient's privacy interests by limiting disclosure of the records to counsel and experts.

The reasoning in *Lora*, supra (Weinstein, Jr..) is persuasive. *Lora* was a civil rights action brought by all black and Hispanic children assigned to certain New York City schools for socially maladjusted and emotionally disturbed children. Plaintiffs sought production of 50 randomly selected diagnostic and referral files that, as in the instant case, included the results of psychological and psychiatric consultations or examinations and other clinical and "intensely personal information." All parties agreed that, if the files were supplied, the names and identifying data would be redacted. The Court compelled disclosure of the records, holding:

*Only strong countervailing public policies should be per-
mitted to prevent disclosure when, as here, a suit is brought
to redress a claim for violation of civil rights under the
Constitution. 42 U.S.C. § 1983. Enforcement is by private
individuals but they are acting in the capacity of (private
attorneys-general.)*

In determining whether disclosure in this case will unreasonably interfere with justifiable privilege expectations of students and their families,
four significant factors must be considered. First, is the identification of
the individuals required for effective use of the data? Second, is the invasion of privacy and risk to psychological harm limited to the narrowist
possible extent? Third, will the data be supplied only to qualified personnel
under strict controls over confidentiality? Fourth, are the data necessary
or simply desirable?

*List the options open to you. That is, answer the question, "What
    could you do?"*

- 
- 
- 
- 

*Choose the best solution from an ethical point of view, justify it, and
    respond to possible criticisms. That is, answer the question,
    "What should you do, and why?"*

- 
- 
- 
- 

*Select one member of your PBL group to role-play as a DMH
    representative and have another member of your PBL group
    role-play as a patient representative. How might the two
    converse about different ways of thinking and techniques for
    conflict management?*

- 
- 
- 
-

*Again, select one member of your PBL group to role-play as a DMH
representative and have another member role-play as a patient
representative. How might the DMH representative use what
is known about stages of change and about motivational
interviewing to solve what you consider the major problem
presented in the case?*

- 
- 
- 
- 

## Part three

Following this analysis, I [the judge in this case] find which is consistent
with the Hampers analytic framework, I find that state law does afford a
privilege to the medical records of the mentally ill, and this privilege is
intrinsically meritorious. Nonetheless, as in *Lora*, plaintiffs have demonstrated that the information is necessary for a full development of the facts
in this litigation.

I allow the motion to compel subject to certain conditions. Plaintiffs have
agreed that all references to the patients' identities will be redacted prior to
production. The protective order, already entered by this Court, seems to
meet the *Lora* criteria. It narrows disclosure to counsel, certain legal and
clerical assistants, and experts; it provides that the information shall be used
only in connection with the preparation and trial of this action; and it contains other protections to minimize the invasion of the other patients' privacy.
However, the Court will consider any proposed modifications to the protective order that defendants consider necessary.

Second, defendants argue that production and redaction of the 210 files
would be overly burdensome. Plaintiffs have proposed limiting production
to the medical records of every fifth person on the list of 210. I order that
defendants produce the medical records for such persons by July 18, 1986.
Thus, defendants will be producing both the redacted medical records and
responsible medical care personnel data for every fifth person on the list of
210. This ruling is without prejudice to plaintiffs seeking additional records
if the class is certified and if the initial production indicates that supplemen-
tation is warranted.

## Discussion

This type of situation raises the question of balancing confidentiality and
optimizing the care undertaken. While the patient has an undeniable right
to privacy concerning personal medical records, there are beneficial consequences to reviewing and monitoring the care to minimize cost and promote

the use of the best treatment available. However, there is often a very thin line in this reviewing process between impartial beneficence and the act of advertising/promoting/monitoring a particular product or treatment.

Patients should demand and are entitled to the best care available. These same patients must be willing, however, to sacrifice some of their autonomy in exchange for that care. It is incumbent on both the health care professional and the patient to be vigilant in ensuring that the thin line between impartiality and promotion for profit does not disappear entirely.

## Conclusion

As this problem-based learning case points out, it is obvious that the rights and responsibilities of both professionals and patients take on various forms when applied to different situations. Often, a compromise must be struck between the rights of the patient and the steps necessary to carry out effective therapy or promote general public health. Benefit to the patient should be the primary concern and the ultimate goal of any decision made by both patient and provider. Real-world situations are rarely as cut and dried as we prefer to encounter, and careful consideration of the rights and responsibilities of all concerned must often be given carefully to arrive at the appropriate decision.

*case three*

# Privacy and confidentiality

This problem-based learning session is based on the following: *Humphreys v. DEA*, No. 96-3099, U.S. Court of Appeals for the Third Circuit, 96 F.3d 658; 1996 U.S. App. Lexis 24339. July 26, 1996, Argued. September 17, 1996, Filed. It is reprinted with permission of LexisNexis.

## Objectives

This exercise explains various aspects of informed consent. These include:

- Information needed to receive informed consent
- Medical and legal dimensions of decisional capacity
- How to proceed if treatment is refused

Only in the last few decades has patient consent become a very prominent aspect of health care. The growing importance of the principles of autonomy, informed consent, and the shift from paternalism in practice require that all health care providers be familiar with the issues of consent and how to proceed if treatment is refused.

## Part one

Humphreys is a Pittsburgh, Pennsylvania, doctor specializing in gastroenterology and internal medicine; prior to this proceeding, he practiced for over 35 years without any disciplinary actions against him. On April 12, 1995, a deputy assistant administrator of the DEA issued to Humphreys an order to show cause why the DEA should not revoke Humphreys' certificate of registration under 21 U.S.C. § 824(a)(4) and deny any pending application under 21 U.S.C. § 823(f) as being inconsistent with the public interest. Specifically, the order to show cause alleged that "from the early 1980s to mid-1993, [Humphreys] prescribed controlled substances to at least four individuals without a legitimate medical need and with knowledge that these individuals were not the ultimate recipients of the controlled substances."

The DEA's action was precipitated by Humphreys' personal and professional relationship with former Pennsylvania Supreme Court Justice Rolf Larson ("Larson") and the criminal investigation of Larson. Humphreys had acted as Justice Larson's personal physician for approximately the past 20 years. In 1993, based on the findings and recommendations of a grand jury, Larson was charged with one count of conspiracy to commit "Acquisition or Obtaining of Possession of a Controlled Substance by Misrepresentation, Fraud, Forgery, Deception, or Subterfuge" and numerous other violations of law. Humphreys was named as an unindicted co-conspirator in the conspiracy count and received immunity in return for his testimony against Larson.

The criminal conspiracy charge against Larson and DEA's regulatory investigation of Humphreys stemmed from Larson's attempts to keep his mental health problems out of public sight. Beginning in the 1960s, Larson visited psychiatrists and psychologists for the treatment of clinical depression and anxiety. These doctors prescribed various tranquilizers and antidepressants, which Larson paid for to preserve his privacy. Beginning in 1981, however, Larson revised his method of ensuring his privacy: he asked Humphreys to prescribe various controlled drugs for Larson in the name of certain of his employees (secretaries and a law clerk). From the early 1980s to mid-1993, Humphreys wrote approximately 34 prescriptions for drugs in this manner, including prescriptions for Valium, Ativan, and Serax.

It is undisputed that the individuals named on the prescriptions always gave the prescription drugs to Larson and did not take the medications themselves or resell them. It is also undisputed that Humphreys was aware of Larson's diagnosed condition, that he believed each medication he prescribed was for an appropriate medical purpose, and that he prescribed the substances in appropriate medical dosage amounts and at acceptable time intervals. Moreover, although Humphreys did not examine Larson each time he prescribed drugs, Humphreys did examine Larson before the first prescription and approximately every 6 months thereafter. Although Humphreys was aware that Larson was continuing to see other doctors, Humphreys was not aware of any other medications prescribed by Larson's other doctors and did not attempt to coordinate his prescriptions with those of these other doctors. Humphreys received no money for writing these prescriptions.

After receiving the order to show cause, Humphreys and his attorney each filed a response to the order. Humphreys' primary defense was that, by prescribing the medication in the names of Larson's close associates, he was attempting to protect Larson's privacy in a manner common and acceptable in standard medical practice for famous patients with mental conditions. Humphreys waived his right to a hearing as he was recovering from a stroke.

On January 23, 1996, the deputy administrator entered his final order based on the investigative record and Humphreys' written statement. The deputy administrator acknowledged that he could revoke Humphreys' registration only if continued registration would be inconsistent with the public interest pursuant to the five factors set forth in 21 U.S.C. § 823(f). The deputy administrator considered, discussed, and relied on each of the five factors except for Factor 3 — Humphreys' conviction record under federal or state laws relating to controlled substances, which was not a relevant factor because he had none — and, based on these factors, determined that the public interest would be best served by revoking Humphreys' registration. The deputy administrator did not discuss, and apparently did not consider, Humphreys' privacy defense. Humphreys appealed, and this court granted a stay of the order pending our disposition of this appeal. We have jurisdiction to hear this appeal under 21 U.S.C. § 877 (1994).

## Analysis

### The standard of review

Agency decisions, such as the deputy administrator's order, may be set aside only if arbitrary, capricious, an abuse of discretion, or otherwise not in accordance with the law. "As a reviewing court, we must accord proper deference to the DEA's expertise but must nonetheless make a 'searching and careful inquiry' of the record to determine whether the agency's decision was based on a consideration of the relevant factors and whether there was a clear error of judgment."

### The regulatory framework

The Controlled Substances Act, as amended by the Dangerous Drug Diversion Control Act of 1984, requires that any person who dispenses controlled substances must first obtain a certificate of registration from the attorney general. The attorney general has delegated the authority to deny, revoke, or suspend registrations to the administrator of the DEA.

Prior to 1984, the DEA could revoke a registration for only three reasons: (1) falsification of an application; (2) felony conviction related to controlled substances; and (3) suspension, revocation, or denial of a state license. In 1984, with the enactment of the Dangerous Drug Diversion Control Act, Congress added a fourth reason for which a registration could be revoked: a finding that the physician had committed "such acts as would render his registration under section 823 of this title inconsistent with the public interest as determined under such section." In determining whether registration would be inconsistent with the public interest, the DEA must consider the following factors:

> *(1) The recommendation of the appropriate State licensing board or disciplinary authority. (2) The applicant's experience in dispensing, or conducting research with respect to controlled substances. (3) The applicant's conviction record under Federal or State laws relating to the manufacture, distribution, or dispensing of controlled substances. (4)*

> Compliance with applicable State, Federal, or local laws
> relating to controlled substances. (5) Such other conduct
> which may threaten the public health and safety.

The five factors are independent, and the deputy Administrator may revoke
a registration based on one factor or a combination of several factors.

### Applicability of the statute to Humphreys and its application

Humphreys raises two primary issues on appeal: whether 21 U.S.C. § 824(a)
can apply to the facts of this case and, if so, whether the DEA properly
applied the five public interest factors to his case and properly considered
his privacy defense.

Initially, we may easily dispose of Humphreys' contention that 21
U.S.C. § 824(a) was never meant to apply to physicians in his circumstances. Citing Trawick, 861 F.2d at 76, Humphreys argues that the legislative history of the 1984 amendment indicates it was meant to apply
only in egregious cases and was specifically directed to those physicians
who prescribed controlled substances to addicts, who then could either
use the drugs themselves or resell them to purchase different drugs, such
as heroin. Humphreys argues that his actions did not fall within the
category of egregious cases. Certainly, there is no allegation here of sales
to addicts.

However, Humphreys, while relying on selected language in the Trawick opinion, has ignored not only the holding of the Trawick decision, but
other language as well. In Trawick, a dentist was indicted on state felony
drug charges, including conspiracy to distribute and distribution of
cocaine, based on acts not related to his patients. The dentist pled guilty
only to misdemeanor possession of cocaine as part of a plea bargain.
Following his conviction, the DEA revoked his registration as being inconsistent with the public interest. The Court of Appeals noted that the legislative history of the public interest standard was much as Humphreys now
suggests, but concluded that the dentist there could not "avoid the plain
statutory language of the amendment merely by showing that Congress,
in enacting it was largely concerned with a situation different from the
instant case." Reasoning that a court must uphold any reasonable agency
construction of a statute it is entrusted to enforce, the court concluded it
was reasonable to interpret the statute to authorize revocation based on a
misdemeanor drug conviction.

Likewise, here there is nothing unreasonable about the DEA's interpretation of the statute as authorizing revocation based on Humphreys' allegedly unlawful and irregular prescription of controlled substances in the
names of individuals other than his patient, Larson. As discussed below,
however, the DEA's application of the statute to the precise situation facing
Humphreys is so deficient as to be an abuse of discretion.

## The privacy defense

In a combined discussion of Factors 2 and 4 under 21 U.S.C. § 823(f), the two factors on which the deputy administrator relied most heavily, the deputy administrator emphasized that Humphreys had engaged in a course of conduct during approximately a 12-year period that clearly violated federal drug-prescribing regulations. Specifically, the deputy administrator concluded that Humphreys' conduct violated 21 C.F.R. § 1306.04(a), which provides that a prescription for a controlled substance "must be issued for a legitimate medical purpose by an individual practitioner acting in the usual course of his professional practice." The deputy administrator concluded that these factors weighed in favor of revoking Humphreys' registration as Humphreys' long practice of issuing prescriptions in the names of individuals unknown to him and not under his care would not meet this criterion.

The central deficiency in the deputy administrator's decision is his complete failure to discuss the one and only defense raised by Humphreys: that prescribing antidepressants and other such drugs for a famous patient in the name of another individual to preserve the privacy of the patient was, in fact, the "usual course" of medical practice in circumstances such as these, and that therefore Humphreys did not violate the federal regulation. Humphreys squarely and intelligibly raised this defense before the deputy administrator, as before us.

Specifically, Humphreys, too ill to appear in person, wrote in a letter responding to the DEA order to show cause that: "The psychiatrist and the neurologist at the trial for Justice Larson testified that they probably would have done the same thing and might have even used the same medications. They indicated that it is common practice, especially in psychiatric patients, to do this." In addition, Humphreys' attorney wrote the following:

> *Separate and apart from Dr. Humphrey's opinion is the sworn testimony of Gerald Sandson, M.D., given in the case of* Commonwealth of Pennsylvania v. Rolf Larson *at #9313844, in which this psychiatrist completely concurred with the need for privacy in the treatment of Justice Larson. . . . Testimony at trial showed that psychiatric patients suffer a stigma in society, and that public figures bear even greater burden.*

> *During the case of* Commonwealth of Pennsylvania v. Larson, *it was established without contradiction, that on a daily basis, psychiatrists on the staffs of at least Allegheny General Hospital and the Western Psychiatric Institute prescribed drugs in names of people for whom the prescriptions were not intended because privacy was an essential part of the treatment of the patient. No prosecutions were ever brought for any of these doctors or hospitals.*

Humphreys' attorney asserted that the sworn testimony at the Larson trial also established that privacy was an essential part of Larson's treatment, that privacy was the reason the drugs were prescribed in the names of others, and that the manner and method of Larson's treatment were not inconsistent with generally accepted medical standards.

The deputy administrator apparently failed to consider any of this evidence, stating instead only that "the trial transcript from Justice Larson's trial was not a part of the investigative record, and the Respondent did not attach a copy of the referenced sections to his Reply." It is true that Humphreys failed to include the Larson trial transcripts he cited in the DEA record. Humphreys should have submitted these transcripts to the DEA for inclusion in the record. However, while the record did not contain these trial transcripts, the deputy administrator was clearly aware of the trial and referred specifically to Humphreys' testimony at a pretrial hearing in the Larson case.

Thus, the deputy administrator did have before him, and took notice of, Humphreys' sworn testimony, observing that:

> *Beginning in 1981 and continuing until 1993, [Humphreys] had issued prescriptions for Schedule IV controlled substances intended for Justice Larson's use, but he had issued the prescriptions in the name of third-parties. . . . [Humphreys] had never met these individuals, and they were not his patients. . . . [Humphreys] testified that he examined Justice Larson about every six months, but not necessarily prior to issuing each of the prescriptions. Rather, Justice Larson would telephone [Humphreys] and tell him what substances he wanted and in whose name to issue the prescription. . . . [Humphreys] was aware of Justice Larson's diagnosed condition. . . and that it was [his] belief that every medication he prescribed for Justice Larson was for a legitimate medical purpose. [Humphreys] testified that he had prescribed the substances in legitimate medical dosage amounts and at appropriate time intervals. He states that he prescribed these controlled substances in this manner in order to preserve his patient's privacy.*

Indeed, nearly the entirety of the administrative record consists of items from Larson's criminal trial, including hearing transcripts and a copy of the complaint, and newspaper reports regarding the trial.

We are troubled by the fact that the deputy administrator went outside the papers submitted by Humphreys for evidence supporting his decision, such as Humphreys' pretrial testimony — evidence that actually indicated that Humphreys acted out of concern for Larson's privacy — yet failed to obtain the public trial transcripts of Dr. Sandson and others from the very same trial, which were cited by Humphreys in his support, or to otherwise consider Humphreys' privacy defense. Such failure is especially egregious when, as here, the record is devoid of any evidence, in the form of affidavits, medical treatises, or anything else, that would support a conclusion that doctors do not prescribe drugs in the name of proxies for famous patients with mental disorders in the usual course of their medical practice. We have not been able to locate any previous published DEA or court decision in which such privacy concerns were raised and rejected. Indeed, at oral argument, the DEA representative acknowledged that she was unaware of any other proceeding in which such a privacy defense had been raised.

An agency's action is arbitrary and capricious if the agency "entirely failed to consider an important aspect of the problem, offered an explanation for its decision that runs counter to the evidence before the agency, or is so implausible that it could not be ascribed to a difference in view or the product of agency expertise." Here, the decision of the deputy administrator, lacking any analysis of Humphreys' privacy defense, is arbitrary and capricious.

In short, the deputy administrator failed both to evaluate and address Humphreys' defense and to resolve the conflict created by the arguments and evidence before him. Humphreys and other trial witnesses asserted that such prescribing occurred in the usual course, and there is no contrary evidence in the record. Thus, there is a conflict between the record evidence and the deputy administrator's tacit assumption about the usual course of medical practice. The deputy administrator nevertheless failed to resolve or even acknowledge this conflict. He neither gave any reasons for rejecting Humphreys' assertions about the usual course nor cited any evidence supporting the conclusion that Humphreys did not act in the usual course. That he avoided this conflict is all the worse given his failure to review the public testimony that Humphreys and his attorney specifically cited, summarized, and asserted would corroborate Humphreys' position.

It may well be that the testimony referred to by Humphreys and his attorney does not, in fact, establish that Humphreys was merely engaging in the usual course of practice. Here, however, the deputy administrator improperly failed to consider Humphreys' privacy concerns and failed to determine whether Humphreys' privacy concerns brought his otherwise allegedly improper prescribing conduct within the usual course. Failing to analyze the privacy defense was an abuse of discretion. Absent such analysis, it was arbitrary and capricious to revoke Humphreys' registration in reliance on the second and fourth factors of 21 U.S.C. § 823(f).

We neither disregard nor minimize the substantial deference to which such agency decisions are always entitled. We also recognize that we must not simply substitute our judgment for that of the agency. However, this is not simply a case for which we disagree with the deputy administrator's application of relevant mitigating aspects of the statutory factors to settled facts. Rather, here the agency improperly failed even to consider the defense put forth by Humphreys. The case must be remanded for proper consideration of that defense.

*Make a list of the major problems presented in this case*

- 
- 
- 
- 

## Hypothesis and mechanism

For the problems in your list above, give a cause or a reason for each to happen:

- 
- 
- 
- 

## Learning issues

Make a list of learning issues in the form of questions. Remember, your goal is to gather the medical, social, and all other relevant facts that may apply to the case.

List the salient features of a "patient bill of rights."
> Access to care regardless of race, creed, sex, national origin, or ability to pay
> Considerate and respectful care
> Privacy
> Know the name and professional status of the individuals providing service
> Obtain from the physician complete information concerning the patient's care
> Refuse treatment to the extent permitted by law
> Information necessary to give consent prior to treatment (except in emergencies)
> Formulate advance directives
> Be informed of medical experimentation affecting the patient's care and have the choice not to participate
> Reasonable continuity of care
> Know which hospital rules apply to the patient's conduct
> Review and resolution of questions and concerns
> Explanation of the patient's bill

What is meant by the term *autonomy*?
> The current APhA code states "a pharmacist respects the autonomy and dignity of each patient."

Defined as the ability to make one's own decisions and act on them.

Related to the principles of informed consent.

Issues may arise when determining whether a patient is autonomous.

What does "refusal of treatment" mean?

Through the Medical Act of 1988, a patient can legally refuse medical treatment.

Treatment is defined as an operation, administration of a drug or other like substance, or any other medical procedure.

However, the Refusal of Treatment form must be filled out and signed for the patient's wishes to be carried out.

Define "decisional capacity."

A person may be capable of making decisions in some areas of life, but not in others. Many times, a mentally ill patient has lost the capacity to make decisions regarding medical treatment. For a person to have the capacity to make a decision involving medical treatment, they must:

1. Understand and remember information about treatment
2. Believe the essential information about treatment
3. Be able to weigh it in balance and arrive at a choice

What is meant by "lack of decisional capacity"?

When a mental illness interrupts decisional capacity and the patient does not have a living will or power of attorney, the attending physician must determine if the patient has a surrogate who can make the decision about the treatment on behalf of the patient. The law ranks the possible surrogates in this order:

1. A court-appointed guardian of the patient
2. The patient's spouse
3. Any adult son or daughter of the patient
4. Any adult brother or sister of the patient
5. Any adult grandchild of the patient
6. A close friend of the patient
7. The guardian of the patient's estate

What are a physician's responsibilities involving a patient lacking decisional capacity?

Discern the patient's full medical prognosis.

Ensure the patient's values and preferences are ascertained.

Inform the family of all alternatives that might be beneficial to the patient.

Proceed with the plan of care that is most in accord with the patient's values when the family and direct caregivers concur.

If the plan of care is not what the patient would have preferred, as long as the family and direct caregivers concur, it should be implemented.

How does a physician proceed if treatment is refused?

Everyday treatment: the attending physician has only two options:
- Comply with the patient's legitimate request.
- Transfer the patient to another physician.

Emergency treatment: the health care provider can only override the patient's decision if it was an emergency treatment for which the lack of treatment could result in death.

## Literature review

To help you get ready to answer certain questions you anticipate being asked during the second part of the case, look in the local medical library and on the World Wide Web for helpful information. Please indicate in the spaces below (1) several helpful articles or books you found and (2) several helpful Web sites you found.

- **Helpful articles/books:**

  Ho, V., Marginal capacity: the dilemmas faced in assessment and declaration, *Can. Med. Assoc. J.*, 152, 259–263, 1995.

  Reich, W.T. (Ed.), *Encyclopedia of Bioethics*, Vol. 13, Macmillan, New York, 1995.

  Sim, M., Legal limits to physician–patient confidentiality, *Can. Med. Assoc. J.*, 155, 859–860, 1996.

  Veatch, R.M. and Haddad, A. (Eds.), *Case Studies in Pharmacy Ethics*, Oxford University Press, New York, 1999.

- **Helpful Web sites:**

  University of Houston Law Center — Health Law Perspectives: www.law.uh.edu/healthlawperspectives

  Rush – Presbyterian – St. Luke's Medical Center, for patients, families, and general public: www.rush.edu/patients/rads/newsletter/1998

  Parkview Medical Center, information for patients: www.parkview-mc.com/geriatric/srguardianshipproxy.html

  Alzheimer's Disease Education and Referral Center: www.alzheimers.org/legal94.html

## *Identify all relevant values that play a role in the case and determine which values, if any, conflict*

Nonmaleficence:

Beneficence:

Respect for persons:

Loyalty:

Distributive justice:

## Learning issues for next student-centered problem-based learning session

- List the options open to you. That is, answer the question, "What could you do?"
- Choose the best solution from an ethical point of view, justify it, and respond to possible criticisms. That is, answer the question, "What should you do, and why?"
- What are the different ways of thinking about the problem? Which conflict management techniques can be used in the situation?

# Part two

## Proceedings on remand

In addition to the deputy administrator's improper reliance on Factors 2 and 4 in the absence of a consideration of Humphreys' privacy defense, the deputy administrator's remaining discussion of the 21 U.S.C. § 823(f) factors contains several additional inconsistencies and problems that should be addressed and corrected on remand.

First, as to Factor 1, the "recommendation" of the appropriate state licensing board or professional disciplinary authority, section 823(f)(1), the deputy administrator noted that the Pennsylvania Bureau of Professional and Occupational Affairs had issued a show cause order alleging that Humphreys had engaged in a 12-year pattern of issuing prescriptions to individuals who were not his patients that, if proven, would violate state law and might justify revoking his medical license. At the time of DEA's decision, however, the only evidence in the record pertaining to the state investigation indicated merely that the show cause order had been issued and that Pennsylvania bore the burden of proving the charges by a preponderance of the evidence. We have no indication whether Humphreys advanced the same defense there as here or what ruling, if any, Pennsylvania made on any such defense. On remand, the DEA should determine whether Pennsylvania, in fact, met its burden and what actions, if any, have actually been taken against Humphreys. If none, then the deputy administrator should consider whether, by merely issuing the order to show cause, Pennsylvania authorities have made any recommendation within the meaning of section 823(f)(1). Only if the deputy administrator properly concludes Pennsylvania has made a recommendation of revocation or other punitive action may any weight adverse to Humphreys be given under Factor 1. Although in this decision the deputy administrator only gave limited weight to Factor 1, it is not clear any weight at all is appropriate.

Second, we note that, as applied by the deputy administrator, any weight under Factor 2, which concerns "experience with dispensing . . . controlled substances," is entirely dependent on the violation of a federal regulation found by the deputy administrator under Factor 4. That is, if Humphreys violated the federal regulation, that he did so for over 12 years is an aggravating factor. However, if his conduct was indeed in the usual course, its duration is irrelevant.

Third, the DEA found that Humphreys' "prescribing of controlled substances to Justice Larson merely upon his request, without seeing him, examining him, or otherwise making a medical evaluation prior to issuing the prescription, demonstrated behavior such that **the patient's demands seemed to replace the physician's judgment**. . . . Such uncontroverted actions on the part of the Respondent are preponderating evidence that he has dispensed controlled substances in violation of federal law." We have reviewed the administrative record and see nothing in the current record that would support this particular finding. While there is some evidence indicating Larson would call Humphreys and request prescriptions for certain drugs or request a change in his prescription, there is absolutely no testimony indicating Humphreys failed to exercise his medical judgment when prescribing medication for Larson. We do not mean to say that the DEA might not be able to prove this fact at a later date on an expanded record — only that it has not done so on this record. Indeed, if anything, the current record indicates Humphreys, in fact, was exercising independent medical judgment. Specifically, Humphreys stated that he would have adjusted the drugs accordingly had he become aware that other doctors were prescribing Larson other drugs. Humphreys also testified that it was his belief that every medication he prescribed for Larson was medically appropriate. In addition, the testimony of Larson himself indicates Humphreys exercised his judgment. Specifically, Larson testified Humphreys performed a full physical evaluation before prescribing drugs for the first time, that the drugs were later changed due to side effects, and that Humphreys was the "ultimate decider" of which particular drugs to prescribe. Thus, it remains unclear how Factor 4 can weigh against Humphreys in this regard.

Fourth, the deputy administrator found, under Factor 5, that the public was at risk from the potential diversion of controlled substances by both Larson, who could have received duplicative prescriptions for controlled substances, and the employees named on the prescriptions, who were prescribed medication they did not intend to ingest and for which they lacked a medical need. The deputy administrator's inferences of a threat of public harm are overly broad and only weakly, if at all, supported by the present record. Indeed, the deputy administrator admitted that no such diversion in fact occurred. The conclusion that substantial risk for diversion existed because Larson or the secretaries and the law clerk might resell the drugs, under these circumstances, is so unlikely as to be unsustainable. The secretaries and law clerk in whose names the prescriptions were written were, after all, trusted employees and responsible adults. They obtained the drugs at Larson's specific requests and under his instruction. Moreover, Larson was aware of which drugs he should receive from each of these individuals and when he should receive them, having contacted Humphreys each time to tell Humphreys which name to use for a particular prescription. Any deviation would have been quickly noticed and, presumably, dealt with appropriately. That such trusted employees were at risk because they might take the drugs or endanger others because they might attempt to resell them, rather than turn them over to Larson, is "implausible."

It is true, as the deputy administrator noted, that the pharmacist filling a prescription could not have checked any available computer data bank for conflicting prescriptions for Larson since the prescriptions for Larson were not in his name. However, the DEA did not establish that the pharmacy or pharmacies patronized by Larson had such a system in place during the relevant time period. Moreover, if Larson frequented more than one pharmacy, the DEA has not shown that problems would have been detected even if all of Larson's prescriptions had been written in his name.

Our discussion of the need on remand to correct the deficiencies in the decision under review should not be construed in any way as suggesting that Humphreys either is or is not entitled to retain his DEA registration. We intimate no view on that issue. Rather, we hold only that the deputy administrator failed to analyze the evidence and decide the issues properly and must do so on remand.

---

*List the options open to you. That is, answer the question, "What could you do?"*

- 
- 
- 
-

*Choose the best solution from an ethical point of view, justify it, and respond to possible criticisms. That is, answer the question, "What should you do, and why?"*

- 
- 
- 
- 

*Select one member of your PBL group to role-play as Dr. Humphreys and have another member role-play as the deputy administrator. How might the two converse about different ways of thinking and techniques for conflict management?*

- 
- 
- 
- 

*Again, please select one member of your PBL group to role-play as Dr. Humphreys and have another member of your PBL group role-play as the deputy administrator. How might Dr. Humphreys use what is known about stages of change and about motivational interviewing to solve what you consider the major problem presented in the case?*

- 
- 
- 
- 

## Part three

Because the DEA utterly failed to consider Humphreys' defense and improperly analyzed some of the evidence, its analysis was so inadequate and prejudicial to Humphreys as to constitute an abuse of discretion and render the revocation order an arbitrary and capricious agency action. Therefore, we vacate and remand.

## Conclusion

A mentally ill patient has the same medical rights as every other patient. Difficulties might arise for the health care provider regarding these patients due to situational factors such as lack of decisional capacity. Informed consent and the right to refuse treatment protect the health care provider and patient involving medical decisions. Working together with these options, the health care provider and the patient can improve the patient's care and quality of life.

## case four

# Ethics committees

This problem-based learning session is based on the following: *Conant v. Walters*, No. 00-17222, U.S. Court of Appeals for the Ninth Circuit, 2002 U.S. App. Lexis 22492. April 8, 2002, Argued and Submitted, San Francisco, California. October 29, 2002, Filed. It is reprinted with permission of LexisNexis.

## Objectives

The objectives of this problem-based learning case are to gain a better understanding of:

- What ethics committees are
- Why they exist
- Who comprises them
- How they function
- When they should be used
- The role of ethics consultants, when and if they should be used, and whether they should function independently or in conjunction with a committee
- Advantages and disadvantages of utilizing these entities
- The future of bioethics and some pivotal goals that must be attained to ensure the perpetuation and progression of ethics committees

## Introduction

In the late 1960s and early 1970s, there came to light some revelations that research physicians were using patients as their subjects without informing the patients of either their participation or the risks involved. In other words, there was no informed consent. This spawned the creation of ethics committees. Meant to protect patients, they were initially viewed as "strangers" or "watchdogs" that were interfering with the physician–patient relationship. In spite of these negative perspectives, these groups have evolved from fledgling beginnings into an entire field known as bioethics.

## Part one

This is an appeal from a permanent injunction entered to protect First Amendment rights. The order enjoins the federal government from either revoking a physician's license to prescribe controlled substances or conducting an investigation of a physician that might lead to such revocation when the basis for the government's action is solely the physician's professional "recommendation" of the use of medical marijuana. The district court's order and accompanying opinion are at *Conant v. McCaffrey*, 2000 U.S. Dist. Lexis 13024, 2000 WL 1281174 (N.D. Cal. Sept. 7, 2000). The history of the litigation demonstrates that the injunction is not intended to limit the government's ability to investigate doctors who aid and abet the actual distribution and possession of marijuana [21 U.S.C. § 841(a)].

The government has not provided any empirical evidence to demonstrate that this injunction interferes with or threatens to interfere with any legitimate law enforcement activities. There is no evidence that the similarly phrased preliminary injunction that preceded this injunction [*Conant v. McCaffrey*, 172 F.R.D. 681 (N.D. Cal. 1997)], which the government did not appeal, interfered with law enforcement. The district court, on the other hand, explained convincingly when it entered both the earlier preliminary injunction and this permanent injunction how the government's professed enforcement policy threatens to interfere with expression protected by the First Amendment. We therefore affirm.

## The federal marijuana policy

The federal government promulgated its marijuana policy in 1996 in response to initiatives passed in both Arizona and California decriminalizing the use of marijuana for limited medical purposes and immunizing physicians from prosecution under California state law. The federal policy declared that a doctor's "action of recommending or prescribing Schedule I controlled substances is not consistent with the 'public interest' (as that phrase is used in the federal Controlled Substances Act)" and that such action would lead to revocation of the physician's registration to prescribe controlled substances. The policy relies on the definition of "public interest" contained in 21 U.S.C. § 823(f), which provides:

> *In determining the public interest, the following factors shall be considered: (1) The recommendation of the appropriate State licensing board or professional disciplinary authority. (2) The applicant's experience in dispensing, or conducting research with respect to controlled substances. (3) The applicant's conviction record under Federal or State laws relating to the manufacture, distribution, or dispensing of controlled substances. (4) Compliance with applicable State, Federal, or local laws relating to controlled substances. (5)*

> *Such other conduct which may threaten the public health and safety.*

The policy also said that the Department of Justice (DOJ) and the Department of Health and Human Services (HHS) would send a letter to practitioner associations and licensing boards informing those groups of the policy. The federal agencies sent a letter 2 months later to national, state, and local practitioner associations outlining the administration's position ("medical leader letter"). The medical leader letter cautioned that physicians who "intentionally provide their patients with oral or written statements in order to enable them to obtain controlled substances in violation of federal law ... risk revocation of their DEA prescription authority."

## Litigation history

Plaintiffs are patients suffering from serious illnesses, physicians licensed to practice in California who treat patients with serious illnesses, a patient's organization, and a physician's organization. The patient organization is Being Alive: People with HIV/AIDS Action Coalition, Inc. The physician's organization is the Bay Area Physicians for Human Rights. Plaintiffs filed this action in early 1997 to enjoin enforcement of the government policy insofar as it threatened to punish physicians for communicating with their patients about the medical use of marijuana. The case was originally assigned to District Judge Fern Smith, who presided over the case for more than 2 years. After Judge Smith received the parties' briefs, she issued a temporary restraining order, certified a plaintiff class, denied the government's motion to dismiss, issued a preliminary injunction, awarded interim attorney's fees to plaintiffs, and set the briefing schedule for discovery.

Judge Smith entered the preliminary injunction on April 30, 1997. It provided that the government "may not take administrative action against physicians for recommending marijuana unless the government in good faith believes that it has substantial evidence" that the physician aided and abetted the purchase, cultivation, or possession of marijuana (18 U.S.C. § 2) or engaged in a conspiracy to cultivate, distribute, or possess marijuana (21 U.S.C. § 846. 172 F.R.D. at 700). Judge Smith specifically enjoined the "defendants, their agents, employees, assigns, and all persons acting in concert or participating with them, from threatening or prosecuting physicians, [or] revoking their licenses . . . based upon conduct relating to medical marijuana that does not rise to the level of a criminal offense." The preliminary injunction covered not only recommendations, but also "non-criminal activity related to those recommendations, such as providing a copy of a patient's medical chart to that patient or testifying in court regarding a recommendation that a patient use marijuana to treat an illness."

The government did not appeal the preliminary injunction, and it remained in effect after the case was transferred more than 2 years later to

Judge Alsup on August 19, 1999. Judge Alsup in turn granted a motion to modify the plaintiff class, held a hearing on motions for summary judgment, granted in part and denied in part the cross motions for summary judgment, dissolved the preliminary injunction, and entered a permanent injunction. The class was modified to include only those patients suffering from specific symptoms related to certain illnesses and physicians who treat such patients. The permanent injunction appears to be functionally the same as the preliminary injunction that Judge Smith originally entered. It provides that the government is permanently enjoined from:

> *(i) revoking any physician class member's DEA registration merely because the doctor makes a recommendation for the use of medical marijuana based on a sincere medical judgment and (ii) from initiating any investigation solely on that ground. The injunction should apply whether or not the doctor anticipates that the patient will, in turn, use his or her recommendation to obtain marijuana in violation of federal law.*

In explaining his reasons for entering the injunction, Judge Alsup pointed out that there was substantial agreement between the parties as to what doctors could and could not do under the federal law. The government agreed with plaintiffs that revocation of a license was not authorized when a doctor merely discussed the pros and cons of marijuana use. The court observed that the plaintiffs agreed with the government that a doctor who actually prescribes or dispenses marijuana violates federal law. The fundamental disagreement between the parties concerned the extent to which the federal government could regulate doctor–patient communications without interfering with First Amendment interests. This appeal followed.

## Make a list of the major problems presented in this case

- 
- 
- 
- 

## Hypothesis and mechanism

For the problems in your list above, give a cause or a reason for each to happen:

- 
- 
- 
-

## Learning issues

Make a list of learning issues in the form of questions. Remember, your goal is to gather the medical, social, and all other relevant facts that may apply to the case.

What were the precursors of the present-day ethics committees?

Institutional review boards (IRBs): implemented by the government in the early 1970s to ensure informed consent of research subjects.

Dialysis patient selection committees (1960s): dealt primarily with resource allocation.

Abortion selection committees (pre-1973, *Roe v. Wade*): determined whether a pregnant woman who had requested an abortion was risking her life or health if the pregnancy was not terminated.

Medical-moral committees in Catholic hospitals:
1. Reproductive issues
2. Terminal illness
3. Use of analgesics

Prognosis committees:
1. Most likely the birth of current-day ethics committees.
2. Born of a mandate by the New Jersey Supreme Court in 1976.
3. A hospital was ordered to convene an ethics committee to corroborate Karen Ann Quinlan's prognosis. If determined by the committee that Ms. Quinlan would not return to a cognitive state, her surrogate (representative, agent, caregiver, etc.) would be permitted to request that treatment be stopped.

What are ethics committees?

Ethics committees are entities that are found in almost all medical care facilities. They have three major functions:
1. Providing ethics consultation
2. Developing or revising clinical ethics policies for a medical institution
3. Facilitating education in the area of clinical ethical issues for employees of medical institutions

What are the goals of an ethics committee?
1. Promote the rights of patients
2. Promote shared decision making between patients (or their surrogates if the patient is decisionally incapacitated) and their clinicians
3. Promote fair policies and procedures that maximize the likelihood of achieving good, patient-centered outcomes
4. Enhance the ethical tenor of health care professionals and health care institutions

Why do ethics committees exist?

In 1991, the Joint Commission on Accreditation of Healthcare Organizations (JCAHO) mandated the establishment of a "mechanism" to consider ethical issues in patient care and to educate health care professionals and patients in these issues:

1. They provide information, review, and guidance when difficult decisions arise.
2. They provide a forum for communication between patients and physicians.
3. They ensure the interests of all parties involved.
4. They exist to give advice, not to make decisions. (This may be viewed as beneficence and returning autonomy to the patient.)

Who comprises ethics committees?

Ethics committees optimally have 8 to 12 members, but membership numbers can vary. A cross section of the population is utilized to provide a broad spectrum of perspectives. Typically found on an ethics committee are the following: 1 or 2 doctors, a nurse, a hospital administrator, an attorney, a member of clergy, a bioethicist, a social worker, and a layperson. These people perform their committee duties on a volunteer basis. They are valued for their different backgrounds and views on life. They are individuals who commit to the responsibility of further educating themselves in the area of ethics. Guests may be allowed to sit in on meetings, and to uphold patient confidentiality, they are usually asked to sign oaths.

How do ethics committees function?

Usually, ethics committees are brought together when a difference in opinion (between patient and physician, patient and family member, physician and physician, physician and nurse, etc.) concerning a patient's care arises. It has been noted that it would be best to introduce the ethics committee early in a patient's stay at a facility if it is foreseen that the patient may not survive the stay.

The ethics committee consults with all parties involved, explores all possible legal options, and presents these options to the parties. Further, it provides insight and guidance as to the pros and cons of each choice.

Again, these committees do not make decisions. They merely help inform those involved of options available to them.

Committees will also meet periodically to develop and review policies of the medical facility. Furthermore, meetings may be called to provide education on ethical issues for committee members.

What is the step-by-step process of an ethical consultation?

A difficult decision concerning patient care arises. Examples include do not resuscitate (DNR) orders, organ donation, level of care for the terminally ill, allocation of resources, disclosure of information, patients who refuse treatment, and many other possibilities.

One of the parties involved asks for outside advice and help on how to deal best with the situation. (They want to know the right answer to the dilemma.)

A member of the ethics committee is sent to talk with all parties involved, define the problem, explore all possible options, and inform those involved of their options.

The representative of the committee reports back to the committee, and the case is reviewed. If the parties involved cannot come to agreement, the committee may have to function in a decision-making capacity. Most often, once those involved are informed of all aspects of the situation, an agreement can be reached.

What is an ethics consultant?

An ethics consultant is a person from any number of different backgrounds (philosophy, law, pastoral care, etc.) who has advanced training in the area of ethics. These individuals provide ethical consultations and educate staff members on ethical issues. They are paid by the medical institution, as opposed to being voluntary committee members, which is why utilization of individual consultants is often restricted by the resources of the medical facility.

What are the three roles that a consultant can assume in resolving conflict?

*Negotiator* — the purpose is to gain a settlement to the agreement that is favorable to the party issuing the invitation

*Mediator* — acts as nonpartisan catalyst who aims for conflict resolution by facilitating discussion

*Arbitrator* — serves as a judge and renders a decision

Committee versus consultant: which should be used?

Use of a consultant may be preferable in the following instances:

When the patient of family prefers a consultant (less intimidating than a committee environment); when the physician prefers a consultant (due to their expertise); when an ethics committee has been unsuccessful; if direct contact with the patient is desired; if repeated contact with the patient is needed; for questions of fact regarding law, policy, or societal consensus; when a consultation is needed on short notice; or for evaluation of the decision-making capacity of the patient

Use of a committee becomes advantageous in the following situations:

When the patient, family, or physician prefers a committee (diverse perspectives or expertise); when the issue has ethical or legal implications for hospital policy, allocation, or credibility; if the issue threatens the hospital or significant relationship within it (physician/physician, nurse/physician, etc.); if the consultant is ineffective; for complex issues for which there is lack of societal consensus; for empowerment of the patient or nonphysician requesting a review (lack of intimidation from expert); when there is a conflict of interest for a consultant; or for surrogate decision making when there is no proxy

What are the advantages and disadvantages of ethics committees and ethics consultants?

Ethics committees:
  Advantages:
    Issues with policy implications better handled by committees
    Broad spectrum of viewpoints
    More appropriate for ethical reflection
    Volunteer status
  Disadvantages:
    Susceptible to adverse effects of group dynamics
    Size of committee is intimidating to those seeking case review
    May have more political power than necessary
Ethics consultants:
  Advantages:
    Direct contact with patient and families
    More flexible and efficient than committees
    Preferred for expertise
  Disadvantages:
    Model conveys that experts should be used for ethical dilemmas
    Use of consultant may allow physician to defer moral responsibilities
    Availability limited by resources

## Literature review

To help you get ready to answer certain questions you anticipate being asked during the second part of the case, look in the local medical library and on the World Wide Web for helpful information. Please indicate in the spaces below (1) several helpful articles or books you found and (2) several helpful Web sites you found.

- **Helpful articles/books:**
  Abramson, M., Ethics committees, *Trends Health Care, Law Ethics*, 7, 32, 1992.
  American Medical Association, *Code of Medical Ethics: Current Opinions with Annotations*, Chicago, 2000, pp. 216–217.
  Fletcher, J.C. and Hoffmann, J.D., Ethics committees: time to experiment with standards, *Ann. Intern. Med.*, 120, 335–338, 1994.

Heilicser, B.J., Meltzer, D., and Siegler, M., The effect of clinical medical ethics consultation on healthcare costs, *J. Clin. Ethics*, 11, 31–38, 2000.

La Puma, J. and Toulmin, S.E., Ethics consultants and ethics committees, *Arch. Intern. Med.*, 149, 1109–1112, 1989.

McIntyre, R.L., The legitimation of ethics consultation, *Trends Health Care, Law Ethics*, 8, 7–10, 34, 1993.

Nelson, W.A., Using ethics advisory committees to cope with ethical issues, *Mo. Med.*, 89, 827–830, 1992.

Orr, R.D. and deLeon, D.M., The role of the clinical ethicist in conflict resolution, *J. Clin. Ethics*, 11, 21–29, 2000.

Ross, J.W. et al., *Health Care Ethics Committees: The Next Generation*, American Hospital Association, 1993, pp. 1–59.

Smith, M.L., The future of healthcare ethics committees, *Trends Health Care, Law Ethics*, 9, 7–10, 1994.

Swenson, M.D. and Miller, R.B., Ethics case review in health care institutions: committees, consultants, or teams? *Arch. Intern. Med.*, 152, 694–697, 1992.

- **Helpful Web sites:**

  Medical College of Wisconsin — Center for the Study of Bioethics: www.mcw.edu/bioethics

  Columbia University College of P & S Complete Home Medical Guide: cpmcnet.columbia.edu/texts/guide/hmg03_0008.html

  Ethics in Medicine — University of Washington School of Medicine: eduserv.hscer.washington.edu/bioethics/topics/ethics.html

*Identify all relevant values that play a role in the case and determine which values, if any, conflict.*

Nonmaleficence:

Beneficence:

Respect for persons:

Loyalty:

Distributive justice:

## Learning issues for next student-centered problem-based learning session

- List the options open to you. That is, answer the question, "What could you do?"
- Choose the best solution from an ethical point of view, justify it, and respond to possible criticisms. That is, answer the question, "What should you do, and why?"
- What are the different ways of thinking about the problem? Which conflict management techniques can be used in the situation?

## Part two

It is important at the outset to observe that this case has been litigated independently of contemporaneous litigation concerning whether federal law exempts from prosecution the dispensing of marijuana in cases of medical necessity. The Supreme Court in that litigation eventually held that it does not, reversing this court [see *United States v. Oakland Cannabis Buyers' Coop.*, 532 U.S. 483, 149 L. Ed. 2d 722, 121 S. Ct. 1711 (2001), rev'g *United States v. Oakland Cannabis Buyers' Coop.*, 190 F.3d 1109 (9th Cir. 1999)]. When the district court entered the permanent injunction in this case, it pointed out that it was doing so without regard to this circuit's decision in the *Oakland Cannabis* litigation (*Conant*, 2000 WL 1281174).

The dispute in the district court in this case focused on the government's policy of investigating doctors or initiating proceedings against doctors only because they recommend the use of marijuana. While the government urged that such recommendations lead to illegal use, the district court concluded that there are many legitimate responses to a recommendation of marijuana by a doctor to a patient. There are strong examples in the district court's opinion supporting the district court's conclusion. For example, the doctor could seek to place the patient in a federally approved, experimental marijuana therapy program. Alternatively, the patient, on receiving the recommendation, could petition the government to change the law. By chilling doctors' ability to recommend marijuana to a patient, the district court held that the prohibition compromises a patient's meaningful participation in public discourse. The district court stated:

> *Petitioning Congress or federal agencies for redress of a grievance or a change in policy is a time-honored tradition. In the marketplace of ideas, few questions are more deserving of free-speech protection than whether regulations affecting health and welfare are sound public policy. In the debate, perhaps the status quo will (and should) endure. But patients and physicians are certainly entitled to urge their view. To hold that physicians are barred from communicating to patients sincere medical judgments would disable patients from understanding their own situations well enough to participate in the debate. As the government concedes, . . . many patients depend upon discussions with their physicians as their primary or only source of sound medical information. Without open communication with their physicians, patients would fall silent and appear uninformed. The ability of patients to participate meaningfully in the public discourse would be compromised.*

On appeal, the government first argued that the recommendation that the injunction may protect is analogous to a "prescription" of a controlled substance, which federal law clearly bars. We believe this characterizes the injunction as sweeping more broadly than it was intended or than as properly interpreted. If, in making the recommendation, the physician intends for the patient to use it as the means for obtaining marijuana, because a prescription is used as a means for a patient to obtain a controlled substance, then a physician would be guilty of aiding and abetting the violation of federal law. That, the injunction is intended to avoid. Indeed, the predecessor preliminary injunction spelled out what the injunction did not bar; it did not enjoin the government from prosecuting physicians when government officials in good faith believe that they have "probable cause to charge under the federal aiding and abetting and/or conspiracy statutes."

The plaintiffs interpret the injunction narrowly, stating in their brief before this Court that, "the lower court fashioned an injunction with a clear line between protected medical speech and illegal conduct." They characterize the injunction as protecting "the dispensing of information," not the dispensing of controlled substances, and therefore assert that the injunction does not contravene or undermine federal law.

As Judge Smith noted in the preliminary injunction order, conviction of aiding and abetting requires proof that the defendant "associated himself with the venture, that he participated in it as something that he wished to bring about, that he [sought] by his actions to make it succeed," 172 F.R.D. at 700 [quoting *Central Bank of Denver, N.A. v. First Interstate Bank of Denver, N.A.*, 511 U.S. 164, 190, 128 L. Ed. 2d 119, 114 S. Ct. 1439 (1994)]. This is an accurate statement of the law. We have explained that a conviction of aiding and abetting requires the government to prove four elements: "(1) that the accused had the specific intent to facilitate the commission of a crime by another, (2) that the accused had the requisite intent of the underlying substantive offense, (3) that the accused assisted or participated in the commission of the underlying substantive offense, and (4) that someone committed the underlying substantive offense" [see *United States v. Gaskins*, 849 F.2d 454, 459 (9th Cir. 1988)]. The district court also noted that conspiracy requires that a defendant make "an agreement to accomplish an illegal objective and [that he] knows of the illegal objective and intends to help accomplish it."

The government on appeal stressed that the permanent injunction applies "whether or not the doctor anticipates that the patient will, in turn, use his or her recommendation to obtain marijuana in violation of federal law" and suggests that the injunction thus protects criminal conduct. A doctor's anticipation of patient conduct, however, does not translate into aiding and abetting or conspiracy. A doctor would aid and abet by acting with the specific intent to provide a patient with the means to acquire marijuana. Similarly, a conspiracy would require that a doctor have knowledge that a patient intends to acquire marijuana, agree to help the patient acquire marijuana, and intend to help the patient acquire marijuana. Holding doctors responsible for whatever conduct the doctor could anticipate a patient *might* engage in after leaving the doctor's office is simply beyond the scope of either conspiracy or aiding and abetting.

The government also focused on the injunction's bar against "investigating" on the basis of speech protected by the First Amendment and pointed to the broad discretion enjoyed by executive agencies in investigating suspected criminal misconduct. The government relied on language in the permanent injunction that differed from the exact language in the preliminary injunction. The permanent injunction order enjoined the government "from initiating any investigation solely on" the basis of "a recommendation for the use of medical marijuana based on a sincere medical judgment" (*Conant*, 2000 WL 1281174). The preliminary injunction order provided that "the government may not take administrative action against physicians for recommending marijuana unless the government in good faith believes that it has substantial evidence of [conspiracy or aiding and abetting]."

[1] The government, however, has never argued that the two injunctive orders differ in any material way. Because we read the permanent injunction as enjoining essentially the same conduct as the preliminary injunction, we interpret this portion of the permanent injunction to mean only that the government may not initiate an investigation of a physician solely on the basis of a recommendation of marijuana within a *bona fide* doctor–patient relationship unless the government in good faith believes that it has substantial evidence of criminal conduct. Because a doctor's recommendation does not constitute illegal conduct, the portion of the injunction barring investigations solely on that basis does not interfere with the federal government's ability to enforce its laws.

[2] The government policy does, however, strike at core First Amendment interests of doctors and patients. An integral component of the practice

of medicine is the communication between a doctor and a patient. Physicians must be able to speak frankly and openly to patients. That need has been recognized by the courts through the application of the common law doctor–patient privilege.

[3] The doctor–patient privilege reflects "the imperative need for confidence and trust" inherent in the doctor–patient relationship and recognizes that "a physician must know all that a patient can articulate in order to identify and to treat disease; barriers to full disclosure would impair diagnosis and treatment" [*Trammel v. United States*, 445 U.S. 40, 51, 63 L. Ed. 2d 186, 100 S. Ct. 906 (1980)]. The Supreme Court has recognized that physician speech is entitled to First Amendment protection because of the significance of the doctor–patient relationship [see *Planned Parenthood of Southeastern Pennsylvania v. Casey*, 505 U.S. 833, 884, 120 L. Ed. 2d 674, 112 S. Ct. 2791 (1992) (plurality), recognizing a physician's First Amendment right not to speak; *Rust v. Sullivan*, 500 U.S. 173, 200, 114 L. Ed. 2d 233, 111 S. Ct. 1759 (1991), noting that regulations on physician speech may "impinge upon the doctor–patient relationship"].

This Court has also recognized the core First Amendment values of the doctor–patient relationship. In *National Association for the Advancement of Psychoanalysis v. California Board of Psychology*, 228 F.3d 1043 (9th Cir. 2000), we recognized that communication that occurs during psychoanalysis is entitled to First Amendment protection. We upheld California's mental health licensing laws that determined when individuals qualified as mental health professionals against a First Amendment challenge. Finding the laws content neutral, we noted that California did not attempt to "dictate the content of what is said in therapy" and did not prevent licensed therapists from utilizing particular "psychoanalytical methods."

Being a member of a regulated profession does not, as the government suggests, result in a surrender of First Amendment rights [see *Thomas v. Collins*, 323 U.S. 516, 531, 89 L. Ed. 430, 65 S. Ct. 315 (1945), "the rights of free speech and a free press are not confined to any field of human interest"]. To the contrary, professional speech may be entitled to "the strongest protection our Constitution has to offer" [*Florida Bar v. Went-For-It, Inc.*, 515 U.S. 618, 634, 132 L. Ed. 2d 541, 115 S. Ct. 2371 (1995)]. Even commercial speech by professionals is entitled to First Amendment protection [see *Bates v. Arizona*, 433 U.S. 350, 382–83, 53 L. Ed. 2d 810, 97 S. Ct. 2691, 51 Ohio Misc. 1, 5 Ohio Op. 3d 60 (1977)]. Attorneys have rights to speak freely subject only to the government regulating with "narrow specificity" [*NAACP v. Button*, 371 U.S. 415, 433, 438–39, 9 L. Ed. 2d 405, 83 S. Ct. 328 (1963)].

In its most recent pronouncement on regulating speech about controlled substances [*Thompson v. Western States Medical Center*, 152 L. Ed. 2d 563, 122 S. Ct. 1497 (2002)], the Supreme Court found that provisions in the Food and Drug Modernization Act of 1997 that restricted physicians and pharmacists from advertising compounding drugs violated the First Amendment. The Court refused to make the "questionable assumption that doctors would prescribe unnecessary medications" and rejected the government's argument that "people would make bad decisions if given truthful information about compounded drugs." The federal government argued in this case that a doctor–patient discussion about marijuana might lead the patient to make a bad decision, essentially asking us to accept the same assumption rejected by the Court in *Thompson*. We will not do so. Instead, we take note of the Supreme Court's admonition in *Thompson*: "If the First Amendment means anything, it means that regulating speech must be a last — not first — resort. Yet here it seems to have been the first strategy the Government thought to try."

[4] The government's policy in this case seeks to punish physicians on the basis of the content of doctor–patient communications. Only doctor–patient conversations that include discussions of the medical use of marijuana trigger the policy. Moreover, the policy does not merely prohibit the discussion of marijuana; it condemns expression of a particular viewpoint (i.e., that medical marijuana would likely help a specific patient). Such condemnation of particular views is especially troubling in the First Amendment context. "When the government targets not subject matter but particular views taken by speakers on a subject, the violation of the First Amendment is all the more blatant" [*Rosenberger v. Rector*, 515 U.S. 819, 829, 132 L. Ed. 2d 700, 115 S. Ct. 2510 (1995)]. Indeed, even content-based restrictions on speech are "presumptively invalid" [*R.A.V. v. St. Paul*, 505 U.S. 377, 382, 120 L. Ed. 2d 305, 112 S. Ct. 2538 (1992)].

[5] The government's policy is materially similar to the limitation struck down in *Legal Services Corporation v. Velazquez* [531 U.S. 533, 149 L. Ed. 2d 63, 121 S. Ct. 1043 (2001)], which prevented attorneys from "presenting all the reasonable and well-grounded arguments necessary for proper resolution of the case." In *Velazquez*, a government restriction prevented legal assistance organizations receiving federal funds from challenging existing welfare laws. Like the limitation in *Velazquez*, the government's policy here "alters the traditional role" of medical professionals by "prohibiting speech necessary to the proper functioning of those systems."

The government relies on *Rust* and *Casey* to support its position in this case (*Rust*, 500 U.S. 173, 114 L. Ed. 2d 233, 111 S. Ct. 1759; *Casey*, 505 U.S. 833, 120 L. Ed. 2d 674, 112 S. Ct. 2791). However, those cases did not uphold restrictions on speech itself. *Rust* upheld restrictions on federal funding for certain types of activity, including abortion counseling, referral, or advocacy (see *Rust*, 500 U.S. at 179–80). In *Casey*, a plurality of the Court upheld Pennsylvania's requirement that physicians' advice to patients include information about the health risks associated with an abortion, and that physicians provide information about alternatives to abortion. The plurality noted that physicians did not have to comply if they had a reasonable belief that the information would have a "severely adverse effect on the physical or mental health of the patient," and thus the statute did not "prevent the physician from exercising his or her medical judgment." The government's policy in this case does precisely that.

The government seeks to justify its policy by claiming that a doctor's recommendation of marijuana may encourage illegal conduct by the patient, which is not unlike the argument made before, and rejected by, the Supreme Court in a recent First Amendment case [see *Ashcroft v. Free Speech Coalition, Inc.*, 122 S. Ct. 1389, 1403 (2002)]. In *Free Speech Coalition*, the government defended the Child Pornography Prosecution Act of 1996 by arguing that, although virtual child pornography does not harm children in the production process, it threatens them in "other, less direct, ways." For example, the government argued pedophiles might use such virtual images to encourage children to participate in sexual activity. The Supreme Court rejected such justifications, holding that the potential harms were too attenuated from the proscribed speech. "Without a significantly stronger, more direct connection, the Government may not prohibit speech on the ground that it may encourage . . . illegal conduct." The government's argument in this case mirrors the argument rejected in *Free Speech Coalition*.

The government also relies on a case in which a district court refused to order an injunction against this federal drug policy [see *Pearson v. McCaffrey*, 139 F. Supp. 2d 113, 125 (D.D.C. 2001)]. The court did so, however, because the plaintiffs in that case did not factually support their claim that the policy chilled their speech. In this case, the record is replete with examples of doctors who claim a right to explain the medical benefits of marijuana to patients and whose exercise of that right has been chilled by the threat of federal investigation. The government even stipulated in the district court that a "reasonable physician would have a genuine fear of losing his or her DEA registration to dispense controlled substances if that physician were to recommend marijuana to his or her patients."

[6] To survive First Amendment scrutiny, the government's policy must have the requisite "narrow specificity" (see *Button*, 371 U.S. at 433). Throughout this litigation, the government has been unable to articulate exactly what speech is proscribed, describing it only in terms of speech the patient believes to be a recommendation of marijuana. Thus, whether a doctor–patient discussion of medical marijuana constitutes a "recommendation" depends largely on the meaning the patient attributes to the doctor's words. This is not permissible under the First Amendment [see *Thomas v. Collins*, 323 U.S. 516, 535, 89 L. Ed. 430, 65 S. Ct. 315 (1945)]. In *Thomas*, the court struck down a state statute that failed to make a clear distinction between union membership, solicitation, and mere "discussion, laudation, [or] general advocacy." The distinction rested instead on the meaning the listeners attributed to spoken words. The government's policy, like the statute in *Thomas*, leaves doctors and patients "no security for free discussion." As Judge Smith appropriately noted in granting the preliminary injunction, "when faced with the fickle iterations of the government's policy, physicians have been forced to suppress speech that would not rise to the level of that which the government constitutionally may prohibit."

Our decision is consistent with principles of federalism that have left states as the primary regulators of professional conduct [see *Whalen v. Roe*, 429 U.S. 589, 603 n. 30, 51 L. Ed. 2d 64, 97 S. Ct. 869 (1977), recognizing states' broad police powers to regulate the administration of drugs by health professionals; *Linder v. United States*, 268 U.S. 5, 18, 69 L. Ed. 819, 45 S. Ct. 446 (1925), "direct control of medical practice in the states is beyond the power of the federal government"]. We must:

> *show respect for the sovereign States that comprise our Federal Union. That respect imposes a duty on federal courts, whenever possible, to avoid or minimize conflict between federal and state law, particularly in situations in which the citizens of a State have chosen to serve as a laboratory in the trial of novel social and economic experiments without risk to the rest of the country.* [*Oakland Cannabis*, 532 U.S. at 501 (Stevens, J., concurring)]

[7] For all of the foregoing reasons, we affirm the district court's order entering a permanent injunction.

Affirmed. Concurring: Kozinski; Circuit Judge, concurring:

I am pleased to join Chief Judge Schroeder's opinion. I write only to explain that for me the fulcrum of this dispute is not the First Amendment right of the doctors. That right certainly exists and its impairment justifies the district court's injunction for the reasons well explained by Chief Judge Schroeder. But, the doctors' interest in giving advice about the medical use of marijuana is somewhat remote and impersonal; they will derive no direct *benefit* from giving this advice, other than the satisfaction of doing their jobs well. At the same time, the *burden* of the federal policy the district court enjoined falls directly and personally on the doctors: By speaking candidly to their patients about the potential benefits of medical marijuana, they risk losing their license to write prescriptions, which would prevent them from functioning as doctors. In other words, they may destroy their careers and lose their livelihoods.

This disparity between benefits and burdens matters because it makes doctors peculiarly vulnerable to intimidation; with little to gain and much to lose, only the most foolish or committed of doctors will defy the federal government's policy and continue to give patients candid advice about the medical uses of marijuana. Those immediately and directly affected by the federal government's policy are the patients, who will be denied information crucial to their well-being, and the State of California, which will have its policy of exempting certain patients from the sweep of its drug laws thwarted. In my view, it is the vindication of these last interests — those of the patients and of the state — that primarily justifies the district court's highly unusual exercise of discretion in enjoining the federal defendants from even investigating possible violations of the federal criminal laws.

In 1996, the people of California, acting by direct initiative, adopted a narrow exemption from their laws prohibiting the cultivation, sale, and use of marijuana. The exemption applies only to patients whose physicians recommend or prescribe the drug for medical purposes. To those unfamiliar with the issue, it may seem faddish or foolish for a doctor to recommend a drug that the federal government finds has "no currently accepted medical use in treatment in the United States" [21 U.S.C. § 812(b)(1)(B)]. But the record in this case, as well as the public record, reflects a legitimate and growing division of informed opinion on this issue. A surprising number of health care professionals and organizations have concluded that the use of marijuana may be appropriate for a small class of patients who do not respond well to, or do not tolerate, available prescription drugs.

Following passage of the California initiative, the White House Office of National Drug Control Policy commissioned the National Institute of Medicine of the National Academy of Sciences (IOM) to review the scientific evidence of the therapeutic application of cannabis (see Institute of Medicine, *Marijuana and Medicine: Assessing the Science Base*, J.E. Joy et al. eds., 1999 [hereinafter IOM Report], available at http://www.nap.edu/books/0309071550/html). The yearlong study included scientific workshops, analysis of relevant scientific literature, and extensive consultation with biomedical and social scientists. It resulted in a more than 250-page report that concluded that "scientific data indicate the potential therapeutic value of cannabinoid drugs, primarily THC, for pain relief, control of nausea and vomiting, and appetite stimulation."

The IOM Report found that marijuana can provide superior relief to patients who suffer these symptoms as a result of certain illnesses and disabilities, particularly metastatic cancer, human immunodeficiency virus/acquired immunodeficiency syndrome (HIV/AIDS), multiple sclerosis (MS), spinal cord injuries, and epilepsy, and those who suffer the same symptoms as side effects from the aggressive treatments for such conditions. As a consequence, the IOM Report cautiously endorsed the medical use of marijuana.

The IOM Report concluded:

> *Short-term use of smoked marijuana (less than six months) for patients with debilitating symptoms (such as intractable pain or vomiting) must meet the following conditions: failure of all approved medications to provide relief has been documented, the symptoms can reasonably be expected to be relieved by rapid-onset cannabinoid drugs, such treatment is administered under medical supervision in a manner that allows for assessment of treatment effectiveness, and [the treatment] involves an oversight strategy comparable to an institutional review board process that could provide guidance within 24 hours of a submission by a physician to provide marijuana to a patient for a specified use.*

The IOM limited its recommendation to 6 months primarily because of health concerns about damage from smoking the drug for a prolonged period of time. This concern may be less alarming to patients suffering critical or terminal illnesses. As Dr. Debasish Tripathy, Assistant Clinical Professor of Medicine at University of California at San Francisco, explains, "Any discussion of adverse consequences appears to focus on the effects of long-term use (e.g., adverse effects on the lungs), and even those concerns are speculative. . . . In populations with short life expectancies, the risks become less imminent and the benefits more paramount." (See also Kassirer, J.P., Federal foolishness and marijuana [editorial], *N. Engl. J. Med.*, Jan. 30, 1997, pp. 366: "Marijuana may have long-term adverse effects and its use may presage serious addictions, but neither long-term side effects nor addiction is a relevant issue in such patients.")

## Appendix: Patient experiences related to this case

From 1978 to 1992, the federal government conducted its medical marijuana program. Today, the government continues to supply individuals who participated in this program with marijuana under its Compassionate Care program; they are among the few people in the country who can use the drug legally. Together with the American Public Health Association and other health care and medical organizations, individuals in this group filed an amicus brief supporting the plaintiffs. The following are their personal statements, taken from that brief.

*Barbara M. Douglass* was diagnosed with multiple sclerosis in 1988 at the age of 22. In 1991, Ms. Douglass began receiving herbal cannabis from the U. S. government on the advice and assistance of her physician. Prior to this date, Ms. Douglass had never tried cannabis. Each month, the government provides her physician with one can containing 300 cannabis cigarettes, each weighing 0.7 ounces. Ms. Douglass and her physician report that herbal cannabis provides relief from pain and spasms and stimulates her appetite to counteract the effects of wasting syndrome, which she suffered prior to using cannabis. Ms. Douglass has never experienced any adverse side effects from marijuana. Without cannabis, Ms. Douglass believes she would not be alive today.

*George Lee McMahon* was born July 22, 1950, with nail patella syndrome, a rare genetic disorder that causes severe pain, nausea, and muscle spasms. Mr. McMahon tried conventional medications to treat his symptoms, but found the side effects of these medications to be intolerable. In the early 1980s, Mr. McMahon discovered that herbal cannabis alleviated his pain, nausea, and spasms; stimulated his appetite; and allowed him to sleep through the night.

In 1988, Mr. McMahon informed his physician that he was successfully self-medicating with cannabis. His physician ordered him to cease his cannabis use and return to prescription medications. Over the following 6 months, Mr. McMahon's health progressively degenerated. Mr. McMahon's physician then helped Mr. McMahon apply to the federal government's Compassionate Care

IND [Investigational New Drug] Program. In March 1990, Mr. McMahon was accepted into the program, and for the past decade has received 300 cannabis cigarettes each month from the U.S. government. Mr. McMahon and his physician believe that without cannabis Mr. McMahon would not be alive today.

*Elvy Musikka* was diagnosed with glaucoma in 1975 at the age of 36. She tried conventional medications to treat her condition, but could not tolerate them. Reluctantly, in 1976, she decided to try herbal cannabis at the advice of her physician. The cannabis provided her immediate relief, substantially lowering her intraocular pressure as no other medication had, with few side effects. Ms. Musikka ingests cannabis by smoking it, as well as eating it in baked goods and olive oil. Fearful of the legal consequences of smoking cannabis, Ms. Musikka underwent several risky surgeries in an attempt to correct her condition, but they were unsuccessful and left her blind in one eye.

In 1988, Ms. Musikka was arrested in Florida and charged with cannabis possession. She challenged her conviction in the Florida Supreme Court, where she prevailed, becoming the first person in that state to establish a medical necessity defense for cannabis. Shortly thereafter, the federal government enrolled Ms. Musikka in its medical cannabis program and has provided her with 1.5 pounds of herbal cannabis on a quarterly basis ever since. Ms. Musikka and her physician believe that if she were deprived of cannabis, she would go blind.

*Irvin Henry Rosenfeld* was diagnosed at age 10 years with multiple congenital cartilaginous exostosis, a disease causing the continuous growth of bone tumors and the generation of new tumors on the ends of most of the long bones in his body. He was told he would not survive into adulthood. In an attempt to treat the painful symptoms of this disease, he was prescribed high doses of opioid analgesics, muscle relaxants, and anti-inflammatory medications. These he took on a daily basis, but they had minimal efficacy and produced debilitating side effects.

In 1971, Mr. Rosenfeld began using smoked herbal cannabis with the approval and under the supervision of a team of physicians. Mr. Rosenfeld found the cannabis highly efficacious in alleviating pain, reducing swelling, relaxing muscles and veins that surround the bone tumors, and preventing hemorrhage. In 1982, the U. S. government, operating under the Compassionate Care IND Program, at the request of his physicians began supplying Mr. Rosenfeld with herbal cannabis to treat his condition.

For the past 19 years, the government has consistently provided him with a 75-day supply of herbal cannabis, totaling 33 ounces per shipment. Mr. Rosenfeld smokes 12 marijuana cigarettes a day to control the symptoms of his disease. In the 30 years that Mr. Rosenfeld has used herbal cannabis as a medicine, he has experienced no adverse side effects (including no "high"), has been able to discontinue his prescription medications, and has worked successfully for the past 13 years as a stockbroker handling multi-million-dollar accounts. Mr. Rosenfeld and his physicians believe that without herbal cannabis Mr. Rosenfeld might not be alive or, at the very least, would be bedridden.

*List the options open to you. That is, answer the question, "What could you do?"*

- 
- 
- 
- 

*Choose the best solution from an ethical point of view, justify it, and respond to possible criticisms. That is, answer the question, "What should you do, and why?"*

- 
- 
- 
- 

*Select one member of your PBL group to role-play as a California physician wishing to prescribe marijuana for a medical purpose and have another member of your PBL group role-play as an ethics consultant. How might the physician converse with the ethics consultant about different ways of thinking and techniques for conflict management?*

- 
- 
- 
- 

*Again, please select one member of your PBL group to role-play as the ethics consultant and have another member of your PBL group role-play as a Department of Justice (DOJ) representative. How might the ethics consultant use what is known about stages of change and about motivational interviewing to solve what you consider the major problem presented in the case?*

- 
- 
- 
-

## Part three

### Discussion

"Conflict is more likely to arise in situations with uncertainty, ambiguity, complexity, stress, and change. Conflict may arise when individuals perceive different facts, hold different values, or experience different emotions. Thus, it is inevitable that there will be situations of conflict in the practice of clinical medicine." Ethics committees and consultants can be of utmost help in these situations. However, there are a few things that the field of bioethics must accomplish to validate its existence and ensure its progression and improvement.

Ethics committees and consultants are experiencing a phenomenon known as "failure-to-thrive syndrome." The characteristics of this syndrome include: parties involved are unsure of the existence of the committee, the function of committee is unclear, attendance at meetings is lower than desirable, lack of expertise can conjure feelings of doubt (for patients and members), and there is lack of networking between facilities to achieve uniformity. If ethics committees are to overcome these deficits, they must strive to achieve the following goals: renewed efforts to educate health care professionals; cooperation and collaboration among ethics committees; networking with community-based ethics groups; clearer delineation of responsibilities and limitations; and continuous quality improvement. "The ability of ethics committees to address successfully these areas of change will determine their future usefulness."

### Conclusion

Ethics committees and ethics consultants can be helpful in resolving conflict in the practice of clinical medicine. A choice must be made as to which model will be most beneficial in a given situation. It is imperative always to bear in mind that these entities exist to provide help, information, and guidance in making difficult decisions. Their primary function is not decision making. Furthermore, ethics committees and ethics consultants need to work toward clarifying their role, achieving industry standards and uniformity, and validating their existence.

*case five*

# Patient privacy

This problem-based learning session is based on the following: *Planned Parenthood of the Rocky Mountains Services Corporation v. Owens*, Civil Action No. 99-WM-60, U.S. District Court for the District of Colorado, 107 F. Supp. 2d 1271; 2000 U.S. Dist. Lexis 12855. August 16, 2000, Decided. August 16, 2000, Filed. It is reprinted with permission of LexisNexis.

## Objectives

The objectives of this problem-based learning case are:

- To understand and discuss how to protect patients' privacy
- To understand and discuss the duty to inform others
- To discuss ways of informing patients of limits of confidentiality
- To identify laws pertaining to requirements of reporting

## Introduction

When it comes to personal matters, privacy and confidentiality become very important and sensitive issues. Most individuals would not like to have their personal matters disclosed; as a result, they tend to keep their personal "data" private. The concepts of privacy and confidentiality should not be confused; they are distinct terms with different definitions.

Alan Westin describes confidentiality as "the question of how personal data collected for approved social purposes shall be held and used by the organization that originally collected it, what other secondary or further uses may be made of it, and when consent by the individual will be required for such uses. It is to further the patient's willing disclosure of confidential information to doctors that the law of privileged communications developed."

There are different definitions of privacy depending on the usage. In the health care context, two main types of privacy exist: informational privacy and decisional privacy. Informational privacy is concerned with the safeguarding of information about an individual; safeguarding can be from the government, research groups, or even family members. Who is an "authorized" person who receives this confidential information can sometimes be a matter of debate. Decisional privacy in the health care profession refers to who has "the right to decide"; that is, it concerns the responsibility for important decisions related to treatments, surgery, and other important medical decisions.

## Part one

The issue of this case is whether the Colorado Parental Notification Act (Act), Colo. Rev. Stat. §§ 12-37.5-101, et seq. (1998), which requires a physician to notify the parents of a minor prior to performing an abortion on the minor, violates the minor's rights as protected by the U.S. Constitution.

The organizational plaintiffs are corporations that provide abortion services to women under the age of 18 years. The individual plaintiffs are physicians who perform abortions in the state of Colorado. The plaintiffs bring this action on behalf of themselves and their minor patients.

Defendant William Owens is the governor of the state of Colorado. The remaining defendants are the district attorneys from the 22 judicial districts of the state of Colorado who handle criminal indictments, information, actions, and proceedings within their respective districts. All defendants are sued in their official capacities.

### The act

The Colorado Parental Notification Act — a citizen-initiated measure — was approved at Colorado's general election on November 3, 1998, and proclaimed law by the governor on December 31, 1998. Its legislative declaration states:

> *That family life and the preservation of the traditional family unit are of vital importance to the continuation of an orderly society; that the rights of parents to rear and nurture their children during their formative years and to be involved in all decisions of importance affecting such minor children should be protected and encouraged, especially as such parental involvement relates to the pregnancy of an unemancipated minor, recognizing that the decision by any such minor to submit to an abortion may have adverse long-term consequences for her.*

*Minor* is defined as "a person under eighteen years of age," but no definition is provided for an "unemancipated" minor.

*Abortion* is defined as "the use of any means to terminate the pregnancy of a minor with knowledge that the termination by those means will, with reasonable likelihood, cause the death of that person's unborn offspring at any time after fertilization."

The Act generally prohibits physicians from performing abortions on an unemancipated minor until at least 48 hours after written notice has been delivered to the minor's parent, guardian, or foster parent [Colo. Rev. Stat. §§ 12-37.5-103(2), 104(1)]. Delivery must be made to both of the minor's parents if they are living or to one parent if only one is living or one "cannot be served with notice." The 48-hour period does not begin to run until actual delivery is accomplished. In lieu of personal delivery, notice may be sent "postpaid certified mail, addressed to the parent at the usual place of abode of the parent, with return receipt requested and delivery restricted to the addressee." Delivery is then presumed to occur at 12:00 noon on the next day of regular mail delivery.

Any person performing or attempting to perform an abortion in willful violation of the Act commits a Class 1 misdemeanor and is also liable for proximate damages. Anyone who encourages a pregnant minor to provide false information to induce a physician to perform an abortion commits a Class 5 felony.

The Act provides two exceptions to the notice requirement:

1. The persons entitled to notice certify they have already been notified.
2. The minor declares she is victim of child abuse or neglect by the persons entitled to notice, and the physician has reported in accordance with the Child Protection Act of 1987.

The Act also provides two affirmative defenses:

1. The physician reasonably relied on representations by the minor as providing true information necessary to comply with the Act.
2. The physician performed the abortion to prevent imminent death, and there was insufficient time to provide the required notice.

Finally, the Act contains a contingent judicial bypass effective in the event the Act is enjoined or restrained for lack of a judicial bypass. Under the bypass procedure, the minor may avoid parental notification if she petitions a judge to dispense with the notice requirements, and the judge determines that such notice is not in her best interest or that the minor is sufficiently mature to make the abortion decision. The proceedings are to be conducted confidentially and decided without undue delay.

## Procedural history and remaining claims

On December 22, 1998, the plaintiffs filed their complaint in state court, asserting six claims for relief:

1. The Act is facially unconstitutional under the U.S. Constitution because it lacks an exception to permit a physician to perform an abortion without notice or a waiting period to protect the health or life of the pregnant minor.

2. The Act fails to provide a judicial procedure to bypass the parental notification requirements in the case of mature, abused, or "best interest" children and thus violates the U.S. Constitution.
3. The contingent judicial bypass provided by the Act does not protect the federal constitutional rights of minors because it lacks adequate procedures to ensure confidentiality, expedition, and appointment of counsel.
4. The Act violates the due process rights guaranteed by the Colorado Constitution.
5. The Act violates the Colorado Constitution's separation of legislative and judicial functions.
6. The Act's definition of abortion unconstitutionally imposes a parental notification requirement on the use of contraceptives.

The plaintiffs seek declaratory relief that the Act violates both the federal and state constitutions and injunctive relief to prevent enforcement of the Act. The federal claims arise under 42 U.S.C. § 1983, asserting the Act is a state action that deprives plaintiffs of their rights and privileges secured by the Constitution. Plaintiffs also claim entitlement to reasonable attorney fees and costs pursuant to 42 U.S.C. § 1988.

On December 23, 1998, a hearing on the plaintiffs' motion for a temporary restraining order was held before Boulder County District Judge Morris Sandstead, who entered a temporary restraining order against the then-lone district attorney defendant, Alex M. Hunter, district attorney for Boulder County.

On January 11, 1999, the then-defendant governor, Roy Romer, and defendant Hunter filed a notice of removal of the action to this court pursuant to 28 U.S.C. § 1446 because four claims for relief were based on the U.S. Constitution [see 28 U.S.C. § 1441(a) and (b)].

On removal, the plaintiffs sought to continue the temporary restraining order. They also filed a motion for certification of a class consisting of all district attorneys in Colorado. Pursuant to the parties' stipulation, the temporary restraining order was extended, but the motion for certification of a class was denied.

As part of the stipulation, the plaintiffs filed an amended complaint naming all of the district attorneys for the 22 judicial districts in the state of Colorado, while the defendants agreed to refrain from enforcing the Act until entry of a final nonappealable judgment.

On my inquiry, all parties recommended against certification of the issues to the Colorado Supreme Court pursuant to Rule 21.1 of the Colorado Appellate Rules. Both sides in essence urged that the issues of this case, including any necessary statutory interpretation of state law, were inextricably tied to issues of federal constitutional law and should be decided in federal court. This is, of course, consistent with the defendants' decision to remove this case to federal court. In any case, a federal litigant need not await a state court interpretation before commencing a federal suit [*City of*

*Lakewood v. Plain Dealer Publishing Co.*, 486 U.S. 750, 108 S. Ct. 2138, 2151, 100 L. Ed. 2d 771 (1988)]. Indeed, certification is inappropriate when the statute at issue is not "obviously susceptible" to a limiting or narrowing construction to preserve its constitutionality [*City of Houston v. Hill*, 482 U.S. 451, 107 S. Ct. 2502, 2513–2515, 96 L. Ed. 2d 398 (1987)].

Given removal to this court, the plaintiffs withdrew their claims of violations of the Colorado Constitution (fourth and fifth claims for relief), and those claims were dismissed without prejudice by minute order, dated January 14, 2000.

On April 26, 2000, and pursuant to the parties' joint motion, I granted defendants' motion for partial summary judgment dismissing plaintiffs' sixth claim for relief, asserting that the Act unconstitutionally defined abortion to require parental notification for prescriptions of contraceptives. This dismissal was based on the undisputed fact that a person prescribing or providing contraceptives, including emergency contraception or the so-called morning after pill, will not know with the statutorily prescribed "reasonable likelihood" that the contraceptives will "cause the death of that person's unborn offspring at any time after fertilization" as defined in the Act. Accordingly, a prescription without parental notification would not violate the Act.

Defendants responded to the plaintiffs' complaint by denying the remaining claims for relief (one through three of the amended complaint) and asserted that the statute is constitutional because: (1) the Colorado Children's Code (Colo. Rev. Stat. § 19-1-101 et seq.) should be incorporated into the Act to protect the health and life of the pregnant minor; (2) a judicial bypass is not constitutionally required for a parental notification act that has an exception for abuse; and (3) the mechanism of the contingent judicial bypass procedure provides for confidentiality and expedition and imposes an obligation on judges to bypass notification if the stated requirements are met.

The parties have filed cross motions for summary judgment asserting that the issues are purely legal and may be decided on the basis of uncontested facts. As to the first claim for relief, I agree.

## Standard of review

Summary judgment is appropriate if there is no genuine issue of material fact, and the moving party is entitled to judgment as a matter of law. The evidence is viewed in the light most favorable to the nonmoving party [*Anderson v. Liberty Lobby, Inc.*, 477 U.S. 242, 249–252, 91 L. Ed. 2d 202, 106 S. Ct. 2505 (1986)]. However, as here, when the parties file cross motions for summary judgment, I need not consider evidence other than that filed by the parties (*James Barlow Family Ltd. Partnership v. David M. Munson, Inc.*, 124 F.3d).

Accordingly, I have limited my review to the evidence the parties have submitted with their many filings as part of their cross motions. Nevertheless, I may still deny summary judgment if dispute remains as to any material fact.

## Factual background

According to records of the Colorado Department of Public Health and Environment, 9183 abortions were performed in Colorado in 1997 (1998 figures were not presented). Of those numbers, 1012 abortions (or approximately 11%) were performed for women under the age of 18 years. The majority of all abortions performed (more than 85%) were performed within 13 weeks of gestation.

With regard to parental knowledge, nationwide statistics indicate that at least 61% of minors seeking abortions do so with the knowledge of at least one parent. There is a strong correlation of parental awareness with age of the minor. The younger the minor, the more likely the parent is aware of the abortion. Nationally, 90% of those minors under 15 years old obtain an abortion with the parent's knowledge.

Planned Parenthood's statistics for Colorado are consistent with national averages. For the 2-year period of 1996 and 1997, 59.2% of minors seen at its facilities informed at least one parent. The statistical gradation by age classification is likewise present: all of the 13-year-olds involved at least one parent; 88.3% of the 14-year-olds did; 70.1% of the 15-year-olds, 58.1% of the 16-year-olds, and 46.9% of the 17-year-olds informed at least one parent. Numerous reasons are given for not involving a parent, including fear of physical or emotional abuse, fear of punishment, fear of worsening already problematic family relationships, fear of losing a boyfriend, and even a desire not to threaten a parent's health.

With regard to health issues, the parties agree that some minors will experience medical conditions during pregnancy that pose serious risks to their health. These conditions include preeclampsia, premature rupture of membranes, and inevitable spontaneous abortion. Some of these conditions require immediate attention to avoid risk of serious health problems or even death. Preeclampsia, for example, calls for immediate action as delay can place the woman at risk for cerebral hemorrhage, liver failure, kidney failure, vision problems, and coma. Therefore, when a pregnant minor presents with one of these urgent medical conditions, delaying aggressive treatment to give notice pursuant to the Act may place the patient's health at risk in circumstances short of imminent death.

*Make a list of the major problems presented in this case*

- 
- 
- 
-

## Hypothesis and mechanism

For the problems in your list above, give a cause or a reason for each to happen:

- 
- 
- 
- 

## Learning issues

Make a list of learning issues in the form of questions. Remember, your goal is to gather the medical, social, and all other relevant facts that may apply to the case.

How has the advancement of information technology affected a patient's privacy?

> Before computer networks were developed, the patients' physical information was in paper format and was held in some central location where access would be given to certain known individuals. However, it was rather cumbersome when access was needed for these records. Computerized networks and the Internet have made this task easier, allowing more efficiency for data collection, which benefits both the patient and the health care professional. The price for this efficiency is the insecure nature of this electronic format, thus threatening patients' privacy. As a result, the health care professional must be more aware of how and where this information is entered in electronic format. In a public setting, the pharmacist's computer monitor, for example, may be in view of customers. Hackers can break into larger World Wide Web networked computers, also leading to a threat to patients' privacy.

How has the passing of OBRA '90 (Omnibus Budget Reconciliation Act of 1990) had an impact on a patients' privacy?

> With the passing of OBRA '90, pharmacists are required to counsel patients receiving prescription drugs under Medicaid coverage. However, to be fair to all patients, this has been extended to include all patients receiving prescriptions. The effect of this on privacy is that most pharmacies do not have a private area where patients can be counseled, and thus there can be a leak of private information to other parties.

Even though the patients' privacy should be protected, when might this not be the case?

When the safety of the patient and others is at risk due to withholding information of the patients' situation, it is in the best interests not to keep that information confidential. One popular case is the duty to inform persons who may be exposed to HIV. In this case, there can be a risk to others if they are not informed, which puts them in significant danger without their knowledge and consent.

What are the limits for which a patient's health records should be kept confidential?

Many believe that there is no potential breach of patient confidentiality when their information is used in some statistical survey or research. It must be emphasized here that there is usually no identity of the specific individual recorded, and it is the results of data from a very large aggregate of patients' records that are used. The data collected for research are used for a variety of purposes; some of them are: to advance basic biomedical science; to know patterns of health, disease, and disability; to reduce public health threats; to understand utilization of health care; to evaluate and improve practices; to make effective innovations; to analyze economic factors and appraise potential markets for products and services.

When can a patient's health information be used for research purposes?

The question of what is considered legitimate research also becomes an issue. Some health care providers claim that they are collecting data for research, but sometimes they act more as businesses; the data that they collect are used for the "market" need and demand aspects of health care and the like. Not only do health care providers use the patients' information for research, but insurance companies also use it to decide what they will cover, prices, and so on.

Describe the Privacy Act of 1974.

There have been attempts to implement a federal minimum standard for the protection of patient health information. In addition to the mandatory federal law, states can and have adopted standards that are even stricter than the federal laws. One of the first of these acts was the Privacy Act of 1974, which required federal agencies to utilize fair information practices with regard to collection and use of records, including patients' records.

Describe the Health Insurance Portability and Accountability Act (HIPAA).

The HIPAA act was originally created to reduce the administrative burden of health care by standardizing the electronic transmission of patients' records. However, as part of this bill, security measures are also to be adopted and passed by legislation to protect private medical information.

Describe the Model State Public Health Privacy Act.

The Model State Public Health Privacy Act was sponsored by several organizations, including the National Conference of State Legislatures (NCSL). The purpose of this act is to develop a model law that addresses the privacy and security issues that arise from the collection, distribution, and use of health information by public health agencies at the state and local levels. This will allow a strict set of rules to be followed by which access to data is provided to a defined set of agencies, and if the use of the information gathered is not defined in the act, then specific penalties will be applied.

## Literature review

To help you get ready to answer certain questions you anticipate being asked during the second part of the case, look in the local medical library and on the World Wide Web for helpful information. Please indicate in the spaces below (1) several helpful articles or books you found and (2) several helpful Web sites you found.

- **Helpful articles/books:**

  Abramson, M., Ethics committees, *Trends Health Care, Law Ethics*, 7, 32, 1992.

  American Medical Association, *Code of Medical Ethics: Current Opinions with Annotations*, Chicago, 2000, pp. 216–217.

  Fletcher, J.C. and Hoffmann, J.D., Ethics committees: time to experiment with standards, *Ann. Intern. Med.*, 120, 335–338, 1994.

  Heilicser, B.J., Meltzer, D., and Siegler, M., The effect of clinical medical ethics consultation on healthcare costs, *J. Clin. Ethics*, 11, 31–38, 2000.

  La Puma, J. and Toulmin, S.E., Ethics consultants and ethics committees, *Arch. Intern. Med.*, 149, 1109–1112, 1989.

  McIntyre, R.L., The legitimation of ethics consultation, *Trends Health Care, Law Ethics*, 8, 7–10, 34, 1993.

  Nelson, W.A., Using ethics advisory committees to cope with ethical issues, *Mo. Med.*, 89, 827–830, 1992.

  Orr, R.D. and deLeon, D.M., The role of the clinical ethicist in conflict resolution *J. Clin. Ethics*, 11, 21–29, 2000.

  Ross, J.W. et al., *Health Care Ethics Committees: The Next Generation*, John Wiley & Sons, New York, 1993, pp. 1–59.

  Smith, M.L., The future of healthcare ethics committees, *Trends Health Care, Law Ethics*, 9, 7–10, 1994.

  Swenson, M.D. and Miller, R.B., Ethics case review in health care institutions: committees, consultants, or teams? *Arch. Intern. Med.*, 152, 694–697, 1992.

- **Helpful Web sites:**
  The role of ethics committees: running and revitalizing: www.mcw.edu/bioethics/lec7.htm
  Ethics committees: cpmcnet.columbia.edu/texts/guide/hmg03_0008.html
  Ethics committees and ethics consultation: eduserv.hscer.washington.edu/bioethics/topics/ethics.html

## Identify all relevant values that play a role in the case and determine which values, if any, conflict

Nonmaleficence:

Beneficence:

Respect for persons:

Loyalty:

Distributive justice:

## Learning issues for next student-centered problem-based learning session

- List the options open to you. That is, answer the question, "What could you do?"

- Choose the best solution from an ethical point of view, justify it, and respond to possible criticisms. That is, answer the question, "What should you do, and why?"
- What are the different ways of thinking about the problem? Which conflict management techniques can be used in the situation?

## Part two

The plaintiffs' first claim for relief is straightforward, namely, that the Act is unconstitutional because it fails to provide an exception to the notice requirement when necessary to protect the health of minors short of imminent death. As to this claim, there is no genuine issue of material fact. As noted, it is uncontested that there are situations when a physician must act promptly to protect the health or life of the minor when the affirmative defense of imminent death would not apply. As a consequence, and as both parties agree, the delay in the abortion inherent in the Act's notification process will result in adverse health consequences for some minors. Accordingly, this issue may be resolved purely as a matter of law, and I begin my analysis with a brief background of the law concerning state regulation of abortions performed on minors as the law existed at the time of the Act's passage.

More than a quarter century ago, the Supreme Court held that women have the constitutional right, with some limitations, to choose abortion [*Roe v. Wade*, 410 U.S. 113, 153, 35 L. Ed. 2d 147, 93 S. Ct. 705 (1973)]. *Roe* provided a trimester framework that permitted limited regulation. As the pregnancy progresses, a woman's right to abortion is subject to increasing regulation to protect both the health of the woman and the state's legitimate interest in potential life. Subsequent to viability, the state may regulate and even prohibit abortion with one exception: "where it is necessary, in appropriate medical judgment, for the preservation of the life or health of the mother." A statute that "excepts from criminality only a life-saving procedure on behalf of the mother . . . is violative of the Due Process Clause of the Fourteenth Amendment."

The Court soon confirmed that these rights applied to minor women as well [*Planned Parenthood of Central Missouri v. Danforth*, 428 U.S. 52, 74–75, 49 L. Ed. 2d 788, 96 S. Ct. 2831 (1976), "Constitutional rights do not mature and come into being magically only when one attains the state-defined age of majority. Minors, as well as adults, are protected by the Constitution and possess constitutional rights"]. Specifically, the Court held that a statute that imposed a blanket parental consent requirement, except when a doctor certified that abortion was necessary to preserve the mother's life, was unconstitutional.

Nevertheless, the Court does recognize the special legal status of the minor and, in particular, her relationship to her parents. In *Bellotti v. Baird* [443 U.S. 622, 61 L. Ed. 2d 797, 99 S. Ct. 3035 (1979)], the Court noted three reasons for not equating the constitutional rights of a minor with those of an adult: "The peculiar vulnerability of children; their inability to make critical decisions in an informed, mature manner; and the importance of the parental role in child rearing." With regard to the role of the parents, the Court referred to several decisions to emphasize its importance to our society, including *Pierce v. Society of Sisters*, 268 U.S. 510, 535, 69 L. Ed. 1070, 45 S. Ct. 571 (1925) (a child is not a mere creature of state; those who raise her have the right and "high duty" to prepare her for "additional obligations"); *Wisconsin v. Yoder*, 406 U.S. 205, 233, 32 L. Ed. 2d 15, 92 S. Ct. 1526 (1972) ("The duty to prepare the child for 'additional obligations' . . . must be read to include the inculcation of moral standards, religious beliefs, and elements of good citizenship"); *Prince v. Massachusetts*, 321 U.S. 158, 166, 88 L. Ed. 645, 64 S. Ct. 438 (1944) ("It is cardinal with us that the custody, care and nurture of the child reside first in the parents, whose primary function and freedom include preparation for obligations the state can neither supply nor hinder"); *Ginsberg v. New York*, 390 U.S. 629, 639, 88 S. Ct. 1274, 20 L. Ed. 2d 195 (1968) ("Deeply rooted in our Nation's history and tradition, is the belief that the parental role implies a substantial measure of authority over one's children"). Accordingly, the state may enact laws to assist parents, who have the primary responsibility for the child's well-being.

However, state support of parents is not without limits. The Court in *Bellotti* invalidated a Massachusetts statute requiring parental consent in all circumstances except when the parent is not available or the abortion need constitutes "an emergency requiring immediate action." Justice Powell, in his plurality opinion, found that children are particularly vulnerable to their parents' efforts to obstruct an abortion and a female child's access to legal help. Accordingly, he established the basic principle that if parental consent is required, the statute must establish an alternative procedure for obtaining an abortion without parental consent to prevent parents from exercising an absolute and possibly arbitrary veto over their children's constitutional rights.

Justice Powell outlined the essentials of such procedures to be that the pregnant minor has access to a proceeding with anonymity and sufficient expedition to allow an abortion by showing either: "(1) that she is mature enough and well enough informed to make her abortion decision, in consultation with her physician, independently of her parents' wishes; or (2) that even if she is not able to make this decision independently, the desired abortion would be in her best interests." These two exceptions are commonly referred to as the "mature" and "best-interest" exceptions.

Since *Bellotti*, parental notification statutes, as opposed to parental consent statutes, have generally passed constitutional muster [*H. L. v. Matheson*, 450 U.S. 398, 67 L. Ed. 2d 388, 101 S. Ct. 1164 (1981), parental notice is constitutional for unemancipated minor who made no claim of maturity; *Ohio v. Akron Center for Reproductive Health*, 497 U.S. 502, 111 L. Ed. 2d 405, 110 S. Ct. 2972 (1990), statute allowed a bypass procedure to prove maturity or best interest]. Compared to parental consent statutes, notification statutes do not grant parents the legal right to make the ultimate decision. "Notice statutes are not equivalent to consent statutes because they do not give anyone a veto power over a minor's abortion decision." In making its rulings, the Supreme Court has expressly reserved the question of whether parental notification statutes require a judicial bypass procedure. Not surprisingly, there is a split in circuit courts whether a parental notification act requires a judicial bypass procedure.

The next important stage of the evolution of this law was the decision of *Planned Parenthood of Southeastern Pennsylvania v. Casey* [505 U.S. 833, 120 L. Ed. 2d 674, 112 S. Ct. 2791 (1992)], which confirmed by plurality opinion the essential holding of *Roe*. The Court concluded that women have a constitutional right, rooted in the Fourteenth Amendment's due process clause, to choose an abortion without unwarranted government interference based on women's right to bodily integrity and privacy. Discounting the trimester approach of *Roe*, the joint opinion ultimately holds that the issue is whether the regulation violates due process by placing an undue burden on a woman's right to choose abortion.

Focusing specifically on the minor's right to abortion, the Court in *Casey* acknowledged the importance of parental involvement and the "quite reasonable assumption that minors will benefit from consultation with their parents and that children will often not realize that their parents have their best interests at heart." The Court, however, recognized there must be exceptions to the requirement of parental consent. In particular, the Court approved the parental consent provision because it had an exception for medical emergencies and a judicial procedure for exempting mature and best-interest minors.

With regard to the plaintiffs' first claim for relief, the Court in *Casey* reaffirmed the state may not regulate or proscribe abortion "where it is necessary, in appropriate medical judgment, for the preservation of the life or health of the mother." Indeed, the Court had previously made plain that the woman's health must be the paramount consideration [*Thornburgh v. American College of Obstetricians and Gynecologists*, 476 U.S. 747, 768–769, 90 L. Ed. 2d 779, 106 S. Ct. 2169 (1986)]. As the Tenth Circuit has noted: "The importance of maternal health is a unifying thread that runs from *Roe* to *Thornburgh* and then to *Casey*. In fact, defendants concede that *Thornburgh*'s admonition that a woman's health must be the paramount concern remains vital in wake of *Casey*" [Jane L. Bangerter, 61 F.3d 1493, 1504 (10th Cir. 1995)]. "The essential holding of *Roe* forbids a State to interfere with a woman's choice to undergo an abortion procedure if continuing her pregnancy would constitute a threat to her health" (*Casey*, at 880, concluding that, given the medical emergency definition exception, there was no undue burden on the woman's abortion right).

With this backdrop in mind, I note that, compared to other notification statutes, the Act is devoid of any such protective exception and, without more, appears unconstitutional on its face.

Most recently, the Supreme Court confirmed the constitutional need for a health exception in both pre- and postviability abortion regulations [*Stenberg v. Carhart*, 530 U.S. 914, 147 L. Ed. 2d 743, 120 S. Ct. 2597, 2609 (2000)]. In effect, the Supreme Court implicitly adopted a *per se* rule that abortion regulations must contain an exception for preservation of the health or life of the mother. Therefore, an abortion regulation that puts a woman's health in jeopardy, regardless of her age or maturity, is unconstitutional. That fact that the threat to health occurs infrequently does not render the statute constitutional because "the state cannot prohibit a person from obtaining treatment simply by pointing out that most people do not need it" (120 S. Ct. at 2611). Thus, an Act that limits its health exception only to those situations when the mother's life is in imminent danger is not sufficient. Accordingly, "[such a] lack of a health exception necessarily renders the statute unconstitutional."

Defendants argue, however, that I should decide, as a matter of statutory construction, that the Colorado Children's Code remains applicable to pregnant minors, and since the code provides an expedited *ex parte* procedure by which a physician can obtain a court order to meet the minor's health needs, the constitutional requirement of a health exception to the Act's regulation of abortion is satisfied. To achieve that interpretative result, the defendants rely principally on two well-recognized rules of construction.

The first is that, if construction is allowed, an interpretation that preserves the constitutionality of the Act should be adopted [*Colorado Ground Water Community Association v. Eagle Park Farms*, 919 P.2d 212, 221 (Colo. 1996); *People v. Zapotocky*, 869 P.2d 1234, 1240 (Colo. 1994)]. The Supreme Court, in a frequently cited case, has stated that the "Court will first determine whether it is fairly possible to interpret a statute in a manner that renders it constitutionally valid."

The second rule of construction is the vehicle by which a health exception would be imported to or superimposed on the provisions of the Act. That rule, known as *in pari materia* construction, holds that when determining the legislative intent of the statute being construed, that statute should be read in conjunction with other statutes relating to the same subject or purpose. Defendants urge that the Children's Code and the Act share common purposes and subject matter, thereby permitting the protection of the minor's health pursuant to the code to be read into the Act, even though the Act contains no mention of those matters. Defendants' arguments, therefore, require that I interpret the Act.

In construing a state statute, a federal court is bound by the state's highest court's interpretation. If, as in this case, none exists, then I must look to the state's rules of statutory construction to determine the legislative intent and the ultimate application of the law.

As is normally the case, I begin the statutory interpretation undertaking with the most basic rule: I must first determine whether ambiguity exists that gives rise to the need for interpretation [see *Colorado v. Nieto*, 993 P.2d 493, 502 (Colo. 2000)]. As the Colorado Supreme Court has repeatedly held, when a statute is unambiguous, the court must apply it as written and must not resort to rules of statutory construction, even to avoid a constitutional conflict [*Van Waters and Rogers, Inc., v. Keelan*, 840 P.2d 1070, 1076 (Colo. 1992)].

A statute is ambiguous if the plain language of the statute permits one or more reasonable alternative interpretations. See *Colorado v. Nieto*, at 502, which explains that a statutory provision is ambiguous if it can be reasonably applied to reach two distinct and opposite results; see also *People v. Terry* [791 P.2d 374, 376 (Colo. 1990)], "The language in the subsections is ambiguous — that is [because] it is susceptible to reasonable, alternative interpretations." Therefore, "where the words chosen by the legislature are unclear in their common understanding, or capable of two or more constructions leading to different results, the statute is ambiguous" according to *Colorado v. Nieto*, 993 P.2d at 500–501 ("[A] statute is ambiguous [if] . . . the words chosen do not inexorably lead to a single result").

The same basic principle remains applicable when a party urges reading another statute *in pari materia* as it is an error to do so when the statute or regulation is unambiguous [*United States v. Fisher*, 456 F.2d 1143, 1145 (10th Cir. 1972)]. Sutherland, the oft-cited authority on statutory construction, states simply that: "Other statutes dealing with the same subject as the one being construed — commonly referred to as statutes *in pari materia* — . . . may not be resorted to if the statute is clear and unambiguous" [2B Sutherland, Statutory Construction § 51.01 at 117 (5th Ed. 1992)]. Accordingly, the threshold issue is whether the Act is ambiguous. Given the long-recognized need for a health exception to abortion regulations, the sharper focus of the ambiguity issue is whether there is any ambiguity concerning exceptions to the Act's notification requirements.

The only specific exceptions to the notice requirement are contained in § 12-37.5–105:

> *(1) The person or persons who are entitled to notice certify in writing that they have been notified.*
>
> *(2) The pregnant minor declares that she is a victim of child abuse or neglect by the acts or omissions of the person who would be entitled to notice, as such acts or omissions are defined in "The Child Protection Act of 1987," as set forth in Title 19, Art. III, of the Colo. Rev. Stat. and any amendments thereto, and the attending physician has reported such child abuse or neglect as required by the said Act.*

Thus, there is no mention of an exception to preserve the health of the minor. It is also noteworthy that, although reference is made to the Colorado Children's Code in the second exception, there is no similar reference to the Children's Code provision that allows expedited *ex parte* emergency orders when the "child's welfare may be endangered" or "emergency medical or surgical treatment is reasonably necessary."

Otherwise, the only other reference to health and life of the pregnant minor is the affirmative defense if "the abortion was performed to prevent the imminent death of the minor child and there was insufficient time to provide the required notice" [§ 12-37.5–106(2)(b)]. Disregarding the fact that an affirmative defense is significantly different from an exception to the reach of a criminal statute, the health exception has never been satisfied only by protection against imminent death. Since 1973, the Supreme Court has emphasized that a law is unconstitutional if its only exception is to preserve the life of the mother [see, e.g., *Roe v. Wade*, 410 U.S. at 163–164 (1973), which states that a statute cannot survive constitutional attack if it is limited to the single reason to save the mother's life; *Planned Parenthood v. Danforth*, 428 U.S. at 68–72]. Therefore, the exception must include preservation of health even though the condition is not life threatening (see *Stenberg v. Carhart*, 120 S. Ct. at 2609–2613).

I therefore conclude that the language of the Act concerning exceptions to its reach is plain and unambiguous. However, even if I were to find ambiguity to allow consideration of rules of interpretation, I would likewise hold that the sole saving interpretation suggested by defendants — reading the Colorado Children's Code health exception *in pari materia* into the Act — would not be appropriate.

In the first instance, the necessary predicate for use of *in pari materia* (namely, that the statutes relate to the same subject or purpose) is not present. The Act's declared purposes are concerned with family life, preservation of the family unit, and the rights of parents. Expression of concern for the minor is limited to the observation that an abortion "may have adverse long-term consequences for her." The Children's Code, on the other hand, although recognizing the importance of family, places primary concern with the child to serve her welfare and the interests of society. As such, the Children's Code is to be "liberally construed to serve the welfare of children and the best interests of society. The emphasis of the Act is on the undeniably important significance of the family and the role of parents. But, it does not assert, even as a subsidiary purpose, a goal to protect the health of minors short of imminent death. Thus, the legislative declaration does not provide any positive indication that the Act should be interpreted in conjunction with the Colorado Children's Code to protect the health of the minor. This legislative omission is carried forward in the Act's two explicit exceptions and two explicit affirmative defenses.

I also observe that the legislative history of the Act addresses only the two specific exceptions found in Colo. Rev. Stat. § 12-37.5–105. The so-called Blue Book, prepared by the Legislative Council of the Colorado General Assembly as an analysis of statewide ballot proposals (defendants' Exhibit A), contains descriptions of the Act and the background to its adoption that may be used to determine the intent of the voters. However, neither the summary description nor the background section makes reference to the legal need to provide an exception to preserve the minor's health, and no part of the Blue Book suggests that the Act would be administered in the context of the Colorado Children's Code.

Further, the defendants' specific *in pari materia* argument — that the provision for an *ex parte* emergency order by a juvenile judge found in the Colorado Children's Code may be imported into the Act to provide the required health care exception — would essentially necessitate rewriting the Act to install a third exception under § 12-37.5–105. Without deciding whether the provisions of the Children's Code for emergency orders would satisfy the constitutional requirements, its importation into § 12-37.5–105 would be inconsistent with the express language that "no notice shall be required" as the imported provision would contradictorily require reasonable efforts for notification. Such inconsistencies do not serve the general purposes of *in pari materia* construction to effectuate legislative intent and "to give consistent, harmonious and sensible effect to all its parts." Thus, importing the Children's Code section creates conflict that would necessitate even further construction to avoid apparent inconsistencies.

Similarly, to import the Children's Code exception would seem inconsistent with the explicit affirmative defense for imminent death, which strongly suggests that health is a consideration only in the most extreme emergency. To incorporate the exception of the Children's Code for reasonably necessary medical treatment would virtually render the affirmative defense meaningless. An interpretation that renders other portions of the Act essentially mere surplus is not proper [see *People v. Terry*, 791 P.2d 374, 376 (Colo. 1990), "Constructions that would render meaningless a part of the statute should be avoided"; see also *People v. Marquez*, 983 P.2d 159 (Colo. App. 1999) (same)]. Accordingly, I conclude that an *in pari materia* interpretation cannot save the constitutionality of the Act.

In sum, I conclude that the Act's language is plain and unambiguous; it does not contain an exception to the notice requirement when it is medically necessary for the preservation of the mother's health to proceed without notice; it is not fairly susceptible to saving or narrowing construction to preserve the Act's constitutionality. Hence, the Act deprives some pregnant minor women of their constitutional rights.

Because their resolution is not necessary to decide this case, I do not address the plaintiffs' other claims.

*List the options open to you. That is, answer the question, "What could you do?"*

- 
- 
- 
- 

*Choose the best solution from an ethical point of view, justify it, and respond to possible criticisms. That is, answer the question, "What should you do, and why?"*

- 
- 
- 
-

*Select one member of your PBL group to role-play as a Colorado physician who performs abortions and have another member of your PBL group role-play as a representative for the Governor. How might the two converse about different ways of thinking and techniques for conflict management?*

- •
- •
- •
- •

*Again, please select one member of your PBL group to role-play as the physician and have another member of your PBL group role-play as a representative of the governor. How might the physician use what is known about stages of change and about motivational interviewing to solve what you consider the major problem presented in the case?*

- •
- •
- •
- •

## Part three

### Order

Families are of vital importance to our society, and laws or regulations designed to support or enhance family relationships — including parental involvement in a minor's decision whether to abort her pregnancy — are understandable objectives of legislation or regulation. It is fundamental to our constitutional system of individual rights, however, that those legitimate legislative objectives cannot be purchased at the expense of individual rights and liberties. No matter how worthy the goals of the Colorado Parental Notification Act, its drafters have overlooked or disregarded the protection of the minor's health. For more than a quarter century, the Supreme Court has required that any abortion regulation have a clear legal exception for an abortion that is medically necessary for the preservation of the mother's health. The Act plainly fails to provide such a health exception, and the facts indisputably show that the delay inherent in the Act's notification requirements will place some women at risk of serious health problems or even death. Therefore, the Colorado Parental Notification Act violates the rights of minor women protected by the Fourteenth Amendment to the United States Constitution.

Accordingly, it is ordered:

1.  Plaintiffs' motion for summary judgment is granted.
2.  Pursuant to the Declaratory Judgment Act, I declare that the Colorado Parental Notification Act, Colo. Rev. Stat. § 12-37.5–101 et seq. (1998) is unconstitutional for the reasons stated.
3.  Effective immediately, the defendants are permanently enjoined from enforcing the Colorado Parental Notification Act, Colo. Rev. Stat. § 12-37.5–101 et seq. (1998).
4.  In accordance with 42 U.S.C. § 1988, the plaintiffs, as prevailing parties in this action pursuant to 42 U.S.C. § 1983, are entitled to reasonable attorney fees.
5.  Plaintiffs, as prevailing parties, may have their costs pursuant to Fed. R. Civ. P. 54(d)(1).

## Conclusion

There are a variety of steps that can be taken to protect a patient's privacy, especially a child's privacy. The most susceptible form of privacy breach is perhaps the electronic form. The first obvious step would be, if possible, to avoid any computerized transactions. However, this option eventually will be phased out. Second, the next thing is for the health care professional always to use secured lines of communications; via the World Wide Web, secure channels can be implemented before transmission of the information.

Pharmacies can also play an important role in the security of confidential information. The counseling area should be as private as possible so that no other individuals can overhear the conversation between the pharmacist and the patient. Also, steps should be taken so that all the workers understand their responsibility to ensure the patient's privacy, and that policies are in place to report violations and misuse of this information.

One legal solution is to impose a set of rules on the collecting organizations concerning which information is collected, how that information is to be used, and the penalties imposed if the rules are abused.

Protecting patients' privacy is of the utmost importance. One cannot rely on laws alone to do this because laws are only now being fully enacted to keep patients' information confidential. The health care individual can take steps to protect patients' privacy, mainly by making sure no one overhears a conversation, by being aware of the insecurities that exist in electronic transactions, and by taking steps to make sure that a transaction is as secure as possible.

There are limits to the confidentiality of the patients' information, and patients should be notified of the possibilities. Most of the information is for useful scientific research that eventually is beneficial, but insurance companies also use some of this information, as do pharmaceutical companies for pricing and supply-related purposes.

There is much harm to the patient that can occur from a breach of this sensitive information, and the free exchange of pertinent medical information between the patient and the health care provider can be inhibited, giving way to a potentially dangerous and life-threatening situation.

## *case six*

# *Truth telling*

This problem-based learning session is based on the following: *Smith v. Cleburne County Hospital*, Nos. 87-2587, 87-2620, 87-2621, 87-2622, U.S. Court of Appeals for the Eighth Circuit, 870 F.2d 1375; 1989 U.S. App. Lexis 2777. November 14, 1988, Submitted. March 8, 1989, Filed. It is reprinted with permission of LexisNexis.

## *Objectives*

The objectives of this problem-based learning case are:

- To discuss the definitions of truth telling and deception and the lack of standardization
- To compare truth-telling attitudes between physicians and pharmacists
- To discuss the importance of autonomy in a culturally diverse country
- To propose a solution to maintain patient autonomy

## *Introduction*

Truth telling is a moral–ethical issue involved in all aspects of providing health care. There is an obligation of every health care provider to give complete autonomy to the patient. Health care providers are also obligated to provide for the best outcome of a patient's therapy; this can cause a conflict of interest, from which arises the issue of "truth telling." A discussion of cultural diversity, patient autonomy, and a physician's (pharmacist's) attitude toward telling the truth helps clarify the issue of truth telling.

## *Part one*

The Cleburne County Hospital is owned and operated by Cleburne County, Arkansas. The business affairs of the hospital are under the supervision of an eight-member board of governors; these members are appointed by the county judge. The county judge is a nonvoting *ex officio* member of the board.

In 1968, Dr. Smith submitted a written application to the Hospital for medical staff privileges. Pursuant to hospital and medical staff bylaws, the medical staff reviews a doctor's application for medical staff privileges, and if the medical staff finds that the applicant has met its established criteria for qualifications, then the medical staff recommends to the board of governors that the doctor be extended privileges. According to this procedure, Smith was given privileges as a member of the active medical staff, which allowed the unlimited admissions of his patients. However, active medical staff privileges were contingent on the assumption of performing rotating emergency room coverage, attending regular medical staff meetings, and submitting a written application annually for renewed staff privileges.

Smith began to criticize the quality of patient care at the hospital, citing perceived problems in nursing, dietary services, and the nursery. By July 2, 1976, Smith's criticism of the hospital's shortcomings prompted his notification to the hospital administration that he had no alternative but to resign from the staff. As of that date, Smith ceased scheduling surgery at the hospital and began referring patients to other hospitals.

Smith was unhappy with the hospital administration's response to his criticisms and found it necessary to address a letter to his patients on November 22, 1976, indicating that, due to the lack of his expected level of patient care, he was quitting use of the hospital in the near future. On the same day, Smith also addressed a different letter to the board of governors criticizing them as political flunkies; he stated he was concerned that negligence at the hospital would cause a person to die, which only then would make them realize that problems existed. Furthermore, he called for a full investigation of his complaints; he indicated that if the investigation showed he was the problem, and not the hospital's poor level of care, then he should not be allowed to remain on the medical staff. This letter was made available to his patients.

Smith met with the board of governors in December 1976 to discuss the hospital's problems. As a result of this meeting, the board requested on December 20 that the Arkansas Department of Health (ADH) conduct an inspection and survey of the hospital facilities and the quality of patient care. Again, Smith was unhappy with this response to his criticisms; on December 29, he wrote personal letters to various board members calling for their resignations because, in his view, they were arrogant and indifferent, failed to learn their duties and perform them, and felt contempt for concerned citizens. In addition, Smith wrote to the *ex officio* member of the board, the county judge, specifically attacking the competency of the hospital administrator and indicating that he felt the biggest problem involving the hospital was the desire on the part of some doctors to be considered gods.

At a regular medical staff meeting on January 3, 1977, Smith gave further response to the board's proposal to have the ADH conduct an investigation; he indicated that his was the only opinion capable of determining whether patients were getting adequate care. Thus, if an investigation was made and the hospital was found to have adequate nursing care, then he would still be unable to live with his conscience and would resign.

On February 1, 1977, the ADH submitted the results of their investigation of Cleburne County Hospital. The department's survey team found 15 deficiencies indicating noncompliance with Arkansas' regulations for hospitals. Items that were found deficient included:

Preparation of food too far in advance of the meal to be served
Incorrect water temperatures for pot washing
Outdated cartons of milk
Phone orders by physicians not co-signed within 24 hours
Outdated drugs
Some controlled substances not in locked storage
Incomplete pharmacy records
Pharmacy stop orders not followed
Irregular pharmacy staff meetings
Improper wiring on some medical equipment
Corridors sometimes obstructed with infant cribs, stretchers, and crash carts
Licensed practical nurses used as circulating nurses during deliveries rather than registered nurses
Refrigerators storing blood not monitored

However, it should be noted the ADH considered the number of deficiencies not unusual for a hospital of comparative size and found the hospital and its staff were dedicated to patient care and safety.

Having found the investigation conducted by the ADH unsatisfactory, Smith announced his candidacy on February 9, 1977, for county judge since the county judge appoints the members of the hospital's board of governors. The election was to be held in November 1978. Smith considered that he needed such an early announcement prior to the election because he felt that the hospital may not be open at the time of the election due to existing financial mismanagement; he also felt it was time to take the issues concerning the hospital to a political platform. In his announcement, Smith criticized the board of governors, the county judge, the medical staff, the hospital administration, and the nursing staff, implying that they collectively contributed to a "rotten political mess" involving petty, corrupt politics and that they had motives similar to crooks, thieves, cheats, and robbers. Smith further called for the resignation of the board.

After concluding that the investigation conducted by the ADH did not support Smith's claim of improper patient care, the medical staff unanimously recommended to the board of governors on February 22, 1977, that the board temporarily suspend Smith's staff privileges pending further investigation by the Arkansas Medical Society. The medical staff specifically disagreed with Smith that the staff physicians operated deceptively and wholly for self-interest. They also disagreed that the overall patient care was poor, or that the medical staff was substandard. Furthermore, because of Smith's request that a full investigation be made and the fact that the ADH's investigation did not support Smith's criticisms, the medical staff determined to make their recommendation to the board in response to Smith's claim on November 22, 1976, that if an investigation demonstrated that he was the problem, then he should not be allowed to remain on the staff.

In response to the medical staff's recommendation, Smith wrote a letter on February 25, 1977, to the hospital administrator, stating:

> *In view of the allegations made by the medical staff, I feel I have no choice but to cease hospital activity until these matters are settled. I have patients in the hospital at this time and will discharge them when they are ready to go and plan no further admissions with the possible exception of an OB patient or possibly two.*

Smith admitted no patients to the Hospital after this date and further refused to comply with rotating emergency room coverage assignments.

The hospital administrator responded to Smith's letter on March 14, 1977, by indicating that he understood Smith's letter was a letter of resignation and would forward it as such to the board of governors. Smith responded by letter on the same day that he had not resigned from the active medical staff. On March 17, the hospital administrator responded to Smith by letter on behalf of the board:

> *As the Board of Governors considers you to be an active member of the medical staff of Cleburne County Hospital, I have been instructed to remind you of the responsibilities a physician must accept to retain this privilege. Of course, this includes emergency room coverage.*

This letter was submitted to Smith after a board of governors' meeting was held on March 16, at which the board also voted to appoint a joint committee comprised of some members of the board and the medical staff to consider further the medical staff's recommendation concerning Smith. Accordingly, Smith responded to the hospital administrator on March 18, 1977, that, on advice of his attorneys, he would not be actively participating in hospital activities.

On March 24, 1977, the joint committee decided to formally request the Professional Relations Committee of the Arkansas Medical Society to investigate and, if possible, mediate the controversy between Smith and the hospital's board and medical staff. After investigation during the following months, the Arkansas Medical Society viewed the controversy as a personality conflict and elected not to participate in further investigation or mediation.

The executive committee of the medical staff officers met for normal business on July 5, 1977. In addition to other business items, the executive committee noted that Smith had missed more than four medical staff meetings and, as a result, according to bylaws had placed himself off the active medical staff and on the courtesy medical staff. As a courtesy medical staff member, Smith could not admit more than six patients per year and held no other staff privileges. No response from Smith was made to this change in medical staff status.

Because the hospital's fiscal year ended yearly at the end of September, each medical staff member was required to submit a yearly application for renewed medical staff privileges prior to the last board meeting of the current fiscal year. Correspondence from the hospital addressed to Smith indicated that he needed to complete the required forms regarding reappointment and return them by August 20, 1977. Smith gave no forms, letters, or notice to the hospital of his intent to obtain reappointment to the medical staff.

No further action was taken by the hospital or the board of governors until the hospital's joint executive committee on October 14, 1981, was ordered by the district court to conduct a hearing on whether Smith should be granted renewed medical staff privileges. This hearing was held to allow Smith to exhaust his administrative remedies before a trial on the merits could be heard. The joint committee concluded that Smith's continued criticisms were detrimental to the public purpose the hospital performs. In addition, they also found that the personality conflicts between Smith and the medical and nursing staffs would disrupt the efficiency of the hospital if Smith's staff privileges were restored. Accordingly, the joint committee unanimously recommended to the board that Smith be denied renewed medical staff privileges.

*Make a list of the major problems presented in this case*

- 
- 
- 
- 

*Hypothesis and mechanism*

For the problems in your list above, give a cause or a reason for it to happen:

- 
- 
- 
-

## Learning issues

Make a list of learning issues in the form of questions. Remember, your goal is to gather the medical, social, and all other relevant facts that may apply to the case.

What is meant by "standardization" to truth telling?
    Truth telling involves the provision of information not simply to enable patients to make informed choices about health care, but also to inform them about their situation.

What are the two types of deception?
    Actively deceiving by lying and using vague speech
    Passively deceiving by nondisclosure, by allowing another to deceive, or by failing to correct a misconception

What are the styles of truth telling?
    Telling what patients want to know
    Telling what patients need to know
    Translation of information into terms that patients can understand

What are the reasons for truth-telling styles?
    Respect for the truth, not necessarily the whole truth
    Patient's right to informed consent
    Doctor's duty to inform, which is one of the responsibilities of a doctor
    Individual contract in patient–doctor relationship

What are the "outcomes" of truth telling?
    Increased patient compliance/concordance
    Improved health outcomes
    Patient autonomy
    Patient's right to know
    Patient's right not to know

## Literature review

To help you get ready to answer certain questions you anticipate being asked during the second part of the case, look in the local medical library and on the World Wide Web for helpful information. Please indicate in the spaces below (1) several helpful articles or books you found and (2) several helpful Web sites you found.

- **Helpful articles/books:**
    Asai, A., Should physicians tell patients the truth? *West. J. Med.*, 163, 36–39, 1995.

Hebert, P.C. et al., Bioethics for clinicians: truth telling, *Can. Med. Assoc. J.*, 156, 225–228, 1997.

Jackson, L.A. et al., Deception and untruths: is lying ever justified? *Hosp. Pharm. Times.*, August 1991, pp. 5–7.

Jackson, R.A. et al., Comparative analysis of pharmacists' and physicians' attitudes toward the use of deception in resolving difficult ethical problems, *Am. J. Pharm. Educ.*, 56, 8–16, 1992.

Marzanski, M., Would you like to know what is wrong with you? On telling the truth to patients with dementia, *J. Med. Ethics*, 26, 108–113, 2000.

Miyaji, N. T., The power of compassion: truth-telling among American doctors in the care of dying patients, *Soc. Sci. Med.*, 36, 249–264, 1993.

Novack, D.H. et al., Physicians' attitudes toward using deception to resolve difficult ethical problems, *JAMA*, 261, 2980–2985, 1989.

Sheldon, M., Truth telling in medicine, *JAMA*, 247, 651–54, 1982.

Surbone, A., Truth telling to the patient, *JAMA*, 268, 1661–1662, 1992.

Surbone, A., Is truth telling to the patient a cultural artifact? *JAMA*, 268, 1734–1735, 1992.

Yaniv, G., Withholding information from cancer patients as a physician's decision under risk, *Med. Decis. Making*, 20, 216–225, 2000.

- **Helpful Web sites:**

American Pharmaceutical Association — Code of Ethics for Pharmacists: www.aphanet.org/pharmcare/ethics.html

Medscape from WebMD: www.medscape.com

*U.S. Pharmacist*: www.uspharmacist.com

*Canadian Medical Association Journal*: www.cma.ca/cmaj

## *Identify all relevant values that play a role in the case and determine which values, if any, conflict*

Nonmaleficence:

Beneficence:

Respect for persons:

Loyalty:



Distributive justice:


## Learning issues for next student-centered problem-based learning session

- List the options open to you. That is, answer the question, "What could you do?"
- Choose the best solution from an ethical point of view, justify it, and respond to possible criticisms. That is, answer the question, "What should you do, and why?"
- What are the different ways of thinking about the problem? Which conflict management techniques can be used in the situation?

## Part two

The district court found that Dr. Smith's medical staff privileges were constructively revoked in retaliation for his engaging in First Amendment protected speech on matters of public concern. We are unable to agree because Smith was not constructively denied medical staff privileges, but rather voluntarily chose to withdraw from participating in required hospital activities necessary to maintain his status on the active medical staff. Furthermore, while certain aspects of Smith's speech were constitutionally protected activity, not all of his activity was such, and thus the protected activity engaged in was not a substantial or motivating factor in the action taken against him.

### Constructive discharge

On February 22, 1977, the medical staff, in accordance with hospital bylaws, unanimously voted to recommend to the board of governors that Smith's staff privileges be temporarily suspended pending further investigation by the Arkansas Medical Society. The medical staff was prompted at this time to make such a recommendation for two reasons. First, the full investigation called by Smith was conducted by the ADH. The results of their investigation indicated that, indeed, there were problems, but they did not rise to the level of the problems Smith was suggesting. Second, Smith indicated to the board on November 22, 1976, that once a full investigation was made and if he was found to be the problem, then he should not be allowed to remain on the staff. The medical staff on February 22, 1977, believed that the ADH report vindicated the hospital against Smith's claims. As such, they felt Smith should be temporarily suspended pending a peer review of his conduct by the ethics committee of the state medical society.

The facts outlined in this opinion lead us to the conclusion that, once Smith received a reaffirmation from the hospital administrator that he was still a member of the active medical staff, he was obligated to fulfill the conditions of his staff privileges. Smith refused to comply with these requirements. In addition, as the facts indicated, Smith also failed to submit the required forms at the end of the hospital's fiscal year for reappointment to the medical staff.

Although Smith and the other medical staff doctors were not employees of the hospital receiving a salary, their conduct and their practice of medicine was within the parameters of the hospital's legitimate interest in promoting the efficiency of the public service it performs. A state-operated hospital has the right, and the duty, to regulate the conduct of its medical staff and maintain the quality of medical care delivered to its patients. The hospital afforded Smith every opportunity to comply with the necessary requirements to maintain his staff privileges. By his inaction in assuming these duties, Smith voluntarily withdrew from the hospital.

A constructive discharge would occur only if the hospital rendered Smith's working conditions intolerable enough to force him to quit. There is nothing in the record that would suggest that the hospital tried to create intolerable working conditions to force Smith to quit. In fact, it is abundantly clear that the hospital and its staff tried to accommodate Smith as much as possible, as demonstrated in their continued efforts to enable Smith to maintain his privileges. In addition, it is noteworthy that the Joint Executive Committee did not take official action against Smith until the court ordered a hearing in 1981. Under the facts of this case, we believe the restraint of the board of governors and the hospital is admirable.

We hold that a state hospital has the right to regulate the requirements of physicians to obtain and continue to maintain medical staff privileges as a legitimate interest in promoting the efficiency of the public service it performs. As such, the hospital had the right and the duty to extend medical staff privileges to any doctor fulfilling the necessary requirements for holding staff privileges according to the hospital bylaws. Once a doctor refuses to comply with these necessary requirements, then the doctor voluntarily withdraws from his association with the hospital. The fact that the hospital reaffirmed Smith's medical staff privileges to dispel any perception that Smith no longer held privileges clearly refutes Smith's claims that he suffered a constructive revocation of privileges.

## First Amendment analysis

Dr. Smith, as a member of the active medical staff of Cleburne County Hospital, was an independent contractor rather than a salaried employee of the hospital. However, the hospital, as a public institution, has the right to regulate its medical staff to ensure the delivery of adequate medical care to its patients. According to the hospital's bylaws, not only were there established guidelines in determining the competency of those making new applications to the medical staff, but there were also guidelines for existing staff members to follow to maintain their privileges. While there is not a direct salaried employment relationship, there is an association between the independent contractor doctor and the hospital that has similarities to that of an employer–employee relationship. For instance, there is an application process for privileges, there are required duties to be performed by both parties, and there are potential liabilities each party is responsible, jointly and severally, for tortious conduct. As a result of these similarities, it is appropriate to consider arguments from both sides of this case.

Smith initiated this action on April 26, 1977, alleging that the defendants terminated his medical staff privileges because he engaged in First Amendment protected speech. The inquiry into whether speech is constitutionally protected is a question of law. A court must first consider whether the speech addresses a matter of public concern to be protected constitutionally. This determination is made by a review of the content, form, and context of the speech.

It is clear that speech on public issues occupies the "highest rung of the hierarchy of First Amendment values and is entitled to special protection." However, when there is a conflict between speech on matters of a public concern and the legitimate interest of a public institution in promoting the efficiency of the public service it performs, a decision taking both matters into consideration needs to be made.

Smith's suit challenged that he was wrongfully terminated from the hospital's medical staff because he engaged in First Amendment speech. Courts reviewing challenges to discharges based on constitutionally protected speech apply a three-step analysis. The Court must determine whether (1) the plaintiff has carried the burden that he or she engaged in constitutionally protected activity; (2) by engaging in such activity, the plaintiff can show that it was a substantial or motivating factor in the action taken against him or her; and (3) the defendant can refute plaintiff's claim by demonstrating that the same action would have been taken in the absence of the protected activity.

Under the first step of analysis, for which Smith must show that he engaged in protected speech, the district court was persuaded that Smith's criticisms were shown to be substantially accurate, as demonstrated by the report submitted by the Arkansas Department of Health. Due to the nature of the complaints, the district court was correct in determining that some aspects of Smith's complaints were a matter of public concern, at least as they were initially made. However, it is clear in the record that Smith's criticisms, when viewed in their cumulative effect, evolved into statements of personal animosity against specific people and further evolved into a pattern of disrupting the public service the hospital performs. Smith went beyond the scope of protected speech when his criticisms became caustic personal attacks on almost every person connected with the hospital, ranging from the county judge (as *ex officio* board member) to staff personnel. These attacks were vindictive and personal and as such are not a matter of public concern.

For instance, Smith began writing letters to his patients and to the board of governors in late 1976 claiming that the hospital could not provide patients with a level of care he feels they should receive. From Smith's view, this was because the members of the board of governors were political flunkies who were arrogant and indifferent, failed to learn their duties, and held contempt toward concerned citizens. The purpose of these letters was not to criticize the hospital constructively, which is a constitutionally protected activity of a matter of public concern. Instead, the letters were disparaging personal attacks against various people, and the letters were written for the ultimate purpose of economically disrupting the hospital.

Under the second part of the three-step analysis, Smith must show that the hospital revoked his medical staff privileges for the substantial or motivating reason that he engaged in protected speech. The district court was persuaded that Smith's revocation of privileges was the direct retaliatory result that the controversy between Smith and the hospital did not remain "in house" and became a public issue. As a result of the controversy becoming public, the district court believed that Smith's public speech on the controversy was the motivating factor in the revocation of his privileges.

Smith's initial criticisms of the hospital, indeed, became a matter of public concern and were given press coverage from the local newspapers. However, when the medical staff unanimously voted to recommend that Smith's privileges be temporarily suspended pending a peer review, the hospital's prepared statement indicated that it was Smith's disruptive attacks on various individuals over a period of 3 to 4 years, even though some of these attacks were publicly made, that were one of the considerations in the medical staff's recommendation. The prepared statement even went on to state further the medical staff's other reason for recommending temporary suspension. For instance, it pointed to the financial impact on the hospital the controversy created; the low morale as a result of Smith's direct attacks on various nurses; the continued disagreement with Smith that the medical staff does not operate deceivingly and wholly for self-interest; the continued disagreement with Smith that the medical staff is substandard; and the lack of support of the nature of his criticisms by the Department of Health's investigation.

The fact that Smith's initial criticisms became a public issue alone is insufficient in Smith's burden to show a causal connection that his public speeches were a substantial or motivating factor for the hospital's alleged revocation of his privileges. That the criticisms became a public issue was not the reason the medical staff voted to recommend that Smith's privileges be temporarily suspended. Instead, it was because the medical staff viewed Smith's behavior over a period of 3 to 4 years as disruptive and argumentative.

The third step of analysis in reviewing challenges to discharges based on constitutionally protected speech is whether the defendants can refute Smith's claim by demonstrating that the same action would have been taken in the absence of the protected activity. Within this analysis, balancing is required between the interests of the person engaged in protected speech on matters of public concern and the interests of the public institution in promoting the efficiency of the public service it performs. Factors needed to be weighed include: (1) the need for harmony in the office or workplace (or hospital); (2) whether the public institution's responsibilities require a close working relationship between the plaintiff and coworkers when the speech engaged in has caused or could cause the relationship to deteriorate; (3) the time, manner, and place of the speech; (4) the context in which the dispute arose; (5) the degree of public interest in the speech; and (6) whether the person engaging in speech is impeded in ability to perform his or her duties.

By the time the medical staff unanimously voted to recommend Smith's temporary suspension, there was a long history of conflict between Smith and various hospital administrators, members of the board, nursing staff, and other personnel. Smith notified the hospital in July 1976 that he was going to resign from the medical staff because of his disenchantment with the quality of patient care. Unhappy with the hospital's response to his criticisms, Smith wrote a letter to his patients in November 1976 saying he was quitting the hospital in the near future. Because Smith had one of the largest patient loads in the hospital, the economic effect of Smith quitting the hospital would surely be felt.

But, Smith was not making mere criticisms of the hospital. He attacked several board members by letter, chastising them as political flunkies. The purpose of these personal attacks, in addition to Smith's letters to his patients, was a calculated effort to disrupt the efficiency of the hospital. Bringing economic coercion against the hospital as a public institution, even when some of Smith's initial criticisms were a matter of public concern, goes beyond the scope of constitutionally protected activity in view of the six factors enunciated above.

There is ample evidence to conclude that the medical staff found other numerous and sufficient reasons for voting to recommend that Smith's privileges be temporarily suspended. Smith was disruptive and a malcontent. He disassociated himself from the efficiency of the hospital because he considered his the only view with merit. Even after a full investigation was made, he rejected the findings of the ADH as insufficient and a cover-up.

We hold that when a person does initially engage in protected First Amendment speech on matters of public concern, they may not use this protection, in the guise of public concern, also to level personal attacks on various officials and employees of a public institution when the attacks cause disruption, disharmony, and dissention and create an adverse economic effect on the public service the institution performs. Because of the course of disruptive behavior, which included personal attacks on various people, by Smith over a period of 3 to 4 years, the medical staff had sufficient foundation to recommend to the board that Smith's privileges be temporarily suspended pending peer review.

*List the options open to you. That is, answer the question, "What could you do?"*

- 
- 
- 
- 

*Choose the best solution from an ethical point of view, justify it, and respond to possible criticisms. That is, answer the question, "What should you do, and why?"*

- 
- 
- 
- 

*Select one member of your PBL group to role-play as Dr. Smith and have another member of your PBL group role-play as a representative of the medical staff. How might the two converse about different ways of thinking and techniques for conflict management?*

- 
- 
- 
- 

*Again, please select one member of your PBL group to role-play as Dr. Smith and have another member of your PBL group role-play as a representative of the medical staff. How might the representative of the medical staff use what is known about stages of change and about motivational interviewing to solve what you consider the major problem presented in the case?*

- 
- 
- 
-

## Part three

The record in this case is voluminous and extensive. However, when the record is reviewed as a matter of law, the progeny of *Pickering* have refined the scope of what is considered protected speech as a matter of public concern and its effect on the public institution's ability to perform its public service. As a result of these refinements, to suggest to those persons engaged in protected speech that they hide behind its protection to also engage in nonprotected personal attacks is clearly beyond the special protection in the hierarchy of First Amendment values on speech of public concerns. We simply cannot allow this to happen in this case.

Dr. Smith did voice initially legitimate concerns. He also voiced personal attacks that, when read in the manner, place, and context in which they were made, are not on matters of public concern. Therefore, when the medical staff voted to make their recommendation to the board of governors, it was for substantial reasons other than to retaliate against Smith for engaging in protected speech.

Smith was not discharged nor did he have his privileges revoked, either in fact or constructively. It was Smith's failure to comply with the necessary requirements to maintain staff privileges that led to his voluntary withdrawal from the Cleburne County Hospital's medical staff. Moreover, even if the hospital constructively revoked Smith's privileges, there are other substantial reasons for the medical staff's recommendation that were not based on Smith engaging in First Amendment protected speech.

## Discussion

Physicians' decisions regarding deceptive behavior are based on their understanding of deception. Truth telling involves the provision of information not only to enable patients to make informed choice about health care, but also to inform them about their situation. Deception involves actively deceiving by lying and using vague speech. Another form of deception involves passively deceiving by nondisclosure by allowing another to deceive or by failing to correct a misconception. Using these very strict definitions, it should be easy for health care workers to solve ethical dilemmas. However, not all physicians see truth telling and deception as being clearly black and white.

In the 1992, edition of the *American Journal of Pharmaceutical Education* (Volume 56, pages 8 to 16) Jackson, Novack, and colleagues illustrate the various shades of gray regarding truth telling. Their research places physicians and pharmacists in certain situations and asks if they would tell the truth or deceive. After making a decision, they were further asked to state the reasons for their decision. The comparison between these two health care provider types showed that both professions did what they thought was best for the patients,  suggesting that, in at least some situations when confronted by conflicting moral values, the majority of respondents are willing to use deception. In evaluating the consequences of their decisions, they appear to place a higher value on their patients' welfare and keeping the patients' confidence than on truth telling for its own sake. These values stem from the Hippocratic oath that is taken by physicians and the code of ethics the pharmacists hold as truth. However, by complying with this value, a patient's autonomy suffers. In medical practice, truth telling can sometimes be based on the practitioner's moral values and beliefs. Over decades, health care providers have sometimes taken a paternalistic role and removed the autonomy from the patient. Different cultures have seen this as either impedance of their freedom or as a benefit.

The decision on what to tell the patient or the family, how much should be told, and in what manner is dependent on several factors. These factors include the patient's age, sex, occupation, character, and religion, among many others.

To respect the patient's right to autonomy, health care providers should respect the patient's right to know as well as the patient's right not to know. The question now becomes who should decide whether a patient wants to be told the whole truth or just enough to keep the patient satisfied. A solution to this problem is first recognizing that the diagnosis affects the life of the patient. Diagnostic information regarding one's body and life belongs to the person to whom it refers, not to family or physicians. Therefore, a patient's wish to know or not to know the truth is the most important factor in determining disclosure.

There is a sample questionnaire that can be modified to let physicians and pharmacists know how much information a patient wants to know. The questionnaire is given to patients during their first appointment, before the physician or pharmacist has seen them so suspicion about health status is not aroused. It follows here.

Would you want to know a diagnosis of an early and potentially curable cancer if it should develop?

Would you want to know a diagnosis of incurable cancer and its prognosis?

We will abide by your answers when we decide what and how much we should tell you. Is this acceptable to you?

Should we tell you a diagnosis of cancer even if your family insists that we not tell you?

Once you decide that a physician should tell a diagnosis of cancer to your family or whomever you choose, but not you, we will discuss your treatment with them and withhold all information from you. Is this acceptable to you?

## Conclusion

Truth telling will remain a moral–ethical issue. With such diverse cultures among and between health care providers and patients, there will remain instances of the using of discretion to disclose information. Disclosure of information will be on a patient-to-patient basis. Standards regarding when and how to implement disclosure will provide guidelines, but not in themselves be the mandate for truth telling.

## case seven

# Reproductive ethics

This problem-based learning session is based on the following: A *Woman's Choice — East Side Women's Clinic et al., Plaintiffs–Appellees, v. Scott C. Newman, Prosecuting Attorney for Marion County Indiana, on behalf of a class of prosecutors et al., Defendants–Appellants,* No. 01-2107 U.S. Court of Appeals for the Seventh Circuit 305 F.3d 684; 2002 U.S. App. Lexis 18840. February 19, 2002, Argued. September 16, 2002, Decided. It is reprinted here with permission of LexisNexis.

## Objectives

The objectives of this problem-based learning case are:

- To present the reproductive ethical dilemmas facing health care providers today
- To discuss behavioral options as they apply to individual interpretations of the oath and the code of ethics
- To discuss the legality of health care providers' actions, if applicable

## Introduction

There are various reproductive issues that the practicing health care providers (including the pharmacist) are confronted with in the course of everyday work. Reproductive ethics involve a variety of issues that challenge pharmacists and the oath they have taken. Reproductive ethical issues include, but are not limited to: abortion, birth control, sterilization, sexually transmitted diseases (STDs), reproductive research, and appropriate referrals. These issues will be compared and contrasted as they pertain to the practicing health care providers.

## Part one

In 1995, Indiana enacted a statute making the woman's informed consent a condition for an abortion. Even though the text of this law is materially identical to one held constitutional in *Planned Parenthood of Southeastern Pennsylvania v. Casey* [505 U.S. 833, 881–887, 120 L. Ed. 2d 674, 112 S. Ct. 2791 (1992)], a federal district court issued a preliminary injunction preventing the statute from taking effect [*A Woman's Choice — East Side Women's Clinic v. Newman* 904 F. Supp. 1434 (S. D. Ind. 1995)]. Two years later, the district court modified this injunction to permit the state to enforce most of the law, but it blocked enforcement of the requirement that information be provided "in the presence of the pregnant woman, [by] the physician who is to perform the abortion, the referring physician or a physician assistant." After four more years had passed, the judge held a trial and made permanent the injunction as modified in 1997.

By requiring information to be supplied "in the presence of the pregnant woman" — rather than by printed brochure, telephone, or Web site — the statute obliges the woman to make two trips to the clinic or hospital. This raises the cost (both financial and mental) of an abortion. On the basis of studies concerning similar laws in Mississippi and Utah, the district court concluded that the higher cost would reduce by 10 to 13% the number of abortions performed in Indiana. Some of these women will travel to states that do not require two trips; others will forego an abortion; some who do have an abortion in Indiana will delay that procedure until the second trimester. These consequences show that the law creates an "undue burden" on abortion, the district judge held. Although by the time the district judge entered the permanent injunction we had concluded that the Mississippi study does not warrant condemnation of Wisconsin's law [which like Pennsylvania's requires two trips to the medical facility and a 24-hour wait; see *Karlin v. Foust*, 188 F.3d 446, 484–488 (7th Cir. 1999)], the district judge wrote that data from the Utah study and a new analysis of the Mississippi data required a different result. The judge also thought that experience in Indiana showing that the demand for abortion did not decline when information was provided on paper or over the telephone implied that the reduction in the number of abortions is attributable to higher cost (a bad reason) rather than to the statutory information (a valid reason).

Indiana's statute reads as follows:

> An abortion shall not be performed except with the voluntary and informed consent of the pregnant woman upon whom the abortion is to be performed. Except in the case of a medical emergency, consent to an abortion is voluntary and informed only if the following conditions are met:
>
> (1) At least eighteen (18) hours before the abortion and in the presence of the pregnant woman, the physician who

*is to perform the abortion, the referring physician or a
physician assistant (as defined in IC 25-27.5-2-10), an
advanced practice nurse (as [\*4] defined in IC
25-23-1-1(b)), or a midwife (as defined in IC 34-18-2-19)
to whom the responsibility has been delegated by the
physician who is to perform the abortion or the referring
physician has orally informed the pregnant woman of the
following:*

*(A)  The name of the physician performing the abortion.*
*(B)  The nature of the proposed procedure or treatment.*
*(C)  The risks of and alternatives to the procedure or treat-
ment.*
*(D) The probable gestational age of the fetus, including
an offer to provide:*
  *(i)  a picture or drawing of a fetus;*
  *(ii)  the dimensions of a fetus; and*
  *(iii)  relevant information on the potential survival of
an unborn fetus; at this stage of development.*
*(E)  The medical risks associated with carrying the fetus
to term.*

*(2) At least eighteen (18) hours before the abortion, the preg-
nant woman will be orally informed of the following:*
*(A)  That medical assistance benefits may be available for
prenatal care, childbirth, and neonatal care from the
county office of family and children.*
*(B)  That the father of the unborn fetus is legally required
to assist in the support of the child. In the case of
rape, the information required under this clause may
be omitted.*
*(C)  That adoption alternatives are available and that
adoptive parents may legally pay the costs of prenatal
care, childbirth, and neonatal care.*

*(3) The pregnant woman certifies in writing, before the abor-
tion is performed, that the information required by sub-
divisions (1) and (2) has been provided.*

When the litigation began, plaintiffs challenged not only the requirement
that advice be delivered in person, but also the medical emergency exception,
which they deemed insufficient because it lacked details found in the Pennsylvania statute. The district court certified the medical emergency issue to
the Supreme Court of Indiana, which interpreted it [see *A Woman's Choice
— East Side Women's Clinic v. Newman*, 671 N.E.2d 104 (Ind. 1996)], to the
district judge's satisfaction. Plaintiffs then dropped this objection, leaving
only the advice requirement as a ground of contention.

Still, to say that a claim is justifiable does not mean that we must ignore
the fact that enforcement has not commenced. Plaintiffs rely on predictions

about what is likely to happen if Indiana's law were enforced as written. Because Indiana has been disabled from implementing its law and gathering information about actual effects, any uncertainty about the inferences based on the experience of other states and how that experience would carry over to Indiana must be resolved in Indiana's favor. This, coupled with doubts about the role of predictions in constitutional analysis, turns out to be important, for reasons explained presently.

*Casey* stated, and *Karlin* reiterated, that an informed consent statute may have effects that differ from the written terms, and that those effects could in principle demonstrate that an innocuous-appearing law actually imposes an undue burden on abortion. But, neither decision explained how such factual arguments are to be evaluated: whether before or after implementation and which standards to use.

Normally, a court asked to say that a statute will have forbidden effects asks only whether a proper outcome is possible; it does not hold a trial — and, if a district judge nonetheless takes evidence and makes findings, the appellate court will reexamine matters with a heavy presumption favoring the law's [*9] constitutional application [see, e.g., *Vance v. Bradley*, 440 U.S. 93, 111, 59 L. Ed. 2d 171, 99 S. Ct. 939 (1979); *National Paint and Coatings Association v. Chicago*, 45 F.3d 1124 (7th Cir. 1995)].

One may say in response that these cases deal with rational basis review, while abortion implicates fundamental rights. But, laws that regulate, not abortion itself, but ancillary issues (such as informed consent) do not affect fundamental rights unless the ancillary rule creates an undue burden on the underlying right. How does the court handle factual disputes that bear on whether an undue burden has been created? It cannot simply assume that a fundamental right has been burdened; that begs the question.

Findings based on new evidence could produce a new understanding, and thus a different legal outcome; the plurality implied this in *Casey*, as we did in *Karlin*. But, if the issue is one of legislative rather than adjudicative fact, it is unsound to say that, on records very similar in nature, Wisconsin's law could be valid (as we held in *Karlin*) and Indiana's law invalid just because different district judges reached different conclusions about the inferences to be drawn from the same body of statistical work. Because the Supreme Court has not made this point explicit, however, and because the undue burden approach does not prescribe a choice between the legislative fact and adjudicative fact approaches, we think it appropriate to review the evidence in this record and the inferences that properly may be drawn at the pre-enforcement stage.

By concluding that the empirical work had been carried out competently, the district judge established (for purposes of this litigation) that abortions dropped in Mississippi, compared to those in South Carolina, during the year after Mississippi enacted a statute requiring two visits. The authors of this study (and its replication in Utah) did not ask how Mississippi compares with Indiana. The study did not include a regression based on the sorts of variables, such as urbanization, income, average distance to an abortion clinic, average price of abortion, and so on, that might enable conclusions drawn from Mississippi to be extrapolated with confidence to other states. That is one reason why we held in *Karlin* that the Mississippi study was a poor basis for predicting what would happen in Wisconsin, which we thought more similar to Pennsylvania than to Mississippi (188 F.3d at 485–486).

That shortcoming could have been fixed in one of two ways. First, the authors could have conducted a more comprehensive study with additional variables and regression coefficients that would reveal their effects. That was not done. Second, the authors (or other scholars) could have gathered data from other states to test whether (and, if so, how) state-specific characteristics affect the results. That was not done either. What has happened in Pennsylvania, Wisconsin, and the other states that have informed consent laws that require two visits? Did Mississippi prove to be a better predictor of Wisconsin than *Karlin* anticipated, or was the outcome in Wisconsin dissimilar? This record is silent on these matters. Mississippi and Utah, two states with a history of hostility to abortion and very few abortion providers (implying long travel times), may be poor models for other states. Indianapolis has multiple abortion clinics; another in Fort Wayne serves the northeastern portion of the state; women in the northwest and southeast can use not only local providers, but also those just across the state lines in Chicago and Louisville. So, just as in *Karlin*, the application of the Mississippi data (and now Utah's data) to a different state would be a leap of faith. This is where the pre-enforcement nature of this suit matters.

Plaintiffs did try to deal with another problem identified in *Karlin*: the original Mississippi study did not try to separate the raw costs of a two-visit requirement from the effects of the information that was provided during the first visit (188 F.3d at 486–488). The Supreme Court's first two encounters with informed consent statutes treated these laws as meddling in the physician–patient relation with no valid purpose and no effect other than to heap pointless costs on women. See *Akron v. Akron Center for Reproductive Health, Inc.*, 462 U.S. 416, 442–449, 76 L. Ed. 2d 687, 103 S. Ct. 2481 (1983); *Thornburgh v. American College of Obstetricians and Gynecologists*, 476 U.S. 747, 759–765, 90 L. Ed. 2d 779, 106 S. Ct. 2169 (1986) in this regard. *Casey* overruled both of these decisions and held that states may try to persuade women not to abort their pregnancies.

Maybe all the Mississippi study reveals is successful persuasion, which we observed in *Karlin*. In this case, the plaintiffs tried to separate the effect of information from the effect of making two visits. Since 1997, Indiana has been able to enforce the portion of its informed consent statute requiring the provision of certain information to women who inquire about abortions. Yet, the number of abortions has not declined. This shows, the district judge wrote, that the law lacks persuasive effect; if a decline in abortions cannot be attributed to persuasion, then the cause must lie in some other and impermissible feature of the law.

Yet, this assumes what is to be proven: Indiana is like Mississippi and Utah, so the number of abortions would decline 10% or more if the law were enforced as written. Maybe what Indiana's experience since 1997 shows is that Indiana differs from Mississippi and Utah and will not experience a substantial decline with or without multiple visits. Or, maybe it shows that presenting the information in person is critical to its persuasive effect. Our education system rests on the premise that information delivered orally, with an opportunity for give-and-take, "takes" better than information delivered exclusively in writing. Otherwise, a university would simply mail a syllabus to the freshman class and ask the students to appear 4 years later for exams. So, the fact that advice delivered in writing or over the phone is uninfluential need not imply that advice delivered in person will be uninfluential. Again, the fact that Indiana has been blocked from enforcing its law as written means that the record does not contain evidence needed for accurate assessment of that statute's effects.

Then, there is an open question regarding what the 10% reduction reflects. Let us suppose that abortions would decline 10% in Indiana if that state's law were fully enforced. What would the decline signify? One possibility is that many women who strongly want an abortion have been blocked by the cost (in money and time) of multiple visits to the clinic or because the more times the woman must be absent, the greater is the likelihood that an abusive parent, spouse, or partner would discover what the woman has planned and intervene notwithstanding the availability of the emergency bypass, which the Supreme Court of Indiana held to encompass any kind of threat to the woman's health or safety. Another possibility is that about 10% of all women who have abortions are on the fence between ending the pregnancy and carrying the pregnancy to term, so that even a modest cost tips the scales. If the former, then a two-visit rule might be deemed an undue burden; if the latter, the two-visit rule would not be an undue burden because only a law that "has the purpose or effect of placing a substantial obstacle in the path of a woman seeking an abortion of a nonviable fetus" is an undue burden. This record does not permit (and the district judge did not make) an inference either way about the reason for the decline in Mississippi and Utah. Perhaps this shortcoming could be rectified by studying the effects of changes in out-of-pocket outlays or travel time as prices change, or clinics open, close, or move locations, but the studies in this record do not address the question.

Since 1992, when the plurality in *Casey* announced the undue burden standard, only two kinds of statute have flunked the test: a law forbidding the "intact dilation and extraction" method of abortion (the subject of *Stenberg*) and a law requiring a woman to notify her husband before obtaining an abortion (discussed in *Casey*). Because the language used to describe the dilation and extraction also could be understood to prohibit other procedures that were common (and perhaps essential) to late-term abortions, *Stenberg* concluded that the law would forbid abortions altogether for substantial numbers of women. The notification statute did not forbid abortions, but the Court feared that it would come to the same thing for those women whose husbands were likely to respond violently to the notice (if not to any contact from an estranged spouse). The plurality explained:

> *The spousal notification requirement is thus likely to prevent a significant number of women from obtaining an abortion. It does not merely make abortions a little more difficult or expensive to obtain; for many women, it will impose a substantial obstacle. We must not blind ourselves to the fact that the significant number of women who fear for their safety and the safety of their children are likely to be deterred from procuring an abortion as surely as if the Commonwealth had outlawed abortion in all cases.*

This is not to say that a two-visit requirement could not create a burden comparable to a spousal notice requirement. Quoting the district court, *Casey*'s plurality assumed that "for those women who have the fewest financial resources, those who must travel long distances, and those who have difficulty explaining their whereabouts to husbands, employers, or others, the 24-hour waiting period will be 'particularly burdensome.'" But, it held these considerations insufficient to condemn the Pennsylvania statute. All that the record in the current case shows is that these costs are positive and have some effect — something that the plurality in *Casey* assumed. Likewise, in *Mazurek* the Court assumed that a statute preventing nurses and other skilled medical personnel whose training falls short of the medical doctor degree from performing abortions would increase the expense (and thus, by the law of demand, reduce the number) of abortions; this again was held insufficient to show invalidity even on the assumption that one legislative purpose was to curtail abortion.

The record in this case does not show that a two-visit rule operates similar to a spousal notification rule by facilitating domestic violence or even inviting domestic intimidation. It shows nothing except a decline in the number of abortions in Mississippi and Utah — leaving open both the extent to which other states would experience the same effect and the reason why the effect occurs. This is not the sort of evidence that permits an inferior federal court to depart from the holding of *Casey* that an informed consent law is valid even when compliance entails two visits to the medical provider. If Indiana's emergency bypass procedure fails to protect Indiana's women from risks of physical or mental harm, it will be a failure in operation; it is not possible to predict failure before the whole statute goes into force.

Justice Souter reached a similar conclusion when denying a request to set aside a post-*Casey* decision enforcing Pennsylvania's statute [see *Planned Parenthood of Southeastern Pennsylvania v. Casey*, 510 U.S. 1309, 127 L. Ed. 2d 352, 114 S. Ct. 909 (1994) (in chambers)]. Like the Third Circuit, the decision of which [14 F.3d 848 (1994)] he declined to disturb, Justice Souter concluded that *Casey* itself had resolved the facial challenge to Pennsylvania's law. What remained was a challenge to the law in application, on a record showing how that law actually operated in Pennsylvania.

What is more, it would be incongruous to hold Indiana's informed consent law invalid on the basis of studies covering Mississippi and Utah that (to the district judge's eyes) imply the unconstitutionality of the Mississippi and Utah statutes, while the laws continued to be implemented in Mississippi and Utah. Relying on *Casey*, the Fifth Circuit has allowed Mississippi to enforce its statute [see *Barnes v. Moore*, 970 F.2d 12 (5th Cir. 1992)], and Utah's statute likewise has been sustained [see *Utah Women's Clinic, Inc., v. Leavitt*, 844 F. Supp. 1482, 1487, 1494 (D. Utah 1994), appeal dismissed in pertinent part for lack of jurisdiction, 75 F.3d 564 (10th Cir. 1995)].

No one has asked these courts to hold the Mississippi or Utah statute invalid on the basis of the local experience; if these laws remain enforceable despite the consequences demonstrated in this record, it is difficult to see why Indiana's law should be unenforceable even though it is unclear whether similar effects would occur there. Indiana is entitled to an opportunity to have its law evaluated in light of experience in Indiana. And, in the event the sort of effects that could make the burden undue — such as women deterred by the threat or actuality of violence at the hands of those tipped off by a preliminary visit — come to light in Indiana, then it will be informed consent laws nationwide that must be reevaluated.

## Make a list of the major problems presented in this case

- 
- 
- 
- 

## Hypothesis and mechanism

For the problems in your list above, give a cause or a reason for them to happen:

- 
- 
- 
- 

## Learning issues

Make a list of learning issues in the form of questions. Remember, your goal is to gather the medical, social, and all other relevant facts that may apply to the case.

Discuss the differences between abortion and sterilization.

The right to refuse the dispensing of controversial drugs is a pertinent issue confronting today's pharmacists. Individual beliefs about abortion, emergency contraception, and chemical sterilization of convicted sex offenders may influence whether a pharmacist will dispense a medication.

What medications are involved with this topic?
RU-486 (Mifeprex™) for the abortion of a fetus
Preven and high doses of various oral contraceptives as emergency contraception and for the prevention of implantation
Depo-Provera injections for chemical sterilization in males
The progression of reproductive research has lead us to various treatments for infertility. *In vitro* fertilization (IVF) and fertility treatments are controversial subjects with which pharmacists have direct contact. Personal beliefs about human reproduction and technology can influence whether a pharmacist will dispense medications involved in the fertility/IVF process. Medications involved include: Clomid and Profasi.

Discuss the issues (pro and con) for the "right to refuse."
Pro:
Employer supports individual right to refuse
Protecting the individual (the unborn child) by refusing to dispense
Protecting the autonomy and dignity of the patient (the sex offender)
Upholding ethical and moral standards
Con:
Employer-mandated dispensing of all drugs
Respect for the patient's autonomy and dignity in reproductive choices
Serving individual and societal needs
Relief of human suffering

Discuss the issues surrounding sterilization.
Informed consent of drug regimen including potential side effects is mandated by OBRA '90. Sterilization is a potential side effect that may inhibit patient concordance or willingness to begin a drug regimen. The issue of complete disclosure may challenge an individual pharmacist if there is concern that the patient may refuse treatment due to sterilization.
Medications involved include common chemotherapy agents such as:
Procarbazine
Cyclophosphamide
Clorambucil
Methotrexate

Discuss the issue of appropriate referrals by pharmacists.
A pharmacist may be challenged ethically by a patient's request for controversial information. The pharmacist may be faced with the decision whether to disclose all available information.

Example: Should a pharmacist try to influence a patient's decision by referring her to a particular facility, such as a religiously affiliated establishment?

Medications/issues involved:

Abortion

Mifepristone

Emergency contraception

Voluntary sterilization

Discuss the pros and cons surrounding the issue of complete disclosure.

Pro:

Respect the autonomy of each patient.

Act with honesty and integrity

Relief of human suffering

OBRA '90 mandated to maintain the highest principles of legal conduct.

Con:

Application of knowledge and skills to ensure optimal drug therapy outcomes

Relief of human suffering.

Service individual needs

What are the issues surrounding "sexually transmitted diseases" and "partner notification"?

The pharmacist may encounter the issue of partner notification when treating an individual for an STD. Partner notification is a public health strategy to prevent the spread of STDs. A pharmacist might be challenged by the issue of patient confidentiality when the patient chooses not to disclose the STD to a partner(s.)

Medications involved might include:

AIDS medications

Acyclovir

Various antibiotics

Partner notification

Pro:

Serves community and societal needs

Welfare of humanity

Promote the good of every patient

Con:

Respect for patient autonomy and dignity

Breach of patient confidentiality

Respect for the covenant between the patient and the pharmacist

## Literature review

To help you get ready to answer certain questions you anticipate being asked during the second part of the case, look in the local medical library and on the World Wide Web for helpful information. Please indicate in the spaces below (1) several helpful articles or books you found and (2) several helpful Web sites you found.

- **Helpful articles/books:**
  Bucci, K. and Stier, D. Infertility in women: an update, *J. Am. Pharm. Assoc.*, 38, 480–486, 1998.

  Code of ethics for pharmacists. Available at: http://www.utex-as.edu/dept/#Pharmacy

  Coffee, A.L., Current issues in infertility, *ASHP Midyear Clin. Meet.*, 1–112, 2000.

  Faxelid, E. and Ramstedt, K., Partner notification in context: Swedish and Zambian experiences, *Soc. Sci. Med.*, 44, 1239–1242, 1997.

  Flanagin, A., Human rights in the biomedical literature: the social responsibility of medical journals, *JAMA*, 284, 618–619, 2000.

  Haddad, A., Fortresses and formularies: response 1, *Am. J. Health Syst. Pharm.*, 57, 856–857, 2000.

  Lachowsky, M., The patient–doctor relationship, *Eur. J. Obst./Gynecol. Reprod. Biol.*, 85, 81–83, 1999.

  Mappes, T. and DeGrazia, D., *Biomedical Ethics*, McGraw-Hill, New York, 1996.

  Massai, M.R., Focus on Fertility, *Calif. J. Health-Syst. Pharm.*, 6–9, 1999.

  McGuffey, E., Contraceptive options for the 1990's, *J. Am. Pharm. Assoc.*, 37, 149–153, 1997.

  Seubert, D., Thompson, I., and Gonik, B., Partner notification of sexually transmitted disease in an obstetric and gynecologic setting, *Obstet. Gynecol*, 94, 399–401, 1999.

  Snyder, K., Ethical hot spots, *Drug Topics*, 141, 41–62, 1997.

- **Helpful Web sites:**
  www.plannedparenthood.org
  www.rxlist.com
  www.ashp.org
  www.worldmedicus.com

## *Identify all relevant values that play a role in the case and determine which values, if any, conflict*

Nonmaleficence:

Beneficence:


Respect for persons:


Loyalty:


Distributive justice:


## Learning issues for next student-centered problem-based learning session

- List the options open to you. That is, answer the question, "What could you do?"
- Choose the best solution from an ethical point of view, justify it, and respond to possible criticisms. That is, answer the question, "What should you do, and why?"
- What are the different ways of thinking about the problem? Which conflict management techniques can be used in the situation?


## Part two

This case again requires me to review the constitutionality of informed consent legislation in the context of the abortion industry. Seventeen years ago, I stated that a 24-hour waiting period enacted by the Illinois General Assembly was a reasonable and lawful means of ensuring that a woman has "at least a brief time to discuss and consider" the numerous moral, social, economic, practical, psychological, and medical factors "involved in reaching a mature, well-informed decision of whether or not to abort the pregnancy." Similarly, I concluded 3 years later in another case from Illinois that the state is empowered to promote childbirth and discourage abortion on demand by requiring abortionists to advise women about the reasonable alternatives to abortion, just as the state may require physicians to notify their patients about the risks and alternatives to many other invasive medical procedures. Accordingly, for more than a decade, there has been authority for the view that a state legislature may require abortion clinics to provide expectant mothers "with a description of the procedure to be performed, an explanation of risks and possible complications, and a discussion of alternatives so that the woman can make a responsible enlightened choice" prior to terminating the life of her pre-born child.

In today's opinion, the majority of this panel embraces the dissenting opinions in *Zbaraz* and *Ragsdale*, rejects the abortion clinics' facial challenge, and allows the state of Indiana to enforce its informed consent statute. Although the dissent criticizes the majority for reversing the district court and "finding flaws with the evidence on which the court based its factual findings" — findings that Judge Wood believes "should stand" regardless of "whether this court is looking at the record *de novo*, under an abuse of discretion standard, or merely for clear error" — I take issue with my colleague's criticism for the undue burden standard applicable in this case may be uniformly applied only if appellate courts independently inquire whether the trial judge's findings of constitutional fact are firmly supported in the record and based on a proper application of the law.

Judge Easterbrook succinctly and forcefully explains that the trial judge's conclusion in this case involves a "leap of faith" that events that may or may not be occurring in Mississippi and Utah will be replicated in Indiana. I add that the trial judge's factual findings in this case are based on a faulty study by biased researchers who operated in a vacuum of speculation. As even the dissent recognizes, the "key" piece of evidence relied on by the district court was a study published in the August 27, 1997, *Journal of the American Medical Association* (*JAMA*) and was coauthored by a statistician employed by the Planned Parenthood-affiliated Alan Guttmacher Institute.

It is most obvious that the study fails to shed any light on the question before us today: will Indiana's abortion statute cause a decline in abortion rates in Indiana? The answer is "no," for the study is riddled with flaws and biases, one of the most serious being its failure to account for the effects that will result from the substantive differences between the scope of the medical emergency exception in the state of Mississippi's statute as contrasted with the state of Indiana's statute. Thus, it is logically impossible to draw on the study of Mississippi's legislation when predicting the future effects of Indiana's legislation.

I initially reject the notion that we must defer to the *JAMA* study because, according to the dissenting judge, the study "meets any conceivable standard for peer-review" and was published in "one of the most highly respected journals in the medical field." A party proffering expert testimony must always establish that it is reliable and relevant to an understanding of the issue before the court [*Clark v. Takata Corp.*, (7th Cir. 1999)], and *JAMA's* peer review policy is no guarantee of reliability. Moreover, the test for admissibility is not whether an article has been reviewed, or even well accepted, by one's peers. According to the Supreme Court:

> *Publication (which is but one element of peer review) is not
> a sine qua non of admissibility; it does not necessarily cor-
> relate with reliability, and in some instances well-grounded
> but innovative theories will not have been published. Some
> propositions, moreover, are too particular, too new, or of too
> limited interest to be published. . . . The fact of publication
> (or lack thereof) in a peer reviewed journal thus will be a
> relevant, but not dispositive, consideration in assessing the
> scientific validity of a particular technique or methodology
> in which an opinion is premised. [Daubert v. Merrell Dow
> Pharmaceuticals, Inc., 509 U.S. 579, 593–594, 125 L. Ed.
> 2d 469, 113 S. Ct. 2786 (1993)]*

Caution regarding the value of "peer review" as a judicial gatekeeper is particularly important in the case of an abortion-related study published in *JAMA*. George D. Lundberg, the editor at the time of publication of the 1997 study relied on by the plaintiffs in this case, has publicly stated that abortion is "a religious issue" that should be decided solely by the woman "after consultation with the father (if possible), members of her family, perhaps a religious adviser, and the woman's physician" (Lundberg, G.D., *JAMA*, abortion and editorial responsibility, *JAMA*, 280, 740, 1998).

Lundberg went on to assert that the abortion decision is "not the business of police, lawyers, courts, the U.S. Department of Health and Human Services, the Congress of the United States, various state legislatures, or anybody else except the individuals named above." The executive vice president of the American Medical Association, an organization that at one time was considered to be the voice of the majority of physicians and surgeons practicing in this nation, stated that Lundberg was terminated for "inappropriately and inexcusably interjecting *JAMA* into a major political debate that has nothing to do with science or medicine" by choosing to publish a study on how college students defined "having sex" in the midst of President Clinton's impeachment proceedings. Relying on these facts, it is apparent that this *JAMA* study must be viewed with a jaundiced eye for it was written by a statistician and published by an editor who are outspoken supporters of "abortion on demand" and thus cannot reasonably be classified as impartial and without prejudice or bias.

Moreover, the faulty *JAMA* article cannot be utilized to serve as a reliable, trustworthy, and independent basis for predicting the effects of the Indiana legislation for the additional reason that neither the article nor anything else in this record accounted for the fact that more Indiana women with medical problems (compared to similarly situated women in Mississippi) will avoid the burdens of Indiana's notice-and-waiting provisions by qualifying for the state's medical emergency exception. The trial judge concluded that the number of Indiana women who will find themselves unable to obtain abortions as a result of the notice-and-waiting provisions will be equivalent to the number of women in Mississippi who supposedly are foreclosed from having an abortion — approximately 10% of the relevant population.

However, as is evident from even a cursory reading of the statute, the exceptions to the notice-and-waiting requirements are far broader in scope and more inclusive in Indiana than they are in Mississippi. As a result, even after attempting to accept the trial judge's notion that properly performed regression analyses have accounted for all other differences between the female population in Indiana and in Mississippi, the breadth of the Indiana exception will obviously result in more Indiana women being excused from the statute's requirements, and thus fewer Indiana women will be burdened by Indiana's requirements than those burdened by the requirements in Mississippi.

The Supreme Court of Indiana in its decision broadly defines the term *medical emergency* as any physical or mental condition that is more severe and prolonged than those "lesser and regular conditions normally associated with pregnancy" [*A Woman's Choice v. Newman*, 671 N.E.2d 104, 109 (Ind. 1996)], while the Mississippi legislature has narrowly defined medical emergency as "that condition which, on the basis of the physician's best clinical judgment, so complicates a pregnancy as to necessitate an immediate abortion to avert the death of the mother or for which a twenty-four-hour delay will create grave peril of immediate and irreversible loss of major bodily function" [Miss. Code Ann. § 41-41-31(b)]. In Indiana, an abortion clinic may disregard the notice-and-waiting requirements if "the attending physician, in the exercise of her clinical judgment in light of all factors relevant to a woman's life or health, concludes in good faith that medical complications in her patient's pregnancy indicate the necessity of treatment by therapeutic abortion" without delay. On the other hand, in Mississippi at the time of the 1997 *JAMA* study, an abortion clinic was allowed to waive the notice-and-waiting requirement only in "medical emergencies to avoid the death of the woman or prevent peril of immediate or irreversible loss of major bodily functions" [*Pro-Choice Mississippi v. Fordice*, 716 So. 2d 645, 656 (Miss. 1998)].

As we pointed out above, because the statutory exception is much more expansive in Indiana than in Mississippi, more Indiana women will be exempt from the limitation of their statute than similarly situated women in Mississippi; thus, I cannot agree that evidence of a 10% reduction in Mississippi's abortion rate predicts that a similar reduction is on the horizon in Indiana.

I cannot understand the dissent's attempt to enlarge the scope of Indiana's medical emergency exception by claiming that "the majority acknowledges [that] Indiana's law has been construed to have an emergency bypass provision that covers any kind of physical or psychological risk to the woman from any of its provisions, including presumably the 'presence' requirement." In doing this, the dissent has mischaracterized the majority opinion as well as the Indiana Supreme Court's construction of the statute before us. We in the majority, when stating that Indiana's emergency bypass has been "held to encompass any kind of threat to the woman's health or safety" are referring to the Indiana Supreme Court's statement that the "medical

emergency exception excuses a woman from the informed consent requirement when there is a significant threat to her life or health, physical and
mental," but that "severe-but-temporary conditions in which an abortion is
not the medically necessary treatment are not covered by the exception"
(Newman, 671 N.E.2d at 111). "Federal courts must interpret a state statute
as that state's courts would construe it" [*Brownsburg Area Patrons Affecting
Change v. Baldwin*, 137 F.3d 503, 507 (7th Cir. 1998)]. In light of *Newman's*
interpretation of the emergency bypass provision, I disagree with the dissent's misinterpretation of the legislature's intent in which it asserts that the
bypass shall apply in situations when the alleged emergency determination
is triggered by simple compliance with the 18-hour notice-and-waiting provisions, which will in turn expose the woman to either: (1) a temporarily
greater risk of harm from an abusive parent, spouse, or partner; or (2) a
temporary period of emotional distress, mental anguish, or trauma.

Furthermore, even if I were to ignore the decision of the Indiana Supreme
Court and the many methodological flaws within the *JAMA* study, it is
evident that the very language of the study disproves the theory that the
effects of Indiana's abortion law will be the same as Mississippi's for the
study's authors admit on the final page of their study that the burdensome
effects of abortion legislation "may be greater in states that have relatively
fewer abortion providers" (Mississippi) than in other states (Indiana).
According to the authors:

> The availability of abortion providers is also important to
> consider. The effect of mandatory delay statutes necessitat-
> ing 2 visits to a provider may be greater in states that have
> relatively few abortion providers. In Mississippi, there were
> only 8 abortion providers in the entire state in 1992 or 1.3
> providers per 100,000 women aged 15 to 44 years. . . . The
> large decline in abortion rates we observed in Mississippi
> may not occur in states with greater availability of abortion
> providers both within the state and among neighboring
> states.

The undisputed evidence in this record establishes that: (1) Indiana has
11 more abortion clinics than Mississippi; (2) Indiana women have much
easier access to clinics in nearby states than Mississippi women; and (3)
Indiana women, on average, live closer to abortion clinics than Mississippi
women. More than 99% of Indiana women — but only 85% of Mississippi
women — live within 100 miles of an abortion clinic. Thus, even if we were
to accept the *JAMA* study at face value, we would be forced to accept the
fact that Indiana's law will be far less burdensome than Mississippi's.

Providing neither support nor an analysis for his ruling, the district judge
found that "the Mississippi results did not correlate at all with distance or
geography" and then somehow concluded that the effects of Indiana's statute
"are likely to be equivalent to the effects of the similar law in Mississippi."

The trial judge's finding is beyond the realm of reasonable speculation and may best be classified as unworthy of credence. Comparing Indiana to Mississippi is like comparing a turnip to a loaf of bread. As the majority observes, neither the Mississippi study nor any other evidence cited by the plaintiffs establishes that the population and demographics of Mississippi and Indiana are similar in terms of "urbanization, income, average distance from an abortion clinic, [or the] average price of abortion." There is also evidence of similarity between Mississippi and Indiana in terms of their availability of social support services, attitudes toward abortion, respective success with adoption and abortion alternative programs, or countless other factors that might allow us to equate the two states with any degree of confidence.

The dissent spends several pages arguing the proposition that "only by ignoring key points such as the number of women" in Mississippi "who willingly undertook the burden of seeking an abortion out-of-state, where they could have the entire procedure accomplished in one visit, rather than staying in-state and enduring the two-visit burden, can the majority come to the result it does." The dissenting judge ignores the key fact that nothing in this record answers the critical question of why some Mississippi women left the state to abort their pregnancy. A woman might very well think twice about her momentous decision if she believed that her identity were to become known within her local community.

On the other hand, we are cognizant of the fact that even a small increase in the cost might dissuade an already vacillating woman living near the poverty level. Since nothing in this record distinguishes "between those incidental effects [e.g., slightly increased cost or time delay] of the statute which make the right to choose more inconvenient or costly and those direct effects which actually prevent women from obtaining an abortion" [*Eubanks v. Schmidt*, 126 F. Supp. 2d 451, 457 (W. D. Ky. 2000)], it is impossible to know whether "the waiting period, as opposed to some other factor or factors, caused the negative abortion trend in Mississippi" [*Karlin v. Foust*, 188 F.3d 446, 488 (7th Cir. 1999)]. It also is impossible to come to a well-reasoned and logical conclusion based on the record before us whether the laws of the state of Indiana will have a similar impact as Mississippi's laws.

For the reasons set forth above, it is apparent that the district court's reliance on Mississippi data to predict the effects of materially different legislation in Indiana (notice and waiting) piles a mountain of speculation on a foundation of quicksand. I am convinced that the district judge erred when he relied on the biased *JAMA* study when searching for a way to enjoin Indiana's abortion control statute [see *General Electric Co. v. Joiner*, 522 U.S. 136, 144–145, 139 L. Ed. 2d 508, 118 S. Ct. 512 (1997), expert studies based on data that were "so dissimilar to the facts presented in this litigation" were irrelevant and inadmissible; *Daubert*, 509 U.S. at 591–592, expert studies that fail to establish "a valid scientific connection to the pertinent inquiry" before the court are irrelevant and inadmissible].

Even if the plaintiffs had somehow been able to produce reliable evidence in support of the trial judge's belief that Indiana's abortion rates will decline 10 to 13% as a result of the state's informed consent laws, Indiana's statute would still pass constitutional scrutiny for a law enacted that seeks to promote a legitimate state interest will be deemed valid unless "in a large fraction of the cases in which the law is relevant, it will operate as a substantial obstacle to a woman's choice to undergo abortion" [*Casey*, 505 U.S. at 895]. Accordingly, I write separately to explain my disagreement with the dissent's contention that "we would still be required to enjoin" Indiana's statute even if it blocked a much smaller percentage of Indiana women — "'only' 1%" of the population — from exercising their "right to choose."

In determining whether Indiana's notice-and-waiting provisions are lawful, we must inquire whether women in Indiana seeking abortions, who are unable to qualify for any of the numerous exceptions to the law, will bear added costs and inconveniences from complying with the notice-and-waiting provision that are so burdensome that they will have the direct effect of preventing a "large fraction" of those women from obtaining abortions. I am of the opinion that the dissenting judge misinterprets *Casey* when she argues that "*Casey* made it clear" that "we would still be required to enjoin [Indiana's statute] if it affected 'only' 1%, the number presumptively affected by the spousal notification rule in Pennsylvania." The *Casey* Court stated that it was enjoining Pennsylvania's spousal notification law because a large fraction or a "significant number" of a subgroup of the 1% of women who feared complying with the law were "likely to be deterred from procuring an abortion" — not because the law imposed some insubstantial burdens on 1% of women in the state.

According to the Court:

> *The analysis does not end with the one percent of women upon whom the statute operates; it begins there. Legislation is measured for consistency with the Constitution by its impact on those whose conduct it affects. . . . The proper focus of constitutional inquiry is the group for whom the law is a restriction, not the group for whom the law is irrelevant. . . . Of course, as we have said [the Pennsylvania statute's] real target . . . is married women seeking abortions who do not wish to notify their husbands of their intentions and who do not qualify for one of the statutory exceptions to the notice requirement. The unfortunate yet persisting conditions we document above will mean that in a large fraction of the cases in which [the statute] is relevant, it will operate as a substantial obstacle to a woman's choice to undergo an abortion. It is an undue burden, and therefore invalid.*

In other words, *Casey* held that Pennsylvania's law was invalid not because it imposed additional burdens on 1% of the state's women, but rather because it effectively prevented a large fraction of women within that group of 1% of women from obtaining abortions altogether.

The *Casey* plurality did not explain, and thus we refuse to peer into the dark abyss of speculation in an attempt to determine at precisely what point a fractional part of a group becomes an impermissibly large fraction and a statute becomes unduly burdensome. "To the extent I can discern any meaningful content in the 'undue burden' standard as applied in the joint opinion, it appears to be that a State may not regulate abortion in such a way as to reduce significantly its incidence." However, even assuming in the case before us that some number of women will be burdened by the law, it is clear that a law that incidentally prevents "some" women from obtaining abortions passes constitutional muster. Indeed, *Casey* upheld a parental notification law despite the district judge's undisputed finding that, in some of the 46% of cases for which a minor can neither obtain the requisite consent of a parent nor avail herself of the judicial bypass provisions, the law "may act in such a way as to deprive [the minor] of her right to have an abortion." Though the requirement was likely to prevent some minors from exercising their right to choose, the Court refused to interfere and ruled that "the one-parent consent requirement and judicial bypass procedure are constitutional."

The dissenting judge pushes the envelope and expounds a new theory of law without the citation of case law upholding the premise that a statute is unconstitutional if it prevents even 1% of the relevant population from obtaining an abortion and stretches the notion of substantive due process beyond reasonable limits. Were we to accept the dissent's argument, we believe the Supreme Court would have found Pennsylvania's parental consent statute to be unduly burdensome. But, the Court chose not to strike down the Pennsylvania statute, and I believe it defies logic to argue that 1% of any group is a large fraction of that group. In light of the justices' repeated use of words such as "a significant number of women" and "many women," the court's estimate that millions of women would be burdened by a spousal notice law, and the most informative comments of Justice Stevens and Justice Scalia that restrictions are impermissible only if they are "severe" and lead to "significant" reductions in abortion rates, I am of the opinion that the challenged legislation before us is constitutional, even though, as the majority observes, the district court concluded that "the statute . . . raises the cost (both financial and mental) of an abortion" and "will reduce by 10% to 13% the number of abortions performed in Indiana."

My belief is further supported by *Casey*'s forceful statements distinguishing between the constitutionality of mandatory informed consent laws (which are lawful) and mandatory spousal notification laws (which are not). Although under *Casey* states may not enact spousal notification laws embodying views that are "repugnant to our present understanding of marriage and of the nature of the rights secured by the Constitution" (*Casey*, 505 U.S.

at 898), "it does not at all follow that the State is prohibited from taking steps to ensure that [the choice to end a pregnancy] is thoughtful and informed." It is incumbent on the federal judiciary to respect basic principles of federalism and give considerable deference to a state legislature's carefully reasoned decision to "enact rules and regulations designed to encourage [the woman] to know that there are philosophic and social arguments of great weight that can be brought to bear in favor of continuing the pregnancy to full term and that there are procedures and institutions to allow adoption of unwanted children as well as a certain degree of state assistance if the mother chooses to raise the child herself."

This record reflects that the Indiana General Assembly held a full panoply of hearings, engaged in extended floor debates, and considered numerous amendments offered by legislators prior to enacting the informed consent law before us today. Absent a clear constitutional violation, neither a federal district court nor an appellate court should ever take it on itself to strike down legislation merely because it disagrees with the legislation enacted by democratically elected state representatives. Informed consent laws having notice-and-waiting periods like Indiana's should thus be upheld for the Supreme Court has held that the "idea that important decisions will be more informed and deliberate if they follow some period of reflection does not strike us as unreasonable, particularly where the statute directs that important information become part of the background of the decision" concerning the life or death of the child [*Casey*, 505 U.S. at 885].

The Indiana General Assembly enacted its notice-and-waiting statute in an effort to alleviate a widespread problem. Witnesses at legislative hearings reported that literally hundreds of Indiana women were suffering serious regret and long-term physical, emotional, and psychological damage as a result of their choice to terminate their pregnancies without being properly informed about the risks, complications, and alternatives to the procedure [*A Woman's Choice v. Newman*, 904 F. Supp. 1434, 1449 (S. D. Ind. 1995)]. The intent of the legislature, according to the Supreme Court of Indiana, was to reduce the risk of abortion by "ensuring that women receive the best information available" regarding the moral, social, psychological, and medical issues relevant to deciding whether to undergo the procedure.

Included in the information that must be provided to the patient is: (1) the name of the abortionist, (2) the nature of the proposed procedure, (3) the risks and alternatives to the procedure, (4) the probable gestational age of the fetus, (4) the existence of medical assistance benefits and abortion alternatives, and (5) the father's legal responsibility to assist in the support of the child if the child is carried to term. I am convinced that the Indiana General Assembly has made a reasonable and lawful decision when enacting this informed consent bill in an effort to ensure that the woman's choice regarding the life or death of her child has been both knowingly and voluntarily made after extended debate and careful reflection.

This legislation will assist women in understanding that abortion is an invasive procedure that may very well have painful psychological, physical, and moral consequences. The woman undergoing the abortion may very well experience serious psychological disorders and mental health problems in the form of depressive psychosis (including the risk of suicide) before, during, and for many years following her decision — perhaps even for a lifetime. Added to this mental strain and anguish are the almost endless number of physical risks involved, including: trauma, permanent damage to reproductive and other vital organs, dysfunction of the cardiovascular or respiratory system, internal bleeding or hemorrhaging, embolism, and allergic reactions. Other medical factors to be considered in making a mature, informed decision include: the type of abortion to be performed; the woman's past medical and psychological history, her physical reaction to previous medical procedures, and her tolerance for certain medications; the likelihood of contracting a uterine infection; the chance that the placenta and fetus will not be completely removed; the potential for future difficulties in bearing children; and even the possibility of sexual sterility.

The Indiana statute requires that the name of the abortionist be made known to the patient, thus giving her an opportunity to review the credentials, qualifications, and experience of the physician, inquiring into whether the physician is a board-certified gynecologist, is accurate in the pregnancy term diagnosis, and is familiar with both the procedure and the myriad complications that may very well arise during the procedure. In making this decision, she is entitled to know whether the abortion procedure is being performed by "a well-trained, qualified surgeon or simply a second-rate surgeon who entered the abortion practice because he was denied hospital staff privileges by a medical peer review committee after questionable medical procedures or inferior surgical technique." Such information is essential to making a responsible decision.

The woman also will receive information regarding economic issues, such as the father's obligation to contribute to the support of the child, the availability of medical benefits and child care, and the right and possibility of giving up the baby to a loving adoptive family. After receiving such information, it also is probable that the best interests of the client would be better served were she to be granted a reasonable period of time to reflect on the information recently made known to her dealing with the possible social and psychological problems arising from the decision. It is hoped that the medical professionals who meet with the woman will be well trained so they might prepare the patient to confront and resolve the possible feelings of anger, fear, depression, and confusion she may encounter toward herself or the father, the onset of guilt and overall withdrawal from society, and the all-too-frequent threat of taking one's life.

It also is reasonable for a state legislature to have believed that the most efficient way to safeguard the health, safety, and well-being of the pregnant woman would be to allow her to receive the above-stated information during a face-to-face meeting with medical professionals. It was most unfortunate and inappropriate for the court to accept the proposition that voluntary consent for an abortion may be insured by a patient dialing an 800 (toll-free) phone number, touching certain digits on her keypad, and then passively taking information through the telephone. Only a direct, face-to-face meeting will serve to allow the patient and the doctor a full and complete understanding of the possible problems that might arise during or after the invasive procedure. This — and only this — type of meeting is the way to determine whether the client is giving an informed consent or is conveying a wish to postpone the procedure. Personal contact is vital to any question of informed consent for it allows the medical expert the best opportunity to observe the verbal and nonverbal behavior of the patient by focusing on reactions and responses to questions, facial expressions, attitude, tone of voice, eye contact, posture and body movements, confused or nervous speech patterns, and countless other factors that are indiscernible by telephone, but may reveal incongruities between what the patient says and what is actually felt or believed.

As a result, a face-to-face consultation occurring a reasonable time before the abortion "may disclose what a telephone interview will mask: whether a woman is apprehensive, uncertain, or equivocal about whether to have an abortion; whether she needs or wishes some additional information; or whether she wishes, but may find it difficult, to ask some additional question or explore some other alternative."

In the Indiana House of Representatives, the chief sponsor of this bill stated during extensive debates that it is important for women to receive this information either in the presence of the abortionist or a well-schooled and well-trained physician's assistant, licensed practical nurse, or midwife because the patient might very well "want to talk personally to the person who may be performing" the procedure and would benefit from personal, face-to-face consultation instead of meeting the professional for the first time "on the operating table" when it is unclear whether "this is the doctor or the person you're supposed to be talking to."

Indeed, the need for an in-the-presence requirement was underscored by testimony at the preliminary injunction hearing, at which a woman who had just recently undergone the procedure at an Indiana abortion clinic testified she never saw her doctor until he began the procedure, never saw his face (for it was covered with a surgical mask), and never learned his name because he never spoke with her. The woman testified as follows: "[A female assisting nurse] said, 'This is your doctor,' and I said, 'Does my doctor have a name?' And he giggled and she smiled, but I don't know who he was. And he did the procedure. He never talked to me. He talked to her. They talked about something, I can't even remember, and it was over. And he left."

Some of the materials that the General Assembly directed the abortionist to provide to the woman so she might be properly informed before making one of the most important decisions of her entire life and to minimize as best as possible the potential for future physical or psychological injuries, cannot be conveyed accurately or easily through other media, as the district judge's injunction requires. The General Assembly was of the opinion that it is essential for the woman to be well informed, among other things, of the "probable gestational age of the fetus" and also be given the option of seeing a picture or drawing of the fetus and its dimensions. It is nearly impossible to provide a picture or drawing of a pre-born child over the telephone unless both the patient and the abortion clinic are equipped with expensive, highly advanced video-conferencing equipment. Furthermore, any attempt to provide an illustration through the mail without having first met with the patient for a physical examination may potentially be misleading and inaccurate. The district judge's refusal to enforce Indiana's requirement of face-to-face meetings between the health care provider and the pregnant woman emasculates the statute and undermines the very intent of the legislature.

In my opinion, it was an abuse of discretion for the district judge to disregard controlling legal authority, cast aside the opinions of qualified medical experts and the judgment of the people of Indiana as represented by the elected members of the Indiana General Assembly, and declare that the in-the-presence requirement is not "reasonably likely to provide any genuine benefit" to Indiana women. Not many judges are versed in the nuances of the practices and techniques of the medical profession. Thus, the judiciary is "ill-equipped to substitute [its] views regarding what is medically adequate, proper, or antiseptic" for those of the legislature, which acts with the full benefit of evidence received through hearings, debates, and meetings with the people of the state.

The trial judge's questionably reasoned *ipse dixit*, pronounced without the support of even one citation to the record, invades the legitimate province of the legislative and executive branches and places a straitjacket on their power to regulate and control abortion practice. As a result, literally thousands of Indiana women have undergone abortions since 1995 without having had the benefit of receiving the necessary information to ensure that their momentous choice is premised on the wealth of information available to make a well-informed and educated life-or-death decision. I remain convinced that the trial judge abused his discretion when depriving the sovereign State of Indiana of its lawful right to enforce the statute before us. I can only hope that the number of women in Indiana who may have been harmed by the judge's decision is small.

In Indiana, according to the preamble to its abortion control statute, "child birth is preferred, encouraged, and accepted over abortion" (Ind. Code § 16-34-1-1). Furthermore, "in America, we respect the sanctity of human life" [*Walsh v. Mellas*, 837 F.2d 789, 798 (7th Cir. 1988)]. Pro-life legislation that fails to pose a substantial obstacle for 87 to 90% of a state's women and may have the incidental effect of reducing the demand for abortions by merely 10 to 13%, is reasonable, sensible, and lawful under the Constitution of the United States and the State of Indiana. Because this is the thrust of Judge Easterbrook's reasoning, I am pleased to join his opinion.

*List the options open to you. That is, answer the question, "What could you do?"*

- 
- 
- 
- 

*Choose the best solution from an ethical point of view, justify it, and respond to possible criticisms. That is, answer the question, "What should you do, and why?"*

- 
- 
- 
- 

*Select one member of your PBL group to role-play as a physician who performs abortions and have another member of your PBL group role-play as a representative of the State of Indiana. How might the two converse about different ways of thinking and techniques for conflict management?*

- 
- 
- 
- 

*Again, please select one member of your PBL group to role-play as the physician and have another member of your PBL group role-play as a representative of the State of Indiana. How might the physician use what is known about stages of change and about motivational interviewing to solve what you consider the major problem presented in the case?*

- 
- 
- 
-

# Part three

## Dissent: Diane P. Wood, Circuit Judge, dissenting

In today's opinion, the majority disregards the standards that were established by the Supreme Court in *Planned Parenthood of Southeastern Pennsylvania v. Casey* [505 U.S. 833, 120 L. Ed. 2d 674, 112 S. Ct. 2791 (1992)] for evaluating laws that impose burdens on a woman's right to seek an abortion, and it brushes aside the painstakingly careful findings of fact the district court made in support of the limited preliminary injunction it issued against Indiana's so-called informed consent law (Ind. Code § 16-34-2-1.1). The careful reader of the majority's opinion will see that the majority regrets the fact that the Supreme Court held in *Stenberg v. Carhart* [530 U.S. 914, 147 L. Ed. 2d 743, 120 S. Ct. 2597 (2000)] that pre-enforcement challenges of abortion statutes, like the one presently before us, are permissible. Nevertheless, *Stenberg* is the law of the land, and we must follow its direction, including its endorsement of the constitutional standards governing abortion legislation first articulated by the *Casey* plurality. That direction is by no means the opaque mess the majority accuses the Supreme Court of creating. In my view, the Court has not left us with "irreconcilable directives" nor has it put courts of appeals "in a pickle." At the most, if we were reviewing legislation in some field unrelated to abortion (or speech), we might be faced with the problems the majority describes. As for abortion regulation, the Court's guidance is crystal clear. In the end, the majority concedes that *Stenberg* governs, which ought to be enough for present purposes to lead to an affirmance of the district court's grant of the injunction.

When one follows the analytical path outlined in *Casey*, it becomes clear that the district court did not abuse its discretion when it concluded that one narrow requirement of Indiana's law had to be enjoined. In support of that conclusion, the court found that, in the particular circumstances faced by Indiana women and on the basis of the expanded factual record that the Supreme Court invited in *Casey*, the law's requirement that women receive certain advice in the presence of "the physician who is to perform the abortion, the referring physician or a physician assistant" [§ 16-34-2-1.1(1)] amounts to an unconstitutional undue burden on the abortion decision. I would affirm the district court's decision.

Before turning to the areas of disagreement that lie between the majority and me, it is important to point out that we also share some areas of agreement. First, it is clear that Indiana's requirement to furnish the statutory information in the presence of the pregnant woman (instead of, for example, mailing written materials, having a telephone conversation, or visiting a local doctor who is neither the referring physician nor the physician who will perform the procedure) is one that raises the cost of obtaining an abortion. This is because the "presence" rule normally necessitates two trips to the abortion facility.

Second, the majority notes, and I agree, that there are both unconstitutional ways in which costs may be raised and constitutional ones: an increased cost is unconstitutional if it is has the purpose or effect of forcing some women to give up their constitutional right to choose abortion; it is constitutional if it genuinely furthers the state's legitimate interest in persuading women not to select abortion when faced with an unwanted pregnancy.

Third, I agree with the majority that the standard of review for constitutional or legislative facts is more searching than the one we use for historical facts. That does not mean, however, that we may disregard the district court's findings of historical fact. To the contrary, the Supreme Court has emphasized that we owe deference to such findings even in constitutional cases. Were we to abandon that rule, many constitutional matters would receive far less restrained review than we presently give them: from possible violations of the Fourth Amendment, to the voluntariness of confessions, to the First Amendment protection accorded to public employee speech.

Turning now to the way in which we should resolve this appeal, it is useful to begin with some reminders about what *Casey* held. (For ease of exposition, I refer to *Casey* alone rather than to "the *Casey* standard as endorsed in *Stenberg*" since the latter formulation, while more accurate, is needlessly cumbersome.) First, *Casey* dictates how to draw the line between permissible state regulation and unconstitutional regulation:

> *Numerous forms of state regulation might have the incidental effect of increasing the cost or decreasing the availability of medical care, whether for abortion or any other medical procedure. The fact that a law which serves a valid purpose, one not designed to strike at the right itself, has the incidental effect of making it more difficult or more expensive to procure an abortion cannot be enough to invalidate it. Only where state regulation imposes an undue burden on a woman's ability to make this decision does the power of the State reach into the heart of the liberty protected by the Due Process Clause.*

The opinion later elaborates on the undue burden standard:

> *A finding of an undue burden is a shorthand for the conclusion that a state regulation has the purpose or effect of placing a substantial obstacle in the path of a woman seeking an abortion of a nonviable fetus. A statute with this purpose is invalid because the means chosen by the State to further the interest in potential life must be calculated to inform the woman's free choice, not hinder it. And a statute which, while furthering the interest in potential life or some other*

> *valid state interest, has the effect of placing a substantial obstacle in the path of a woman's choice cannot be considered a permissible means of serving its legitimate ends.*

Applying this standard, the Court struck down the Pennsylvania statute's spousal consent requirement and the record-keeping requirement relating to spousal notice; it upheld the statute's parental consent requirement (which contained the necessary one-parent and judicial bypass provisions), the medical emergency provisions, the rest of the record-keeping requirements, and the informed consent requirement. Knowing both what failed the new test and what passed it gives litigants a road map of the kind of claims that are likely to succeed, and the kind of evidence they must present. It also gives us concrete guidance on the critical questions now before us:

1. Under the *Casey* test, must the statute create an undue burden for every single woman, or is it enough that it creates an undue burden for some women?
2. To what extent are we dealing with empirical, fact-specific issues and to what extent with "legislative" issues?
3. How must the statute allow for flexible compliance with the state's broader goals?

The first question — how many women must be affected — is really another way of putting the question about facial challenges that the majority addresses. In this connection, despite its disclaimers, one is left with the strong impression that the majority is applying either *United States v. Salerno* [481 U.S. 739, 95 L. Ed. 2d 697, 107 S. Ct. 2095 (1987)] or something very close to it. In essence, it holds that a state statute like the one before us now would be unconstitutional only if there was "no set of circumstances" under which it was valid — by which it seems to mean that not a single woman in Indiana would find the law's burdens tolerable. This is an impermissible back-door application of *Salerno*. Worse yet, it assumes the answer to the question before us: will the system Indiana wants to put in place unduly burden Indiana women? Since the pertinent part of the statute has never gone into force, the majority indulges in the presumption that the law imposes no burden at all. But, this presumption is found nowhere in our jurisprudence, at least for laws implicating fundamental constitutional rights. Furthermore, this methodology is inconsistent with *Casey.*

Part V-C of *Casey* addressed the spousal notification requirement of the Pennsylvania law, also under circumstances in which enforcement had not yet begun. The district court had found, and the Supreme Court accepted, that "the vast majority of women consult their husbands prior to deciding to terminate their pregnancy" (505 U.S. at 888). We can assume, therefore, that the spousal notification requirement was not an undue burden, or any kind of burden, for that vast majority of women; they are already doing what the statute specified. But, the Court went on to consider the plight of women who were not already consulting the putative father: the 2 million women a year who are the victims of severe assaults by their male partners. As for those women — "the victims of regular physical and psychological abuse at the hands of their husbands" — matters were different. The Court found, based on "the limited research that has been conducted with respect to notifying one's husband about an abortion, although involving samples too small to be representative" that the spousal notification requirement was "likely to prevent a significant number of women from obtaining an abortion." Later, to underscore the point, it reiterated that "the analysis does not end with the one percent of women upon whom the statute operates; it begins there."

That takes us to the second critical question: is the reduction in abortions performed the result of the law's persuasive force or the consequence of the impermissible placement of obstacles in the path of a woman's right to choose? One may assume, for the sake of argument, that fewer women in Indiana will forego an abortion than did women in Mississippi, according to the studies in the record. One may further assume that a larger percentage of women in Indiana who forego an abortion will do so because they were persuaded by the law's informational requirements, contrary to their sisters in Mississippi. This is no matter: under *Casey*, our focus must be on those women who, like those affected by the spousal notification requirement in Pennsylvania, will forego the abortion because of the burden and not because of persuasion.

I cannot imagine a more resounding repudiation of the *Salerno* approach than the *Casey* opinion gave. The majority opinion in *Stenberg* makes it clear that this was no accident or oversight. We must therefore look at the effect of the in-the-presence requirements on the Indiana women on whom the statute operates: the approximately 10% (as the record suggests and as the district court found) who will no longer be able to obtain abortions under the new regime. (Note that the 10% number could be off by an order of magnitude, and we would still be required to enjoin this part of the law if it affected "only" 1%, the number presumptively affected by the spousal notification rule in Pennsylvania.)

But, the majority responds, the Supreme Court in *Casey* upheld something almost exactly like the Indiana in-the-presence requirement when it found that Pennsylvania's informed consent rules passed muster. Informed consent at the most general level, of course, was not the issue either in our case or in *Casey*; under the injunction the district court entered, every Indiana woman is furnished with the information the state deems helpful, and when she shows up for the abortion procedure, the doctor can again be assured that the patient's consent is informed. Our concern is with the specific way in which the state wants the information to be transmitted.

The majority suggests that *Casey* has already answered this question insofar as it addressed a regulatory regime with a similar two-visit rule. But, a look at the *Casey* opinion shows that the Court was not writing so broadly; to the contrary, the Court took great pains not to rule on informed consent/

two-visit rules either in general as a matter of fact or as a matter of law. Instead, it explicitly limited its holding to the record before it. It stated that there was "no evidence on this record that requiring a doctor to give the information as provided by the statute would amount in practical terms to a substantial obstacle to a woman seeking an abortion." There is no reason to treat the phrases "on this record" and "in practical terms" as casual insertions. The Court thought that the waiting period question was a close one, particularly because it would often translate into a two-visit requirement. The Pennsylvania district court had not made the necessary findings of fact to show that a two-visit requirement would amount to an undue burden [largely because that court had applied the old trimester test from *Roe v. Wade*, 410 U.S. 113, 35 L. Ed. 2d 147, 93 S. Ct. 705 (1973) and had invalidated the rule for other, less factually sensitive, reasons]. If there could be any doubt remaining on the question whether the Court was restricting its ruling to the record before it, the following passage from *Casey* should set it to rest:

> *And the District Court did not conclude that the waiting period is such an obstacle even for the women who are most burdened by it. Hence, on the record before us, and in the context of this facial challenge, we are not convinced that the 24-hour waiting period constitutes an undue burden.*

*Casey*, therefore, establishes the following guidelines for the present case:

1. We must evaluate the Indiana law based on those on whom it is operating, which is to say the set of women who will be burdened by the in-the-presence requirement.
2. If there were no evidence before the court tending to show that this requirement, like the spousal notification rule considered in *Casey*, is "likely to prevent a significant number of women from obtaining an abortion" (505 U.S. at 893), then we would be required to uphold Indiana's rule on this facial challenge.
3. Since there is evidence that is at least as reliable — if not much more so — than the evidence on which the *Casey* opinion relied in evaluating the spousal notification rules, we must look at what that evidence shows, deferring to the district court's findings of historical fact, just as the Supreme Court did in *Casey*.

I now turn to the evidence before the district court.

Initially, it is necessary briefly to consider what we mean by the term "fact" and how a fact may be established. The majority has tried to explain how and why it is reversing the district court, even while it accepts such critical findings of fact as: (1) abortions dropped in Mississippi after enactment of a two-visit rule, as compared to those in South Carolina, which did not have a two-visit rule; and (2) the number of abortions performed in

Indiana has not declined because of the advice given to women pursuant to the statute. Even though these facts support the district court's finding, the majority argues that the ultimate finding of an undue burden cannot be sustained, largely because the Supreme Court did not find such a burden in *Casey* for a similar rule, nor did this court in *Karlin v. Foust* [188 F.3d 446 (7th Cir. 1999)], the decision on which the majority places most of its reliance. With respect, I believe this approach confuses two fundamentally different inquiries: the first concerns the way in which a certain fact must be established; the second asks whether this fact will logically vary from case to case, or if once properly established, it is "legislative" in nature such that it cannot be questioned over and over again.

*Casey*, as the preceding discussion makes clear, was focused on the first of those questions. The Court there decided that the existence of an undue burden had not been established on the record then before it. It left the door open, however, for later parties to present more evidence that would cure the gaps in the record that existed. This point can be illustrated by an analogy to new drug approval. Suppose a pharmaceutical company approaches the Food and Drug Administration (FDA) with an application for approval of a new drug, Alpha. Naturally, it submits supporting information to the agency. If, however, the FDA deems that information insufficient, it will reject the application.

This does not mean that the company cannot reapply later, after it conducts more clinical studies or otherwise cures the deficiencies in the earlier record. Based on a fully supported application, the FDA will decide whether Alpha should be approved as safe and effective for the designated uses. Our situation is exactly the same. We now have in this case the "reapplication" for a finding whether a rule that requires two visits to the clinic (here, Indiana's "presence" requirement) constitutes an undue burden. Are there, in other words, women for whom this rule has the "effect of placing a substantial obstacle in the path of . . . seeking an abortion of a nonviable fetus"?

To answer that question, we must evaluate the evidence presented in this particular case. Before doing so, however, it is also useful to note where the concept of "legislative facts" — on which the majority relies — legitimately applies in this case and where it does not. Skipping over the crucial question about the way in which facts must be established, the majority treats this case as one in which the factual record is identical to the record in *Karlin* and then assumes that, if there was nothing unconstitutional about a two-visit rule in *Karlin*, there can be nothing unconstitutional here. Burdens are burdens, no matter what state a court is considering. Furthermore, reasons the majority, that is how the Supreme Court treated efforts to regulate the late-term abortion procedure at issue in *Stenberg*, and thus it must be the way to treat all facts relating to the abortion issue.

With all due respect, the majority has failed to take into account significant differences in the record that was compiled in this case, as compared with the record before the *Karlin* court, and it has made assumptions about interstate differences that are unsupported in this record (and, I suspect, unsupportable).

What is important here is to recognize that this evidence is highly pertinent to the case. A central reason why the majority treats this as a "failure-of-proof" case, to the extent it does, is that it assumes that studies done in Mississippi, Utah, or North Carolina have nothing to do with Indiana. This assumption is mysterious. What we are considering, after all, is a simple matter of human reactions to sets of incentives or disincentives: will a particular measure be seen as a disincentive at all; if so, will the obstacle be a mere inconvenience, or will it effectively ban a particular option? In the field of economics, we assume that people will react in similar and predictable ways to incentives. (And, sometimes it takes more than one study to ascertain what the incentive effects of a particular measure are, even if, once understood, those effects are presumed to be universal.)

Consistent with that well-accepted proposition, there is every reason here to assume that Indiana women will react to proven incentives and disincentives in the same way women from other states (e.g., Mississippi) have been shown to respond. The law of demand is based on generalized assumptions about human behavior and rationality, and there is no reason to waste time trying to prove that people in one area are exceptions to these rules.

The Supreme Court relied on the same idea in *Stenberg*: faced with high uncertainty about which procedures were legal and which were not, coupled with draconian penalties for an incorrect guess, it was safe to assume that all doctors, everywhere, would err on the side of caution and refuse altogether to perform certain kinds of late-term abortions. Maybe the Court should have carved out an exception for doctors in places famous for attracting gamblers, like Las Vegas or Atlantic City, but for obvious reasons, it did not.

The majority acknowledges that, under the law of demand, higher prices for abortion will decrease the number demanded, but (as it also appears to recognize) that is not the difficult question here. It is instead whether the observed increase in price caused by the in-the-presence or two-visit rule is a permissible one under the undue burden analysis. That is precisely the issue that the Court identified in *Casey* as an empirical point, for which a different result was possible on a more complete record. It is unclear at best to me why the two judges in the majority on this panel think that they know better than the district court judge, who heard all the testimony and weighed all the evidence, what the answer is to the question whether a critical number of Indiana women would experience the in-the-presence rule as such a significant burden that it would effectively prevent them from exercising their constitutionally protected choice. Instead of respecting the district court's extensive work, the majority finds flaws with the evidence on which the court based its factual findings. It thinks, for instance, that the evidence in the record should have taken into account factors like degree of urbanization, average distance to abortion clinics, and income levels.

But, this simply leads to the majority's second misunderstanding about the legal significance of the differences between Mississippi and Indiana that these factors might reveal. At best, studies incorporating these variables at a greater level of detail will indicate that there are some women in Indiana for whom the in-the-presence rule is not a problem, just as there were many women in Pennsylvania who did not anticipate any problem with spousal notification.

Surely, the majority does not think that every woman in Indiana lives close to a clinic; like all states, Indiana has significant rural areas and significant numbers of people living far from a reproductive health services facility. (There are 11 abortion clinics in Indiana [see Indiana Family Institute, Fact sheet: abortion in Indiana, at http://www.hoosierfamily.org/FactSheet13.html], which covers a territory of some 36,000 square miles [see U.S. Census Bureau, State and county quickfacts, at http://quickfacts.census.gov/qfd/states/18000.html]. That adds up to 1 abortion clinic on the average for almost every 3,300 square miles. And, needless to say, it is quite unlikely that these clinics are distributed with perfect geographical regularity; to the extent the clinics are concentrated around major cities like Indianapolis, that means that other women in rural Indiana will live substantial distances away from the nearest facility.) At most, the details the majority demands might suggest that more Indiana women can withstand the burdens of the Indiana statute than their counterparts in Mississippi could.

But, the question is not, for example, whether Indiana women as a group live closer to abortion clinics. It is whether an Indiana woman living 60 miles away from a clinic in Indiana who cannot afford (either financially, socially, or psychologically) to make two visits will respond the same way a Mississippi woman living 60 miles away from a clinic in Mississippi with similar constraints did. To repeat, *Casey* made it clear that the set of women we must consider are those who are burdened by the law, and it found 1% enough to justify striking down the spousal notification rule. Maybe 10% of the women in Mississippi have that problem, and only 3% of women in Indiana do. No matter. The district court was quite reasonable to find that women in Indiana are like all other people, and that their responses will be the same as those of women elsewhere.

Or, it could be that the majority thinks that women in Indiana are more likely to be persuaded by the in-the-presence requirement than are women in Mississippi, so that the decrease in abortions due to the requirement could be attributed to the constitutionally permissible persuasive force of the law. Again, however, all the previous criticisms apply: the question is not whether more women in Indiana are persuaded than are women in Mississippi (bearing in mind that there was no evidence before the district court indicating why that should be the case). It is instead whether a sufficient number of Indiana women (something akin to the 1% delineated in *Casey*) are not so persuaded and yet are among those who will be forced to forego their right to choose.

The majority rejects wholesale the relevance of the Mississippi studies (and several other studies) by implying that the district court clearly erred in its decision that Indiana women would react to burdensome two-visit requirements in the same way, and for the same reasons, as Mississippi women did. But, even in this context, it offers no reason at all to believe that Indiana women are so idiosyncratic, and in my view it could not. The Supreme Court has consistently endorsed the use of studies from other states or areas — shared experience is exactly how the "laboratories" in the several states ought to work. In this regard, see, for instance, *Renton v. Playtime Theatres, Inc.*, 475 U.S. 41, 51–52, 89 L. Ed. 2d 29, 106 S. Ct. 925 (1986) (in the First Amendment context, no requirement that "a city, before enacting such an ordinance, conduct new studies or produce evidence independent of that already generated by other cities, so long as whatever evidence the city relies upon is reasonably believed to be relevant to the problem that the city addresses").

Turning now to the evidence demonstrating that the Indiana in-the-presence rule indeed constitutes an undue burden, we find detailed and meticulous findings from the district court to support that proposition. This evidence was entirely competent to support the district court's decision; *Casey's* discussion of the spousal notification rule makes it clear that evidence on undue burden does not have to meet some heightened standard of perfection. To the contrary, the Court there relied on "limited research that has been conducted with respect to [the issue at hand, their notifying one's husband about an abortion], although involving samples too small to be representative" (505 U.S. at 892) to support its conclusion about spousal notification.

We have more than zero, and less than perfection, when it comes to information about the burden the Indiana statute places on the women affected by the two-visit rule. The majority, in effect, has not only demanded perfection, but also wants a showing that some number of Indiana women significantly larger than the number the Court accepted in *Casey* are unduly burdened by the law. Every time the plaintiffs come back with more studies and more information (as they have surely done here, in comparison with the record they created in *Karlin*), the majority raises the bar higher and tells them to come back another day — even though this court has specifically held that "the biases of one study in one case may be avoided or reversed in the next" [*Mister v. Illinois Cent. Gulf R.R. Co.*, 832 F.2d 1427, 1437, n. 3 (7th Cir. 1987) (Easterbrook, J.)].

In this case, we have evidence, and importantly, we have significant new evidence that has been developed since *Karlin* that answers precisely the kinds of questions that *Karlin* directed future plaintiffs to address. The district court relied on this evidence to conclude that the in-the-presence part of the Indiana law would indeed impose an undue burden on enough Indiana women seeking abortions that this part of the statute had to be enjoined. The Supreme Court has consistently endorsed the use of the type of evidence that was presented here and has analyzed it in the "factual context of each case in light of all the evidence presented by both the plaintiff and the defendant" [*Bazemore v. Friday,* 478 U.S. 385, 400, 92 L. Ed. 2d 315, 106 S. Ct. 3000 (1986)].

Key among this evidence before the court was a new (post-*Karlin*) study published in the *JAMA,* one of the most highly respected journals in the medical field and one that meets any conceivable standard for peer review. The *JAMA* study is a time series and regression analysis designed to assess the effect of the Mississippi law on the abortion and birth rates of Mississippi residents in two ways: first through a retrospective analysis of those rates before and after the passage of the statute and second through a comparison between Mississippi and two similar states, Georgia and South Carolina, neither of which had an in-the-presence requirement in effect at the relevant time, but were otherwise similar in the relevant respects. Regression analyses are an important tool in much of social science research, as well as in law.

To this extent, see *McCleskey v. Kemp* [481 U.S. 279, 293–294, 95 L. Ed. 2d 262, 107 S. Ct. 1756 (1987)], which discusses their role in Title VII of the Civil Rights Act of 1964 cases and in sentencing context. See also *Bazemore v. Friday* (478 U.S. at 398–401) concerning additional regression analyses conducted in response to criticisms and suggestions by the district court, all of which confirmed, and some of which even strengthened, the study's original conclusions, further concluding that multiple-regression analysis need not include every conceivable variable to establish a party's case and chiding the court of appeals because it "failed utterly to examine the regression analyses in light of all the evidence in the record." See *Arlington Heights v. Metropolitan Housing Development Corporation* [429 U.S. 252, 266 n. 13, 50 L. Ed. 2d 450, 97 S. Ct. 555 (1977)], which discusses jury selection context.

The difficulty here is that there is no single independent variable that will show undue burden. The only way to prove that a particular part of a law is imposing an undue burden on abortion choice is to hypothesize that it might constitute an undue burden and then show that no other reasonably related variable (i.e., the phenomenon that is being tested) satisfactorily explains the drop in abortion rates — essentially a process of elimination. This is a methodology we have approved before [see *In re Oil Spill by Amoco Cadiz,* 954 F.2d 1279 (7th Cir. 1992) (*per curiam*)].

In that case, this court endorsed the use of simple linear regressions as a way to draw out all other plausible explanations, leaving only the hypothesized one as a reason for which part of a loss in business was attributable to a massive oil spill. We expressed satisfaction there with this way of getting "a better grip on the relation between dependent and independent variables" and reaching "an inference of causation, and of the size of the effect."

Indeed, the latest pronouncement by the Supreme Court in First Amendment matters endorses a study by the city of Los Angeles aimed at demonstrating the connection between its ban on multiple-use adult establishments and its interest in reducing crime — a connection that can only be shown by ruling out some (but clearly not all) of the other potential independent variables that could have contributed to the effect on crime [see *City of Los*

*Angeles v. Alameda Books, Inc.*, supra, U.S., 122 S. Ct. 1728 (plurality opinion)]. Dealing with the nature of such studies, the plurality concluded that a party "does not bear the burden of providing evidence that rules out every [other] theory." The study, however imperfect, was respected for its probative value precisely because of the lack of evidence presented by the other side to rebut its finding. As in this case, once the point was made, the opponent had to produce concrete evidence on the other side; it was not enough merely to point out an alleged imperfection in the study.

That is exactly what the *JAMA* study did. It was tailored to explore the question (unanswered in the record in *Karlin*) whether the decrease in abortions in Mississippi was an effect not of the persuasive power of the law, but rather of its burdensome qualities. And, it showed that the latter explanation was the correct one. The principal outcome measures in the study were birth rates, abortion rates, the percentage of late abortions, and the percentage of abortions performed outside the state. The researchers found that the resident abortion rates declined 12% more in Mississippi than they did in South Carolina after the passage of the law, and they declined 14% more in Mississippi than they did in Georgia. Limited to Caucasian adults, abortions declined 22% more in Mississippi than in South Carolina and 20% more in Mississippi than in Georgia.

Abortions performed after the 12-week gestation mark increased 39% more in Mississippi than in either South Carolina or Georgia. The percentage of abortions performed out of state increased 42% more among women in Mississippi relative to women in South Carolina.

The *JAMA* study also showed that, in the 12-month period after the law took effect, the total rate of abortions for Mississippi residents decreased by approximately 16%; the proportion of Mississippi residents traveling to other states for an abortion increased by about 37%; and the number of second trimester abortions increased by some 40%. The study concluded that these statistics "suggest that Mississippi's mandatory delay statute was responsible for a decline in abortion rates and an increase in abortions performed later in pregnancy." The researchers who conducted the study testified before the district court that the only salient difference among Mississippi, Georgia, and South Carolina for these purposes was that only Mississippi had a two-trip requirement. Otherwise, the laws regulating abortions in the three states were functionally the same, and no other statistically significant events had taken place in the various states.

The district court realized that it needed to address one final, but critical, question of fact: were declines observed in abortions in Mississippi because women in Mississippi had been persuaded to forego abortions, or were the declines because the new law was impermissibly burdening the right to seek an abortion — precisely the inquiry mandated by *Karlin*? The court found that the latter explanation was the correct one, for several reasons, all amply based on the evidence in the record. First, the "persuasive power" hypothesis was severely undercut by the evidence showing that Mississippi women were leaving the state to have their abortions elsewhere and having more second trimester abortions. Those women quite evidently had not been persuaded to carry their pregnancy to term; they aborted their pregnancies, but they did it outside the state of Mississippi or at a later and riskier time. (Certainly, we must assume that the Mississippi legislature was trying to persuade women to forego abortion rather than to persuade them to travel out of state for the procedure or to postpone it to a riskier time.) Second, the court looked at evidence from Indiana that showed no changes in abortion rates from the information standing alone (a part of the statute that the court permitted to take effect, stripped only of the in-the-presence requirement). The court discussed other evidence as well, and I commend its thorough analysis, particularly its evaluation of similar studies conducted in Utah and Louisiana.

In the end, its conclusion was that the "sum of this evidence, and the absence of evidence of any persuasive effect, shows convincingly that the predicted reduction in abortion rates would result not from persuasion but from restrictions posing a substantial obstacle for some women's ability to obtain abortions." As mentioned, even if the relative numbers of women who were persuaded versus burdened are different in Mississippi and Indiana, the study conclusively reveals that a significant number of Indiana women will be unduly burdened by the in-the-presence requirement. And, those women — not those who are persuaded, unaffected, or not even contemplating an abortion — are those on whom the majority should have concentrated under *Casey* and *Stenberg*.

Whether this court is looking at the record *de novo*, under an abuse-of-discretion standard, or merely for clear error, the district court's findings should stand. I find nothing in the majority's speculation that comes close to refuting the evidence on which the court relied. Only by disregarding key points such as the number of women who willingly undertook the burden of seeking an abortion out of state, where they could have the entire procedure accomplished in one visit rather than staying in state and enduring the two-visit burden, can the majority come to the result it does.

Finally, although not necessary to my analysis, it is worth noting that *Casey* said that "[a] finding of an undue burden is a shorthand for the conclusion that a state regulation has the purpose or effect of placing a substantial obstacle in the path of a woman seeking an abortion of a nonviable fetus" (505 U.S. at 877). The majority considers only the "effect" part of that disjunctive test, perhaps thinking that this court's dismissal of the "purpose" half in *Karlin* was binding on the Supreme Court. I am under no such illusion. I believe, therefore, that it is appropriate to take a brief look at the purpose Indiana offered for this regulation to see if it might help either to save the statute or to condemn it.

The district court found that "there is no evidence tending to show how the 'in the presence' requirement actually furthers the state's legitimate interests in maternal health or in protecting potential life." It said this, importantly, after the plaintiffs had made an extensive *prima facie* showing that the statute furthered neither legitimate interest; in the sense of a burden of production, the court was concerned that Indiana had offered nothing to the contrary. (Indiana argues strenuously that the district court imposed an impermissible shift in the ultimate burden of proof, but it is clear from the court's opinion as a whole that it did no such thing; it was simply addressing the evidentiary vacuum on Indiana's side in the face of the plaintiffs' evidence.)

Indeed, my search of the legislative history of the Indiana statute reveals no reason whatsoever for imposing a two-visit requirement for the dissemination of the required information. Acting as if it were conducting rational basis review, the majority speculates that some Indiana legislator might have thought that absorption of information occurs more effectively when it is transmitted in person. Maybe so, but that does not explain why the state could not simply have said that at the point of checking into the clinic, the previously transmitted information must be reiterated in person. The change from an oral communication to an in-the-presence requirement was added by a floor amendment that was marked by scant debate in the House of Representatives. After some members of the House suggested that the in-the-presence requirement was intended as an obstacle to abortion, its chief sponsor stated instead that the concern was that unless the information was given in person, "How do you know this is the doctor or the person you're supposed to be talking to. . . . I would think you would want to talk personally to the person who may be performing that and know . . . that they are the person indeed that they [say they] are." A special concern with impostor doctors, or generally with practitioners not being who they say they are over the telephone, is not a problem that is specific to abortion — or at least there were no such findings other than a statement that this possibility (of talking to an impostor) "is very dangerous, especially when you're talking about the symptoms and consequences of an abortion." Literally the only other scrap of evidence from the legislature seems to reflect a fear that women would receive the information while they were under sedation on an operating table.

But, that cannot be what the legislature really feared for the simple reason that this concern is already addressed in Indiana's law of "informed consent," which cannot be given by persons already under anesthesia. I would be surprised if many Indiana doctors were in the habit of obtaining consent for medical procedures from unconscious or drugged patients; they would risk loss of their medical license if they did, whether they were performing an appendectomy, knee surgery, a vasectomy, a prostate removal, or an abortion. The law of informed consent is consistent across the spectrum of surgeries and procedures: if no reason is given why heightened consent is needed in the abortion context, then this cannot be accepted as the reason for the in-the-presence requirement.

For all these reasons, I believe that the majority has seriously misapplied the *Casey* test. It has substituted its factual assumptions for evidence that is in the record; it has failed to focus on the women for whom that statute will create problems; and it seems to think that the *Casey* Court was not serious when it emphasized the lack of evidence in the record before it by implying that the result in *Casey* dictates the result here. I respectfully dissent.

## Conclusion

It may be concluded that there were no right or wrong answers to any of these questions. The most important lesson we learned from this is that every individual has an opinion, and that as professionals, we must learn to respect their ideas. Acting ethically and morally allows an individual to feel good about the job that they do and, in turn, allows them to achieve self-actualization.

*case eight*

# Genetic screening

This problem-based learning session is based on the following: *Tiemann v. U.S. Healthcare, Inc.*, Civil No. 99-5885, U.S. District Court for the Eastern District of Pennsylvania, 93 F. Supp. 2d 585; 2000 U.S. Dist. Lexis 502. January 11, 2000, Decided. January 11, 2000, Filed. January 11, 2000, Entered. It is reprinted here with permission of LexisNexis.

## Objectives

The objectives of this problem-based learning case are to discuss the following:

- Genetic screening: mandatory or voluntary
  Who decides what tests should be given?
  Cost versus benefit
  Screening for newborns
- Treatment decisions for seriously ill neonates
  Treatment options
  Who should receive aggressive treatment regardless of condition?
  Choices: who lives, who dies, who decides?
- Ethical dilemmas
  Patient autonomy
  Genetic discrimination
- Policy-making decisions
- Ethical councils

## Introduction

New technology and advanced diagnosis and treatment methods have brought with them many ethical issues. One of these is genetic screening, more specifically, genetic screening and the subsequent treatment options for seriously ill newborns. Before the advent of screening and treatment, many of these problems were left to chance and nature, while now many decisions must be made concerning the welfare of the child and the mother. The ethical problems stem from the fact that access to information pertaining to a newborn's diagnosis of or propensity to certain medical conditions or diseases may induce concerns about the child's welfare and worth as a human being. Other concerns stem from availability of treatment options in certain health care settings and the risk these options pose to the mother and her baby. These issues are increasingly being recognized and addressed as newer information becomes available. Many ethical councils have been formed, and policies are being made regarding how the issues should be handled by each specific health care facility. Yet, these problems will not be solved easily and may only become more complicated as technology progresses.

## Part one

Robert Tiemann and Thelma Tiemann, his wife ("Plaintiffs"), originally brought this action in the Court of Common Pleas of Philadelphia County on June 10, 1999, by the filing of a praecipe to issue writ of summons and a writ of summons. It was subsequently removed to the U.S. District Court for the Eastern District of Pennsylvania. Defendants have filed a motion with this court to have the action dismissed for failure to state a claim on which relief can be granted; Plaintiffs have filed a motion with this court to have the action remanded to the Court of Common Pleas.

### Facts

Between 1991 and 1995, Plaintiff Robert Tiemann was an employee under a group health insurance plan provided by defendants U.S. Healthcare, Inc.; Corporate Health Administrators, Inc.; and Health Maintenance Organization of Pennsylvania (the "Moving Defendants") through Plaintiff's employment. Moving Defendants, in exchange for premium payments, provided such group health insurance coverage to Mr. Tiemann pursuant to a group health insurance policy (the "Plan").

The other parties' defendant, the individual physicians and Family Medical Associates of Abington, Inc. (the "Physician Defendants" and, together with the Moving Defendants, the "Defendants"), were participating physicians and primary health care providers of the Plan and rendered medical treatment and health care services to Mr. Tiemann in return for compensation received from Moving Defendants pursuant to the Plan.

During the course of the provision of such services, Defendants learned, by September 1991, that Mr. Tiemann suffered from emphysema and the progression of the emphysematous condition of his lungs. Plaintiffs allege either the failure of Defendants to disclose the nature of his medical condition, the misrepresentation of Mr. Tiemann's condition, or both. Mr. Tiemann has suffered from a genetic disorder, alpha-1 antitrypsin deficiency disorder, a chronic, progressive disease that caused emphysema and irreversible lung damage in Mr. Tiemann.

In late 1998, Mr. Tiemann was first notified of this diagnosis. Mr. Tiemann has required and sought medical treatment, including alpha-1 antitrypsin replacement therapy and placement in a lung transplant program.

As a result of Defendants' malfeasance and nonfeasance, Mr. Tiemann's medical condition has deteriorated irreversibly. Early detection of Mr. Tiemann's genetic disorder would have permitted the implementation and rendition of necessary medical treatment, including the rendition of alpha-1 antitrypsin replacement therapy that would have prevented the deterioration of the condition of [Mr. Tiemann's] lungs and the extent of irreversible lung damage, which now requires or which in the future will require the rendition of lung transplantation for survival.

Plaintiffs further allege, *inter alia*, physical pain, suffering, mental anguish, financial loss, loss of life's pleasures, and loss of earnings, both now and in the future. Their complaint lists counts of negligence, breach of contract, and loss of consortium.

## Procedural history

On June 10, 1999, Plaintiffs filed a praecipe to issue writ of summons and a writ of summons in the Court of Common Pleas, Philadelphia County. On June 22, 1999, Moving Defendants were served by the sheriff of Montgomery County. The Physician Defendants were served with original process as well.

As a result, counsel for the Physician Defendants entered their appearances in this matter from the end of June to mid-August. On August 25, 1999, the Court of Common Pleas entered a case management order, which scheduled a case management conference for October 1, 1999. However, the Moving Defendants had still not entered their appearances.

On September 9, 1999, Plaintiffs filed their complaint with the Prothonotary's Office and forwarded a copy of the filed complaint, along with a copy of the scheduling order and case management conference memorandum to all counsel of record and to all unrepresented parties (i.e., the Moving Defendants).

On September 27, 1999, Plaintiffs' counsel made certain discovery requests to Defendants, and on October 1, 1999, all counsel of record attended the case management conference. Subsequent to the conference, the Court of Common Pleas issued a case management order. On October 15, 1999, Plaintiffs' counsel responded to Physician Defendants' discovery requests. These parties began planning a deposition schedule. The Physician Defendants filed preliminary objections to Plaintiffs' punitive damages and breach of contract claims; Plaintiffs filed replies on November 8 and 12, 1999.

On October 26, 1999, Plaintiffs' counsel was telephoned by Tarleton David Williams, Jr., who identified himself as the Moving Defendants' attorney in this matter and requested a faxed copy of the complaint. Plaintiffs' counsel fulfilled this request and forwarded all other relevant documentation by overnight courier. On November 15, 1999, two other attorneys, Charles M. O'Donnell and Michael A. Bowman, entered their appearances on behalf of U.S. Healthcare, Inc.

On November 23, 1999, Bowman, on behalf of the Moving Defendants, filed a notice of removal of this lawsuit from the Court of Common Pleas to the U.S. District Court, Eighth District (E.D.), of Pennsylvania, on the basis of certain questions of federal law being implicated. The next day, November 24, 1999, Bowman filed a praecipe to enter the notice of removal with the Court of Common Pleas, Philadelphia County, and followed with the filing in federal court of "Defendants' U.S. Healthcare Systems, Inc. and Corporate Health Administrators Inc.'s Motion to Dismiss Plaintiffs' Complaint" on Rule 12(b)(6) grounds ("Motion to Dismiss"), claiming federal preemption. "Plaintiffs' Response to Defendants U.S. Healthcare Systems, Inc. and Corporate Health Administrators, Inc.'s Motion to Dismiss Plaintiffs' Complaint" ("Plaintiffs' Response") was filed on December 16, 1999. Plaintiffs followed this with a motion of their own: "Plaintiffs' Motion for Remand and Application of Sanctions," filed December 22, 1999 ("Motion for Remand"). On December 29, 1999, two Physician Defendants filed a "Motion to Dismiss of Defendants, Evan Kessler, D.O. and Anthony G. Wydan, M.D. for Failure to State a Claim Upon Which Relief Can Be Granted as to Plaintiffs' Claim for Punitive Damages." Finally, Moving Defendants filed "Defendants' U.S. Healthcare Systems, Inc. and Corporate Health Administrators Inc.'s Reply in Support of Their Motion to Dismiss Plaintiffs' Complaint" ("Moving Defendants' Reply"), which was filed on January 6, 2000.

For the reasons stated below, Defendant's Motion to Dismiss will be denied and Plaintiff's Motion for Remand will be granted in its entirety. The Physician Defendants' Motion to Dismiss will be denied as moot.

## Standard of review

Moving Defendants are before this court with their Motion to Dismiss Plaintiffs' action pursuant to Federal Rule of Civil Procedure 12(b)(6). In addition, Plaintiffs, through their Motion for Remand, have moved to send this case back to the Court of Common Pleas, Philadelphia County.

As we find that removal was improper, we shall grant Plaintiffs' Motion for Remand. For the reasons discussed in connection with our granting of Plaintiffs' Motion for Remand, infra, we shall also deny Moving Defendants' Motion to Dismiss pursuant to Federal Rule of Civil Procedure 12(b)(6). Nonetheless, we briefly review the standard for dismissal for failure to state a cause of action on which relief can be granted.

### Rule 12(b)(6)

Under Rule 12(b)(6), a defendant bears the burden of demonstrating that a plaintiff has not stated a claim on which relief can be granted. When considering such a motion to dismiss, we must "accept as true the facts alleged in the complaint and all reasonable inferences that can be drawn from them. Dismissal under Rule 12(b)(6) . . . is limited to those instances where it is certain that no relief could be granted under any set of facts that could be proved."

Under the present circumstances, Moving Defendants bear the burden of demonstrating that Plaintiffs have not stated a claim on which relief can be granted (*Cohen*, 45 F. Supp. 2d). Further, we are bound to "accept as true the facts alleged" in Plaintiffs' complaint "and all reasonable inferences that can be drawn from them" (*Powell*, 1998 WL 804727). Based on the analysis revealed in our discussion of the lack of ERISA (Employment Retirement Income Security Act of 1974) complete preemption, infra, we do not believe that "no relief could be granted under any set of facts that could be proved." Therefore, for reasons that will become eminently clear, we deny Moving Defendants' request for dismissal under Rule 12(b)(6).

### Remand standard

The statute that prescribes removal procedure states:

> the notice of removal of a civil action or proceeding shall be filed within thirty days after the receipt by the defendant, through service or otherwise, of a copy of the initial pleading setting forth the claim for relief upon which such action or proceeding is based, or within thirty days after the service of summons upon the defendant if such initial pleading has then been filed in court and is not required to be served on the defendant, whichever period is shorter.

Under the subsequent section, "Procedure after removal generally":

> [a] motion to remand the case on the basis of any defect other than lack of subject matter jurisdiction must be made within 30 days after the filing of the notice of removal under section 1446(a). If at any time before final judgment it appears that the district court lacks subject matter jurisdiction, the case shall be remanded. An order remanding the case may require payment of just costs and any actual expenses, including attorney fees, incurred as a result of the removal.

Further, ignoring an exception not apposite to the case at bar, "an order remanding a case to the State court from which it was removed is not reviewable on appeal or otherwise" [28 U.S.C. § 1447(d)]. The U.S. Supreme Court has clarified this statutory language in holding that only "remand orders issued under [28 U.S.C. § 1447(c)] and invoking the grounds specified therein . . . are immune from review under § 1447(d)" [in re *U.S. Healthcare*, 159 F.3d 142, 146 (3d Cir. 1998), quoting *Thermtron Products, Inc., v. Hermansdorfer*, 423 U.S. 336, 346, 46 L. Ed. 2d 542, 96 S. Ct. 584 (1976)]. In other words, for our decision to remand a case to be immune from review, it would have to be issued due to a defect in removal procedure or the lack of subject matter jurisdiction. Of course, it would be for the Third Circuit Court of Appeals (the "Third Circuit") to decide this question in any appeal.

We also note that "removal statutes are strictly construed and all doubts are resolved in favor of remand" [*Weinstein v. Paul Revere Insurance Co.*, 15 F. Supp. 2d 552, 555 (D. N.J. 1998); see also *Batoff v. State Farm Insurance*, 977 F.2d 848, 851 (3d Cir. 1992) and *Miller v. Riddle Memorial Hospital*, 1998 U.S. Dist. Lexis 7752, No. 98-392, 1998 WL 272167 (E.D. Pa., May 28, 1998), both cited by *Weinstein*]. We shall not lose sight of this legal standard in our review of the facts in the case at bar.

There would appear to be a patent defect in removal procedure in the case at bar. Moving Defendants filed their Notice of Removal on November 23, 1999, much later than the 30-day period prescribed by statute [see 28 U.S.C. § 1446(b)]. One might conclude that, under no interpretation of that statutory provision, could the notice of removal have been proper after October 11, 1999, the first business day following the date 30 days after the date the Plaintiffs filed their complaint with the Prothonotary's Office and forwarded copies to all counsel of record and to all unrepresented parties [see Plaintiffs' Response; 28 U.S.C. § 1446(b); see also Fed. R. Civ. P. 6(a)].

Plaintiffs, on the other hand, filed their Motion for Remand within the 30-day window prescribed by Section 1447(c). They filed their Motion for Remand on December 22, 1999, which was within 30 days of the date of "the filing of the notice of removal under section 1446(a)" [28 U.S.C. § 1447(c)].

Under this analysis, as it would be the procedure that Moving Defendants followed that was defective, while Plaintiffs' procedure was proper, we would be confident that our holding would not be scrutinized with the lens of detraction.

However, we shall not rest our holding on these statutory grounds. We recognize that in, Moving Defendants' Reply, they contest Plaintiffs' assertion that removal was not timely. Moving Defendants maintain that, contrary to Plaintiffs' representations, they did not receive a "copy of the initial pleading setting forth the claim for relief" [28 U.S.C. § 1446(b)] until October 26, 1999 [see Moving Defendants' Reply; see also Declaration of Tarleton David Williams, Jr.]. As our holding in the case at bar does not rely on a defect in removal procedure, but rather on a lack of federal subject matter jurisdiction, we shall not delve further into this issue and now proceed to the question of ERISA preemption.

### ERISA preemption

Moving Defendants argue in their Motion to Dismiss that Plaintiffs' claims against Moving Defendants are preempted by ERISA (Motion to Dismiss, at 3–8). Plaintiffs argue to the contrary and move to remand the case on the basis of a lack of federal question subject matter jurisdiction.

*Complete preemption doctrine.* Generally, a federal claim must appear "on the face of a well-pleaded complaint in order to confer federal question jurisdiction for removal under section 1441" [*Weinstein*, 15 F. Supp. 2d at 555, citing *Dukes v. U.S. Healthcare, Inc.*, 57 F.3d 350, 353 (3d Cir. 1995)]. However, there is an exception to this well-pleaded complaint rule, known as the "complete preemption exception" [see *Metropolitan Life Insurance Co. v. Taylor*, 481 U.S. 58, 95 L. Ed. 2d 55, 107 S. Ct. 1542 (1987)]. There, the Supreme Court recognizes that Congress has the authority to "completely preempt certain causes of action under state law so that 'any civil complaint raising this select group of claims is necessarily federal in character'" (*Weinstein*, 15 F. Supp. 2d at 555, quoting *Metropolitan Life Insurance.*, 481 U.S. at 63–64). The question for us to decide is whether the complete preemption exception would apply in the instant case, notwithstanding the common law tort and breach of contract causes of action advanced by Plaintiffs.

We note that the complete preemption doctrine is utilized when:

> *the pre-emptive force of [the federal statutory provision] is so powerful as to displace entirely any state cause of action [addressed by the federal statute]. Any such suit is purely a creature of federal law, notwithstanding the fact that state law would provide a cause of action in the absence of [the federal provision].*

To begin, we assume that the Plan in question here falls within ERISA's coverage. When ERISA is concerned, the complete preemption exception applies to state law causes of action that fall within ERISA's civil enforcement mechanism, which is described at 29 U.S.C. § 1132.

The civil enforcement provision of the ERISA statute allows plan participants or beneficiaries to bring an action "to recover benefits due to [a participant or beneficiary] under the terms of [such person's] plan, or to clarify . . . rights to future benefits under the terms of the plan" [29 U.S.C. § 1132 (a)(1)(B), ERISA section 502(a)(1)(B)]. Therefore, "state law claims which fall outside the scope of ERISA section 502(a)(1)(B) are still governed by the well-pleaded complaint rule and, therefore, are not removable under the complete-preemption principles" (*Dukes*, 57 F.3d at 355).

*Preemption versus removal.* That the complete preemption exception may apply in a given circumstance, namely, "for state law claims which fit within the scope of § 502, by no means implies that all claims preempted by ERISA are subject to removal" (id.). "Removal and preemption are two distinct concepts" [id., quoting *Warner v. Ford Motor Co.*, 46 F.3d 531, 535 (6th Cir. 1995)]. That is because there is another provision within ERISA that deals with preemption more generally, which covers a broader swatch of the ERISA fabric, but does not have the effect of overturning the well-pleaded complaint rule. That rule is nullified only by complete preemption under ERISA's civil enforcement mechanism. As *Dukes* states:

> *Section 514 of ERISA defines the scope of ERISA preemption, providing that ERISA supersede[s] any and all State*

> *laws insofar as they may now or hereafter relate to any employee benefit plan described in [§ 4(a) of ERISA] and not exempt under [§ 4(b) of ERISA].* The Metropolitan Life *complete-preemption exception, on the other hand, is concerned with a more limited set of state laws, those which fall within the scope of ERISA's civil enforcement provision, § 502. State law claims which fall outside of the scope of § 502, even if preempted by § 514(a), are still governed by the well-pleaded complaint rule and, therefore, are not removable under the complete-preemption principles established in* Metropolitan Life.

*Dukes* continues its detailed discussion of the distinctions between these two ERISA provisions:

> *The difference between preemption and complete preemption is important. When the doctrine of complete preemption does not apply, but the plaintiff's state claim is arguably preempted under § 514(a), the district court, being without removal jurisdiction, cannot resolve the dispute regarding preemption. It lacks power [**19] to do anything other than remand to the state court where the preemption issue can be addressed and resolved.* Franchise Tax Board, 463 U.S. at 4, 27–28; Allstate, 879 F.2d 90 at 94; Warner, 46 F.3d at 533–35; Lupo, 28 F.3d 269 at 274.

(*Dukes*, 57 F.3d at 355). In other words, when preemption is based only on § 514, we are without removal jurisdiction and must remand to the state court for resolution of the dispute.

## Make a list of the major problems presented in this case

- 
- 
- 
- 

## Hypothesis and mechanism

For the problems in your list above, give a cause or a reason for each to happen:

- 
- 
- 
-

## Learning issues

Make a list of learning issues in the form of questions. Remember, your goal is to gather the medical, social, and all other relevant facts that may apply to the case.

What does (newborn) genetic screening entail?
> Newborn genetic screening tests are tools used to evaluate the possibility of an infant having or developing certain diseases. These tests may detect in the infant or parent an abnormal genotype that predisposes the infant to potential health problems.

Should genetic screening be mandatory or voluntary?
> Mandatory if early detection and intervention can improve the outcome of a disease.
> Tests beyond those mandated could and should be offered according to the judgment of the health professional if the results of the test would result in a positive outcome of the disease.

Who should decide which tests should be given?
> Government versus parent versus health care professional

What are the costs-versus-benefit issues involving genetic screening?
> Cost associated with impact is not clear. For the most part, common newborn screening tests improve quality of life and are cost-effective.
> Genetic testing for particular diseases offers a clear benefit to patients and society by reducing the impact of disease, improving the health of the population, and lessening the burden on our health care system.

What are some of the specific genetic screening tests/programs?
> Newborn screening programs (NBS)
>> NBS tests for phenylketonuria, congenital hypothyroidism, congenital adrenal hyperplasia, biotinidase deficiency, sickle cell anemia, galactosemia, maple syrup disease, homocystinuria.
> Tandem mass spectrometry (TMS)
>> Diagnoses fatty acid oxidation disorder, amino acid disorder, organic acid disorder, and it can add to the NBS program.
> Bloodspot technology applications
> Important notes: Newborn genetic screening tests are tools used to evaluate whether an infant will have or develop certain diseases. The results of these tests can be used for diagnosis, prognosis, and epidemiology. With the increase in technology, many questions have arisen regarding genetic screening. The first question is whether certain genetic tests should be mandatory or voluntary. Many experts agree that, if early detection and intervention can

improve the outcome of a disease, genetic screening for those diseases should be mandatory. Voluntary genetic screening tests should be offered if the results of the test would result in a positive outcome of the disease. Who should decide which tests should be performed? It is unclear in some situations who has this right. The government has recommended that certain genetic screening tests should be mandatory. In a voluntary situation, for example, the genetic testing can sometimes confirm a diagnosis and expel anxiety of the parents concerning diseases that have no known treatment or method of prevention. Health care professionals can be mediators in such situations. Ultimately, the costs, benefits, and risks of genetic screening need to be evaluated. Mostly, newborn screening tests that are common improve quality of life and are cost-effective. Education is critical in helping everyone understand the meaning of the possible outcomes, risks, and benefits.

What are the treatment decisions that need to be made when genetic problems are encountered?

Treatment should be given to prevent mental retardation, severe illness, and premature death and to minimize false-positive results.

The options are:

Many of the congenital diseases have treatments.

Most are costly and long term.

In the future, as technology advances, many more diseases will be treatable and preventable.

Should all receive aggressive treatment regardless of the condition?

Physically disabling conditions and mentally disabling conditions raise similar issues that must be taken into consideration: cost of long-term care, quality of life, ability to function in society.

Choices: who lives, who dies, who decides?

Substituted judgment: if the infant were competent to make its own decision, what would he or she do?

Parents make decisions on behalf of their child.

Decisions must be based on all available information.

Health care professionals must be able to educate parents fully on the options in question.

Parents must put themselves fully in the child's position to decide which decision is in the best interest of their child.

Important notes: Treatment should be given to prevent mental retardation, severe illness, and premature death and to minimize false-positive results. Many of the congenital diseases have treatments, but most of these are costly and long term. Because of the cost of long-term care, the question has to be asked whether all patients should receive aggressive treatment regardless of the condition and the patient's quality of life.

Which ethical dilemmas revolve around genetic screening?

Patient autonomy, social equality, and respect for human life and dignity are ethical principles that should guide decisions about genetic testing.

Patients should be free to make their own reproductive or lifestyle decisions or even ignore medical advice after being provided with education and counseling about the risks and benefits of genetic testing.

Genetic discrimination:

Genetic testing that appears inappropriate and unjustified in circumstances for which genetic enhancement or discrimination may result should not be done.

Respect for patient autonomy and the confidentiality of test results must be strictly enforced to avoid abuse of genetic information. The U.S. Equal Employment Opportunities Commission declared genetic discrimination unfair, unjustified, and illegal under the Americans with Disabilities Act. Such legislation may help reduce the threat of abuse in genetic testing.

Important notes: The two main ethical dilemmas are patient autonomy and genetic discrimination. Autonomy refers to an individual's existence as an independent moral agent who has the capacity to make moral decisions and act on them. With respect to genetic screening, patients should be free to make their own reproductive or lifestyle decisions after being provided with education and counseling about the risks and benefits of the genetic tests. This stems from the difference in ethical views between individuals. Genetic discrimination can result from lack of confidentiality. For example, insurance companies may use the results of genetic tests to withhold payment for treatments. To ensure the protection and confidentiality of patients, confidentiality of genetic test results must be strictly enforced to avoid abuse of genetic information.

Which entities are involved with policy making involving genetic screening?

Public health infrastructure

Newborn screening a public health agency role

Federal agencies to strengthen the public health infrastructure

HRSA (Health Resources and Services Administration

CDC (Centers for Disease Control and Prevention)

HCFA (Health Care Financing Administration)

AHRQ (Agency for Healthcare Research and Quality)

NIH (National Institutes of Health)

Public's role in newborn screening process

Recommended by the Task Force on Genetic Screening

CORN (Council of Regional Networks for Genetic Services), NAS (National Academy of Sciences), and IOM (Institute of Medicine)

Important notes: Policy making for genetic screening tests starts with the public health infrastructure, for which newborn screening becomes a public health agency role. Some federal agencies that are responsible for strengthening the infrastructure include HRSA, CDC, HCFA, AHRQ, and NIH. The Task Force on Genetic Screening, through reports made by CORN, NAS, and IOM, make recommendations regarding the adoption, introduction, and use of new, predictive genetic tests. In the early 1970s, the CDC saw a need for improving quality assurance of genetic screening. The Newborn Screening Quality Assurance Program was founded. It is a voluntary, nonregulatory program to help state health departments and their laboratories maintain and enhance the quality of test results. In 1985, CORN published newborn screening system guidelines that defined a five-part system of screening, follow-up, diagnosis, treatment/management, and evaluation. The American Academy of Pediatrics (AAP) convenes a national task force on newborn screening. Its purpose is to review issues and challenges for newborn screening programs. With the continued advances in genetic screening, these ethical councils will continue to play a major role.

Which ethical councils are involved with genetic screening?

The Newborn Screening Quality Assurance Program (early 1970s), started by the CDC (and has other funding) because CDC saw the need for improving quality assurance.

CORN (1985), published newborn screening system guidelines that defined a five-part system of screening, follow-up, diagnosis, treatment/management, and evaluation.

AAP convenes a national task force on newborn screening with the purpose of reviewing issues and challenges for newborn screening programs.

State newborn screening systems.

Guidelines linked to legal, ethical, and social considerations: three reports emphasize the criteria:

NAS: *Genetic Screening: Programs, Principles, and Research* (1975)

IOM: *Assessing Genetic Risks: Implications for Health and Social Policy* (1994)

Task Force final report: *Promoting Safe and Effective Testing in the United States: Final Report of the Task Force on Genetic Testing* (1997)

The President's Commission for the Study of Ethical Problems in Medicine and Biomedical and Behavioral Research, which makes recommendations such as "Screening and Counseling for Genetic Considerations" (1993).

## Literature review

To help you get ready to answer certain questions you anticipate being asked during the second part of the case, look in the local medical library and on the World Wide Web for helpful information. Please indicate in the spaces below (1) several helpful articles or books you found and (2) several helpful Web sites you found.

- **Helpful articles/books:**

  Allan, D., Ethical boundaries in genetic testing, *Can. Med. Assoc. J.*, 15, 241–244, 1996.

  Dunst, J., Screening for fetal and genetic abnormality: social and ethical issues, *J. Med. Genet.*, 25, 290–293, 1988.

  Evans, J.A., Screening for fetal anomalies: old habits, new challenges, *Can. Med. Assoc. J.*, 156, 805–806, 1997.

  Gillon, R., Ethics of genetic screening: the first report of the Nuffield Council on Bioethics, *J. Med. Ethics*, 20, 67–68, 92, 1994.

  Hogge, J.S. and Hogge, W.A., Preconception genetic counseling, *Clin. Obstet. Gynecol.*, 39, 751–762, 1996.

  Holtzman, N.A., Medical and ethical issues in genetic screening — an academic view, *Environ. Health Perspect.*, 104(Suppl. 5), 987–990, 1996.

  Mennuti, M.T., Prenatal diagnosis — advances bring new challenges, *N. Engl. J. Med.*, 320, 661–663, 1989.

  Newborn screening fact sheets, American Academy of Pediatrics, Committee on Genetics, *Pediatrics*, 98(3, Pt. 1), 473–501, 1996.

  Serving the family from birth to the medical home, Newborn screening: a blueprint for the future — a call for a national agenda on state newborn screening programs, *Pediatrics*, 106(2, Pt. 2), 389–422, 2000.

  Shapiro, D., The ethics of genetic screening: the first report of the Nuffield Council on Bioethics: another personal view, *J. Med. Ethics*, 20, 185–187, 1994.

- **Helpful Web sites:**

  University of Oregon — Department of Biology: biology.uoregon.edu/Biology_www

  The Family Internet: familyinternet.com

  The Arc of the United States: TheArc.org

  Columbia University Health Sciences: cpmcnet.columbia.edu/texts/guides

## *Identify all relevant values that play a role in the case and determine which values, if any, conflict*

Nonmaleficence:

Beneficence:

Respect for persons:

Loyalty:

Distributive justice:

## Learning issues for next student-centered problem-based learning session

- List the options open to you. That is, answer the question, "What could you do?"
- Choose the best solution from an ethical point of view, justify it, and respond to possible criticisms. That is, answer the question, "What should you do, and why?"
- What are the different ways of thinking about the problem? Which conflict management techniques can be used in the situation?

## Part two

Moving Defendants maintain that Plaintiffs' state law claims fall within the scope of 29 U.S.C. § 1132(a)(1)(B), thus allowing the complete preemption doctrine to permit removal. We are not inclined to agree.

*Dukes* assumed, without deciding, that the plan benefits are not merely "the plan participants' or beneficiaries' memberships in the respective HMOs . . . [, but rather, that the plan benefits encompassed] the medical care provided . . . for the purposes of ERISA" (*Dukes*, 57 F.3d at 356). We, too, shall assume that Moving Defendants arrange for the delivery of Plan benefits, such that "removal jurisdiction would exist if the plaintiffs were alleging that the [Moving Defendants] refused to provide the services to which membership entitled them."

As in *Dukes*, we, too, conclude nevertheless that removal was improper here. When, as here, the Plaintiffs' claims (a) attack the quality of benefits received, and not the quantity (i.e., a "claim that the plan erroneously withheld benefits due") of benefits received; (b) do not ask for the enforcement of their rights under the terms of the plan; and (c) do not ask for clarification of their rights to future benefits, we shall find that Plaintiffs' claims have fallen outside the scope of ERISA's civil enforcement provision, and we shall remand to the Court of Common Pleas, Philadelphia County [see id.; 29 U.S.C. § 1132(a)(1)(B)]. As we do not believe that either Item (b) or (c) listed above is implicated in the instant case, and Moving Defendants do not appear to argue for anything other than Item (a) (alleging that Plaintiffs' claims attack the quantity of benefits received), our analysis focuses on Item (a).

## No claim of failure to provide benefits due

As in *Dukes*, there is no allegation in Plaintiffs' complaint that Plan benefits due were erroneously withheld. Nearly all of the claims made in Plaintiffs' complaint concerning the Moving Defendants center around common law negligence, resulting either directly or through agency principles (see complaint, at pp. 24–28) and breach of contract allegations (see complaint, at pp. 29–32). Plaintiffs do not aver that the Moving Defendants refused to provide certain tests because the Plan would not pay for such tests. Nor do they claim that Robert Tiemann's poor health is the result of the Plan's "refusal to pay for or otherwise provide for medical services" (*Dukes*, 57 F.3d at 357). We find the situation in the case at bar closely parallels *Dukes*:

> *Instead of claiming that the welfare plan in any way withheld some quantum of plan benefits due, the plaintiffs … complain about the low quality of the medical treatment … actually received and argue that the … HMO should be held liable under agency and negligence principles. (Dukes, 57 F.3d at 357).*

This kind of claim is not a claim under the ERISA civil enforcement provision to "recover benefits due … under the terms of [the] plan" [see 29 U.S.C. § 1132(a)(1)(B)].

The Third Circuit gives a detailed explanation of the importance of respecting an existing state regulatory scheme safeguarding the quality of plan benefits, while recognizing the strictly federal terrain of deciding whether the benefits due under a plan were in fact provided:

> *Nor does anything in the legislative history, structure, or purpose of ERISA suggest that Congress viewed § 502(a)(1)(B) as creating a remedy for a participant injured by medical malpractice. When Congress enacted ERISA it*

*was concerned in large part with the various mechanisms and institutions involved in the funding and payment of plan benefits. That is, Congress was concerned "that owing to the inadequacy of current minimum [financial and administrative] standards, the soundness and stability of plans with respect to adequate funds to pay promised benefits may be endangered" [§ 2, 29 U.S.C. § 1001(a)]. Thus, Congress sought to assure that promised benefits would be available when plan participants had need of them and § 502 was intended to provide each individual participant with a remedy in the event that promises made by the plan were not kept. We find nothing in the legislative history suggesting that § 502 was intended as a part of a federal scheme to control the quality of the benefits received by plan participants. Quality control of benefits, such as the health care benefits provided here, is a field traditionally occupied by state regulation and we interpret the silence of Congress as reflecting an intent that it remain such. See, e.g., Travelers Ins. Co., 514 U.S. 645, 115 S. Ct. 1671 at 1678–79, 131 L. Ed. 2d 695 (noting that while quality standards and work place regulations in the context of hospital services will indirectly affect the sorts of benefits an ERISA plan can afford, they have traditionally been left to the states, and there is no indication in ERISA that Congress chose to displace general health care regulation by the states).*

## Complaint pp. 27(c)–(d), 31(c)

We recognize that a few of Plaintiffs' claims in their complaint do, indeed, present a much closer question for us. Specifically, Plaintiffs aver that Moving Defendants' negligence consisted, *inter alia*, of:

*the promulgation of rules, regulations and standards for participating physicians and health care providers that penalized participating physicians and/or health care providers for referring patients for additional required medical treatment, where the [Moving] Defendants knew and/or should have known that the enforcement of the stated rules, regulations and/or standards would lead to the rendition of substandard medical care and deviations from the applicable standard of care with resulting patient injuries [and] the promulgation of rules, regulations and standards for participating physicians and health care providers that rewarded participating physicians and health care providers for decreasing and/or minimizing required medical services, treatments, diagnostics and referrals to specialists where the*

> *[Moving] Defendants knew and/or should have known that*
> *the enforcement of such rules, regulations and/or standards*
> *would lead to the rendition of substandard medical care and*
> *deviations from the applicable standard of care with result-*
> *ing patient injuries.*

Further, Plaintiffs also claimed that Moving Defendants "breached their contractual obligation to provide medical and primary care services" by, *inter alia*:

> *promulgating, implementing and/or following a schedule of*
> *rules, regulations and/or standards in the rendition of med-*
> *ical and primary care services that violated applicable in-*
> *dustry standards and applicable law.*

Specifically, Moving Defendants refer to these paragraphs of Plaintiffs' complaint in their Motion to Dismiss, maintaining that by their nature "these claims are completely preempted by the civil enforcement mechanism set forth in Section 502(a) of ERISA" (Motion to Dismiss, at pp. 15–16).

### § 514 Preemption analysis

Moving Defendants would have been more likely to persuade this court to accept its position that Plaintiffs' claims should be preempted by ERISA had this case been brought during the 1980s or early 1990s. During that period, there were several Supreme Court cases that gave the ERISA preemption provision a broad reach. The words of that provision were to be given their "broad common-sense meaning, such that a state law 'relate[s] to' a benefit plan in the normal sense of the phrase, if it has a connection with or reference to such a plan."

Here, we are dealing with a question of Section 514 of ERISA, rather than Section 502(a), which is the complete preemption exception. Nonetheless, we find the shift in this area that came in the mid-1990s not to be without significance in the complete preemption context (see infra).

The Supreme Court altered its previous approach in *New York State Conference of Blue Cross and Blue Shield Plans v. Travelers Insurance Company*, 514 U.S. 645, 131 L. Ed. 2d 695, 115 S. Ct. 1671 (1995). As Pappas relates:

> *The Court recognized that "if 'relate to' were taken to extend*
> *to the furthest stretch of its indeterminacy, then for all*
> *practical purposes pre-emption would never run its course,*
> *for 'really, universally, relations stop nowhere.'" Id. at 655.*
> *. . . The Court reasoned that the language of the preemption*
> *provision is so extensive that if the Court were to look merely*
> *to the bare language of the provision, the provision would*
> *for all intents and purposes be without limit — an intent*
> *which the Court would not ascribe to Congress.*

(Pappas, 724 A.2d at 892, citing the *Travelers* case). Importantly for us, "pre-emption does not occur . . . if the state law [i.e., negligence/breach of contract] has only a tenuous, remote, or peripheral connection with covered plans, as in the cases with many laws of general applicability" (*Travelers*, 514 U.S. at 661). The Supreme Court noted that "nothing in the language of [ERISA] or in the context of its passage indicates that Congress chose to displace general health care regulation, which historically has been a matter of local concern" (id.).

Subsequent Supreme Court cases have solidified the *Travelers* approach [see, e.g., *California Division of Labor Standards Enforcement v. Dillingham Construction, NA., Inc.*, 519 U.S. 316, 136 L. Ed. 2d 791, 117 S. Ct. 832 (1997); *De Buono v. NYSA-ILA Medical and Clinical Services Fund*, 520 U.S. 806, 138 L. Ed. 2d 21, 117 S. Ct. 1747 (1997)]. For this reason, *Pappas* concluded that negligence claims against an HMO (health maintenance organization) do not "relate to" an ERISA plan and thus are not preempted by ERISA (*Pappas*, 724 A.2d at 893). "As noted by *Travelers*, Congress did not intend to preempt state laws which govern the provision of safe medical care" (id., citing *Travelers*, 514 U.S. at 661). In sum:

> *Claims that an HMO was negligent when it provided contractually-guaranteed medical benefits in such a dilatory fashion that the patient was injured indisputably are intertwined with the provision of safe medical care. We believe that it would be highly questionable for us to find that these claims were preempted when the United States Supreme Court has stated that there was no intent on the part of Congress to preempt state laws concerning the regulation of the provision of safe medical care.*

We find the situation in the instant case closely, though not entirely, related to the *Pappas* circumstances. Further, we note that, based on *Travelers* and its progeny, Moving Defendants' reliance on *Kearney v. U.S. Healthcare, Inc.*, 859 F. Supp. 182 (E.D. Pa. 1994), is misplaced.

### § 502 Complete preemption analysis

As we discussed above, *Pappas* did not directly deal with the complete preemption doctrine of ERISA § 502(a), but rather with § 514, which defines ERISA preemption outside ERISA's civil enforcement context. However, a recent Third Circuit decision, *In re U.S. Healthcare, Inc.*, 193 F.3d 151 (3d Cir. 1999), touches on precisely the question we are facing in the instant suit: how far *Dukes'* quantity versus quality of benefits distinction will take us.

In *U.S. Healthcare*, participants in an ERISA plan brought a state court medical malpractice action against an HMO after the death of their newborn child. The HMO removed the action to the U.S. District Court, District of New Jersey, where one count was dismissed, and the remaining counts were remanded to state court. Both parties appealed. The Third Circuit held that none of plaintiffs' claims was completely preempted by ERISA and remanded all counts to the state court.

*U.S. Healthcare* is instructive in clarifying that the particular role an HMO assumes will determine whether the complete preemption provision of ERISA is implicated. As a complicating matter, an HMO "may have assumed both the role as a plan administrator and the separate role as a provider of medical services." It is necessary as a preliminary matter to determine which role an HMO assumed to determine whether complete preemption is found. The Third Circuit provides much guidance in solving this problem:

> *As an administrator overseeing an ERISA plan, an HMO will have administrative responsibilities over the elements of the plan, including determining eligibility for benefits, calculating those benefits, disbursing them to the participant, monitoring available funds, and keeping records. As we held in* Dukes, *claims that fall within the essence of the administrator's activities in this regard fall within section 502(a)(1)(B) and are completely preempted.*

In contrast, as noted by the secretary, when the HMO acts under the ERISA plan as a health care provider, it arranges and provides medical treatment, directly or through contracts with hospitals, doctors, or nurses [see *Dukes*, 57 F.3d at 361; see also *Corcoran v. United HealthCare, Inc.*, 965 F.2d 1321, 1329–1334 (5th Cir. 1992), recognizing that HMOs act as both health care providers and plan administrators]. In performing these activities, the HMO is not acting in its capacity as a plan administrator, but as a provider of health care, subject to the prevailing state standard of care.

The Third Circuit found it "significant that none of these three counts as pled alleges a failure to provide or authorize benefits under the plan, and the Baumans do not claim anywhere in these counts that they were denied any of the benefits that were due under the plan." We find, likewise, that Plaintiffs have not claimed that they were denied any of the benefits that were due under the Plan in the case at bar.

The count in *U.S. Healthcare* that deals with the HMO's policy of presumptively discharging newborns within 24 hours "charges U.S. Healthcare with both direct negligence for the adoption and implementation of the policy and with vicarious liability for the negligence of [the doctor and the hospital]." This count, like all the others in *U.S. Healthcare*, was held to have been not completely preempted by ERISA. We do not see how the situation in *U.S. Healthcare* differs in any material way from what the Tiemanns have alleged in paragraphs 27(c), 27(d), and 31(c) of their complaint. There, Plaintiffs charge:

> *Moving Defendants with promulgating rules, regulations and standards . . . that [discouraged physicians and partic-*

> *ipating health care providers from] referring patients for additional required medical treatment [and encouraged them to] decrease and/or minimize required medical services, treatments, diagnostics and referrals to specialists where the [Moving] Defendants knew and/or should have known that the enforcement of such rules, regulations and/or standards would lead to the rendition of substandard medical care and deviations from the applicable standard of care with resulting patient injuries [i.e., negligence/medical malpractice].*

[complaint, at P 27(c)–27(d)]. The breach of contract count of Plaintiffs' complaint is of a similar nature, alleging:

> *promulgating, implementing and/or following a schedule of rules, regulations and/or standards in the rendition of medical and primary care services that violated applicable industry standards and applicable law . . .*

The Third Circuit explains its holding in *U.S. Healthcare* with respect to the 24-hour discharge policy:

> *With respect to the direct negligence claim, the Baumans' challenge to* U.S. Healthcare's *twenty-four-hour discharge policy is directed at the HMO's actions in what we characterized in* Dukes *as an HMO's role in "arranging for medical treatment" rather than its role as a plan administrator determining what benefits are appropriate.* Dukes, 57 F.3d *at 360. Thus, it is the HMO's essentially medical determination of the appropriate level of care that the Baumans claim contributed to the death of their daughter. This is not a claim that a certain benefit was requested and denied. As the Secretary points out, under the facts as pleaded in the complaint,* U.S. Healthcare's *policy and incentive structure were such that "the Baumans never had the option of making an informed decision as to whether to pay for the hospitalization themselves," as would occur in a situation in which coverage is sought and denied. . . . Accordingly, this claim fits squarely within the class of claims that we identified in* Dukes *as involving the quality of care. Here, as in* Dukes, *"the plaintiffs . . . are attempting to hold the HMO liable for [its] role as the arranger of their [decedent's] medical treatment."* Dukes, 57 F.3d *at 361.*

(*U.S. Healthcare*, 193 F.3d at 162–163). We believe that, as in *U.S. Healthcare*, Moving Defendants were acting in their role as an arranger of medical treatment, rather than as plan administrator "determining what benefits are appropriate" (id. at 162, citing *Dukes*, 57 F.3d at 360). Further, as in *U.S. Healthcare*, we find that Moving Defendants' "policy and incentive structure were such that [Plaintiffs] never had the option of making an informed decision [regarding treatment], as would occur in a situation in which coverage is sought and denied" (see 193 F.3d at 163). Thus, we, too, conclude that Plaintiffs' claims — even those most subject to challenge on complete preemption grounds — are claims that go to the quality of care received under the *Dukes* standard.

To the extent that Plaintiffs allege that Moving Defendants acted with knowledge or reckless indifference to the possibility that their policies would result in substandard medical care, our conclusion is not affected. Like the negligence claim, this allegation "goes to the quality of care . . . received rather than an administrative decision as to whether certain benefits were covered by the plan." These charges "do not raise the failure of [Moving Defendants] to pay for a benefit or process a claim for benefits as the basis for the injury suffered." Therefore, they are not completely preempted by ERISA.

The similarities between *U.S. Healthcare* and the case at bar are placed in further relief by a claim of plaintiffs in *U.S. Healthcare* that the Third Circuit identified as demonstrating the HMO's role as a provider or arranger of medical services, as opposed to a plan administrator role:

> as the Baumans allege, the HMO adopted policies that "encouraged, pressured, and/or directly or indirectly required" their participating physicians to discharge newborn infants and that also discouraged physicians to readmit newborn infants when the appropriate standard of care required otherwise under state law. . . . Assuming these allegations are true, as we must when considering a motion to dismiss, the Baumans seek recovery for decisions that U.S. Healthcare made in providing and arranging medical services, decisions that adversely influenced the medical judgment of its participating physicians.

Our Plaintiffs have essentially made the same allegations regarding the Moving Defendants as the plaintiffs made of their HMO in *U.S. Healthcare*. Therefore, we are compelled to reach the same conclusion with regard to complete preemption as the Third Circuit reached in *U.S. Healthcare*. We find that there is no complete preemption here.

## Beyond rejection of complete preemption

Interestingly, the court in *U.S. Healthcare* goes beyond accepting the well-pled complaint rule, which it held was not usurped by the complete preemption exception. In one instance, the Third Circuit appears to permit plaintiffs to recharacterize an ambiguously worded count that the district court had held was completely preempted and had therefore dismissed. There, plaintiffs alleged that the HMO was negligent in "not providing for [an in-home] visit by a participating provider [a pediatric nurse], despite assurances under its L'il Appleseed program that such a visit would be provided and despite a telephone call . . . from the Baumans requesting this service, which the district court interpreted as stating a claim that fits under section 502(a)."

We have no analogous claim by Plaintiffs in the instant case. Our Plaintiffs' complaint nowhere alleges that Plaintiffs requested a service that was denied them. Rather, the gravamen of their complaint is one of failure to diagnose and disclose Mr. Tiemann's medical condition in a timely manner, thus allowing his physical deterioration. Nonetheless, we find it instructive to see the extent to which the Third Circuit went to avoid trumping Plaintiffs' state law causes of action. The Third Circuit declared, "we cannot say that the District Court was unreasonable in so holding [that plaintiffs' claim was completely preempted]" but nonetheless accepted Plaintiffs' interpretation of their complaint. Their interpretation was that the complaint stated a cause of action "for violating a tort duty to provide [plaintiffs] adequate medical care, rather than a violation of a [contractual] promise . . . made to them in their ERISA plan."

The Third Circuit went beyond anything we are called on to do in the instant case, as seen in their discussion:

> The mere fact that [plaintiffs] referred in their complaint to a benefit promised by their health care plan does not automatically convert their state-law negligence claim into a claim for benefits under section 502. If, as [plaintiffs] contend, U.S. Healthcare failed to meet the standard of care required of health care providers by failing to arrange for a pediatric nurse in a timely manner, [this count] sets forth an ordinary state-law tort claim for medical malpractice.

Ours is not even as close a case. Our Plaintiffs aver that they did not know of the actual nature of Mr. Tiemann's illness due to the Defendants' alleged negligence. Thus, Plaintiffs' complaint does not allege that they requested a particular service for which they were subsequently rejected by Moving Defendants.

*U.S. Healthcare* also deals with preemption under ERISA section 514(a). The Third Circuit concludes that it is up to the state court to decide that question, as the district court is without jurisdiction to make such a determination, based on *Dukes*:

> *After it concluded that it had subject matter jurisdiction over Count Six, the District Court dismissed that count as expressly preempted by section 514(a), 29 U.S.C. § 1144(a), on the force of its determination that the count was completely preempted. Inasmuch as we conclude that Count Six was not completely preempted, the District Court did not have subject matter jurisdiction over the complaint and should have remanded it to state court under 28 U.S.C. § 1447©. As we stated in* Dukes, *"when the doctrine of complete preemption does not apply, but the plaintiff's state claim is arguably preempted under 514(a), the district court, being without removal jurisdiction, cannot resolve the dispute regarding preemption."* Dukes, 57 F.3d at 355.

In keeping with this line of cases, we conclude that the Court of Common Pleas shall be the arbiter of this preemption issue.

*List the options open to you. That is, answer the question, "What could you do?"*

- 
- 
- 
- 

*Choose the best solution from an ethical point of view, justify it, and respond to possible criticisms. That is, answer the question, "What should you do, and why?"*

- 
- 
- 
- 

*Select one member of your PBL group to role-play as Robert Tiemann's physician and have another member of your PBL group role-play as Mr. Tiemann. How might the two converse about different ways of thinking and techniques for conflict management?*

- 
- 
- 
-

*Again, please select one member of your PBL group to role-play as
    Mr. Tiemann's physician and have another member of your
    PBL group role-play as his health care administrator. How
    might the physician use what is known about stages of change
    and about motivational interviewing to solve what you
    consider the major problem presented in the case?*

- 
- 
- 
- 

## Part three

For all of the reasons set forth above, Moving Defendants' Motion to Dismiss
will be denied and Plaintiffs' Motion for Remand will be granted in its
entirety. To the extent that we have not dealt directly with those counts in
Moving Defendants' Motion to Dismiss that do not concern ERISA preemption — specifically, failure to exhaust ERISA's mandatory grievance procedure and an ERISA bar against punitive damages — we find that in light of
our analysis regarding ERISA preemption, these counts do not require our
further review. The Motion to Dismiss of the physician–defendants will be
denied as moot. The parties shall bear their own costs. An appropriate order
follows.

## Order

Now, this 11th day of January 2000, on consideration of Defendants' U.S.
Healthcare Systems, Inc. and Corporate Health Administrators Inc.'s Motion
to Dismiss Plaintiffs' Complaint and Memorandum of Law Supporting Their
Motion to Dismiss Plaintiffs' Complaint and Exhibits thereto, filed on
December 2, 1999; Plaintiffs' Response to Defendants U.S. Healthcare Sys-
tems, Inc. and Corporate Health Administrators, Inc.'s Motion to Dismiss
Plaintiffs' Complaint and Memorandum of Law Contra Defendants' Motion
to Dismiss Plaintiffs' Complaint and Exhibits thereto, filed on December 16,
1999; Plaintiffs' Motion for Remand and Application for Sanctions, filed on
December 22, 1999; Motion to Dismiss of Defendants, Evan Kessler, D.O.,
and Anthony G. Wydan, M.D. for Failure to State a Claim Upon Which Relief
Can Be Granted as to Plaintiffs' Claim for Punitive Damages, and Memorandum of Law in Support of Their Motion to Dismiss for Failure to State a
Claim Upon Which Relief Can Be Granted and Exhibits thereto, filed December 29, 1999; and Defendants' U.S. Healthcare Systems, Inc. and Corporate
Health Administrators Inc.'s Reply in Support of Their Motion to Dismiss
Plaintiffs' Complaint and Exhibit thereto, filed on January 6, 2000; it is hereby
ordered consistent with the foregoing Memorandum that:

1. Defendants' Motion to Dismiss, filed December 2, 1999, is denied without prejudice in its entirety.
2. Plaintiffs' Motion for Remand, filed December 22, 1999, is granted; however, the application for sanctions is denied.
3. This matter is remanded to the Court of Common Pleas, Philadelphia County, where the parties shall continue to proceed in the case commenced on June 10, 1999.
4. The Motion to Dismiss of Defendants, Evan Kessler, D.O., and Anthony G. Wydan, M.D., for Failure to State a Claim Upon Which Relief Can Be Granted as to Plaintiffs' Claim for Punitive Damages, filed December 29, 1999, is denied without prejudice as moot.
5. This case is closed.

## Conclusion

The ethical issues of genetic screening are among those that may never be solved. As technology and information become increasingly available, it is important for health professionals to be aware and knowledgeable of these important issues. If health professionals fail to address these items with their patients, their patients will turn to less accurate sources, such as their peers, the Internet, or the media. It is also important for health professionals to address these issues among the various health care disciplines to present united and clear ideas to their patients. While these issues may always remain unsettled to the general public, on an individual level, health professionals can help their patients to address these in an informed, confident manner. Only then can health professionals provide and maintain the best care for their patients and their patients' offspring.

*case nine*

---

# Seriously ill neonates

This problem-based learning session is based on the following: *Tarpeh-Doe v. United States*, Civil Action No. 88-0270-LFO, U.S. District Court for the District of Columbia, 771 F. Supp. 427; 1991 U.S. Dist. Lexis 12843. July 24, 1991, Decided. July 24, 1991, Filed. It is reprinted here with permission of LexisNexis.

## Objectives

The objectives for this problem-based learning case are:

- To determine what ethical issues are involved in prolonging life for seriously ill neonates
- To find what approaches are used in deciding to withdraw or withhold treatment
- To understand who is legally and morally responsible for making treatment decisions
- To determine if there are guidelines decision makers can follow when making treatment decisions

## Introduction

Seriously ill neonates and their treatment are matters of extreme concern for both the physician and the parents, who are the ultimate decision makers. Although this is a very personal and private dilemma, there is much discussion as to the ethical and appropriate treatment decision for the child. There are many different aspects that need to be considered before these difficult decisions are made. They include, but are not limited to, family values, available treatments, and the outcomes that these treatments provide.

## Part one

Plaintiffs Linda Wheeler Tarpeh-Doe and Marilyn Wheeler seek relief for injuries suffered by Nyenpan Tarpeh-Doe pursuant to the Federal Tort Claims Act ("FTCA") [28 U.S.C. §§ 1346(b) and 2671 et seq.]. Tarpeh-Doe is the mother of Nyenpan, an 8-year-old boy who is blind and suffers from severe neurological damage. Nyenpan is a long-term patient and resident at the Wheat Ridge Regional Center in Wheat Ridge, Colorado, where he receives constant and complete care. Marilyn Wheeler, a Colorado resident, is Nyenpan's grandmother and legal guardian.

Linda Wheeler Tarpeh-Doe is employed by the U.S. Agency for International Development (AID). The State Department Office of Medical Services in Washington, D.C., has responsibility for the provision of health care worldwide to employees of the State Department, AID, and other government agencies. With respect to overall medical policy, the Uniform State/AID/USIA Regulations provide that:

> *The general medical policy of the Department of State is to assist all American employees and their dependents in obtaining the best possible medical care. This includes personnel of the Department and all agencies participating in the medical program by agreement. This policy extends to the most remote parts of the world, so that no employee need hesitate to accept an assignment to a post where health conditions are hazardous, medical service poor, or transportation facilities limited. Principal and administrative officers, and their designees, and principal representatives of participating agencies are cautioned to be alert to any medical and health problems of employees and their dependents and to take appropriate action promptly.*

In 1981, AID assigned Tarpeh-Doe to a post in Monrovia, Liberia. At that time, Dr. Theodore E. Lefton was the regional medical officer assigned to the embassy in Monrovia. Dr. Lefton had been stationed in Monrovia for 4 years (two 2-year terms) and was scheduled to remain for an indefinite period. However, in March 1982, a routine State Department inspection at the Monrovian embassy revealed widespread dissatisfaction with Dr. Lefton's attitude and lack of availability. Following the inspection, William Swing, then U.S. Ambassador in Liberia, and Jerome M. Korcak, then Medical Director of the Office of Medical Services at the State Department in Washington, D.C., decided to curtail Dr. Lefton's assignment to Monrovia because of his poor attitude and availability.

Swing preferred curtailing Dr. Lefton's assignment as early as possible. However, Dr. Korcak was reluctant to support that preference and was not overly concerned about Dr. Lefton's provision, or more accurately lack of provision, of medical services. On May 17, 1982, following discussions in late April and early May 1982 (including discussions with Dr. Lefton), Korcak and Swing came to an agreement to permit Dr. Lefton to remain at the post until November 1, 1982. There is no evidence that Dr. Korcak gave any special instructions to Dr. Lefton or placed his service under heightened scrutiny, despite the deficiencies in his services that prompted the decision to terminate his assignment. There is no evidence of any special effort by Dr. Korcak to expedite selection and assignment of either a temporary or a permanent replacement for Dr. Lefton.

On May 18, 1982, while stationed with AID in Monrovia, Linda Wheeler Tarpeh-Doe delivered Nyenpan. Within 3 weeks of birth, the baby contracted a bacterial infection that developed into what was ultimately diagnosed as spinal meningitis. On June 5, 1982, Tarpeh-Doe brought the baby to the health unit at the U.S. embassy in Monrovia. On Saturday, June 5, 1982, Nyenpan was examined at the embassy health clinic by Dr. Lefton, who forthwith referred the mother and child to an American pediatrician, Dr. David E. Van Reken. Dr. Van Reken was employed in Monrovia by an American mission not affiliated with the embassy. The baby remained under Dr. Van Reken's care at local hospitals for the next 12 days. On June 17, 1982, Nyenpan, his parents, and an embassy nurse were evacuated to the United States to enable the family to seek additional medical treatment for Nyenpan. By that time, however, he was beyond hope of recovery.

Plaintiffs claim that the Department of State in Washington, D.C., violated its duty to provide Nyenpan, a dependent of its employee, with the "best possible medical care" and "to be alert to any medical and health problems of . . . dependents and to take appropriate action promptly" as required by the Uniform State/AID/USIA Regulations. Specifically, plaintiffs allege that the following acts or omissions of defendants constituted negligence.

First, plaintiffs assert that the State Department failed to inform Tarpeh-Doe that her health benefits included the option to travel to Europe or the United States to deliver her child. Second, plaintiffs claim that the State Department and its Office of Medical Services, acting concurrently with the ambassador, negligently retained Dr. Lefton even after it learned of the widespread dissatisfaction with the doctor's attitude and availability. In addition, plaintiffs contend that the Office of Medical Services in Washington negligently failed to supervise Dr. Lefton adequately, especially once it was on notice of complaints about his attitude and availability, and that his term had been curtailed at the time he treated Nyenpan. Third, plaintiffs allege that the State Department negligently failed to deliver to Monrovia a message from Dr. Schroeter, a neonatologist in Colorado who had been contacted by Marilyn Wheeler in preparation for evacuation, who felt that it was imperative he speak with the treating physician in Liberia. Finally, plaintiffs claim that the Office of Medical Services in Washington negligently conducted the wrong test on a sample of spinal fluid sent to it from Monrovia for laboratory tests. Plaintiffs contend that defendants' negligence proximately caused Nyenpan's injuries. At a trial held on November 26 through December 4, 1990, the parties produced through testimony and designated deposition transcripts the factual evidence summarized below.

## The inspection

The Inspector General's office of the State Department routinely investigates embassies every 3 to 5 years. In February and March 1982, a team of five or six inspectors from that office visited Monrovia, Liberia, as part of an inspection tour that included visits to four embassies in West Africa. The inspection of the Liberian embassy took place from February 22 to March 5. With respect to health services, the inspectors wrote in their final report:

> *The medical facility is totally inadequate. It is crowded, dingy, and anti-therapeutic, among other shortcomings. . . .*

> *The Medical Unit must also improve its image and responsiveness. The inspectors received numerous complaints about it. Health units should make a positive contribution to morale and welfare, and the unit in Monrovia does the opposite.*

> *Complaints about the quality of official US health services have been so widespread that it may be the single most significant non-environmental negative factor affecting morale at this post.*

When the inspectors returned to Washington, they met to report the results of the inspection with administrators of the Office of Medical Services, including Dr. Jerome Korcak, then medical director. In the debriefing, the inspectors explained to Dr. Korcak and others that employees on post had complained in particular about Dr. Lefton's attitude and availability. On April 6, 1982, soon after returning from the inspection tour, Ambassador John J. Crowley, the leader of the inspection team, visited Dr. John Beahler, then deputy medical director, because he felt on a personal and professional basis that he should inform Beahler of the situation. Crowley told Beahler that, "There is 'widespread' discontent with Dr. Lefton's performance as RMO in Monrovia." On April 27, members of the inspection team met with Dr. Korcak. The team informed Dr. Korcak that "'a majority of personnel' in responses on questionnaires and in spontaneous oral complaints indicated their dissatisfaction with Dr. Lefton's attitude and availability." They told him that, "The magnitude and intensity of the complaints was unprecedented in their experience."

Ambassador Crowley believed that "there was a remarkable level of discontent with the medical officer at this post" compared with other inspections. Crowley (who emphasized that the team was not qualified to evaluate Dr. Lefton's medical competence from a technical standpoint) explained further that the general trend of complaints about Dr. Lefton were his "insensitivity, aloofness, lack of sympathy, lack of . . . bedside manner, and also frequent unavailability." Herbert W. Schultz, a member of the inspection team, also stated that the intensity and magnitude of the complaints about Dr. Lefton's attitude and availability were unprecedented. Schultz believed that the problem was that Dr. Lefton did not care and was not available outside the hours of 8:00 a.m. to 5:00 p.m.

Dr. Lefton was unavailable at times because he traveled out of Liberia for long vacation weekends. He was able to obtain free travel on Pan American Airlines because his wife worked as a flight attendant for Pan Am. Dr. Korcak was aware of these trips because, following these weekends, on Monday mornings, Dr. Lefton would sometimes drop by Dr. Korcak's office in Washington. He did not approve of them.

Moreover, Dr. Korcak and others in the Office of Medical Services were informed by the inspection team and embassy officials of several incidents illustrative of Dr. Lefton's poor attitude and lack of availability that revealed an even more serious adverse effect on medical services. For example, in February or March of 1982, a U.S. Marine was injured in a car accident 30 to 40 miles outside Monrovia. Dr. Lefton was asked to go to the scene of the accident to administer medical care. He refused. Ambassador Swing felt that Dr. Lefton's refusal was unreasonable and ordered Lefton to go to the scene of the accident. In addition, Dr. Lefton refused a request to make a house call to administer care to a sick child on at least one occasion. In another incident, Dr. Lefton failed to accompany an American who suffered from burns to the airport to be evacuated. Ambassador Swing felt this was inappropriate and went to the airport himself to show support. In general, Dr. Lefton was unwilling to respond to urgent situations.

Ambassador Swing was aware of problems with Dr. Lefton even before the inspectors visited. Either he or the Office of Medical Services had proposed curtailing Dr. Lefton's assignment in Monrovia earlier than March 1982. Following the inspection, Ambassador Swing, Dr. Korcak, and Dr. Lefton entered into a series of discussions that led toward the termination of Dr. Lefton's assignment in Monrovia. On April 6, following Beahler's meeting at the Office of Medical Services in Washington with Crowley, at which Crowley reported that the complaints about Dr. Lefton were unprecedented, Beahler called Dr. Lefton, who was also in Washington at the time for training.

Beahler related to Dr. Lefton the complaints Crowley had reported to him. Beahler suggested that Dr. Lefton discuss the situation with Ambassador Swing when he returned to Liberia to try to resolve the problem. He did not instruct Dr. Lefton to make himself more available to his patients in Liberia, and he did not establish reporting requirements to ensure that the Office of Medical Services would be apprised of any serious problem there (see memorandum to the file from Jerome M. Korcak on the subject of

"Complaints Regarding the Performance of Theodore E. Lefton, M.D., Regional Medical Officer, Monrovia" recording Korcak's summary of meetings and telephone calls from April 6, 1982, to April 28, 1982). On April 12, Dr. Lefton sent a letter to Swing acknowledging some of the problems and proposing certain remedies, including a reduction in the time patients were required to wait to be seen at the health unit and improved communications procedures to ensure that Dr. Lefton received messages and that patients could locate him.

On April 16, Korcak in Washington received a telephone call from Swing and Dr. Lefton in Monrovia. First, Korcak was advised by Swing that he and Dr. Lefton had worked out a "gentleman's agreement" that Lefton would be reassigned rather than continue his assignment in Monrovia. Then, Korcak informed Dr. Lefton (who took the phone) that he could be reassigned to Sanaa or Islamabad. Dr. Lefton requested leave without pay for a year. Korcak responded that he could not authorize leave without pay if Lefton had no other reason for it than that he did not want to work in the posts offered. Dr. Lefton said he would have to think about it.

On April 26, Korcak met in Washington with Dr. Lefton (who accompanied an evacuee to the United States). At that time, Korcak was told by Dr. Lefton of his intention to resign because Pan Am did not fly to either of the available posts, so that his wife would not be able visit him if he accepted the assignments offered. Korcak advised Dr. Lefton that if he (Lefton) could persuade Swing to permit him to stay in Monrovia until June 1983, more opportunities for reassignment would be available. Dr. Lefton then spoke in Washington to a Mr. Mandersheim. Mr. Mandersheim called Ambassador Swing to urge a compromise. On April 27, Korcak received a call from Swing, who told him he had spoken with Mr. Mandersheim, and that he understood that Dr. Lefton wanted to revise the gentleman's agreement. Korcak told Swing that the assurances he had given Swing previously that the Office of Medical Services would replace Dr. Lefton promptly had been contingent on Dr. Lefton's acceptance of another assignment. Since Dr. Lefton wanted to resign instead, Korcak did not believe a doctor could be located to replace Dr. Lefton in Monrovia until the following spring, a year away. Ambassador Swing told Korcak he would reconsider his decision.

On the afternoon of April 27, Korcak met with members of the investigation team, who informed him of the widespread complaints about Dr. Lefton. On April 28, Korcak phoned Ambassador Swing and told him that the inspectors' briefing had given him "a greater appreciation for the magnitude of the difficulties associated with Dr. Lefton's tenure at post." Korcak suggested that Swing make Dr. Lefton's continuing assignment contingent on resolution of the difficulties. He assured Swing, however, that if the circumstances continued, the Office of Medical Services would proceed "with all deliberate speed" to find a replacement. Swing responded that this proposal was "the most attractive available to him."

However, on April 30, Ambassador Swing called Korcak again. He stated that, following another meeting with Dr. Lefton, he had "reached the conclusion that Dr. Lefton's reputation at post is sufficiently tarnished that an extension of his tenure beyond September 1982 would be in the interest of neither the post nor Dr. Lefton" (defendants' Exhibit 2). He informed Korcak that he would permit Dr. Lefton to stay until September 1982 because he did not want the post to be without a physician and "because Dr. Lefton [had] requested this time so he could have a visit from his daughter." Swing further informed Korcak that he thought the post could tolerate being without a physician for 2 or 3 months thereafter.

In further telephone conversations, Swing and Korcak reached a compromise that permitted Dr. Lefton to remain in Monrovia until November 1, 1982. Swing confirmed this agreement in writing in a letter to Korcak dated May 17, 1982 (defendants' Exhibit 4). Swing explained that the rationale for this decision was "(a) to give M/MED a reasonable period in which to find a replacement for Dr. Lefton; (b) to meet some of Dr. Lefton's concerns including a visit this summer by one of his children to Liberia; and (c) to provide Monrovia and the other posts in his area of jurisdiction adequate coverage until a replacement can be located and placed." In addition, Swing expressed concern in light of Dr. Lefton's forthcoming departure about additional responsibilities that had been given to Dr. Lefton to provide emergency coverage to Dakar and areas around it when another doctor would be on leave in August (id.).

On June 15, 1982, Korcak wrote a letter to Dr. Lefton in which he again raised the issue of reassignment (see Defendants' Exhibit 5, [partially illegible copy]). On June 16, Korcak wrote to Ambassador Swing and informed him of the letter to Dr. Lefton. He added, in response to Swing's concern about the decision to add coverage of Dakar to Dr. Lefton's responsibilities, that he did not believe that Dr. Lefton's planned departure constituted reason to reconsider that decision (defendants' Exhibit 6; plaintiffs' Exhibit 53 [partially illegible copy]). Korcak further noted that he was under a recent "modified hiring freeze," raising additional concerns about approval of a replacement (id.).

Korcak made several attempts to reassign Dr. Lefton rather than accept his resignation. At no time did Dr. Korcak instruct Dr. Lefton to make himself more available to his patients, to attend more closely to his patients' medical needs, or to report immediately any serious medical situation in Monrovia to the Office of Medical Services. This was true despite the fact that Korcak had "learned over the years that [problems with medical officers] rarely involved medical competence . . . but when we did have problems, it involved physicians' attitudes, what was expected of them."

Korcak's uncritical response to the inspectors' reports of complaints about Dr. Lefton and to Ambassador Swing's dissatisfaction with Lefton's performance is possibly explained by Korcak's otherwise high impression of Dr. Lefton. Throughout the period of discussions, he viewed Dr. Lefton as "very positive and upbeat." When Korcak first received complaints, he was not overly concerned because he knew Dr. Lefton as a "bright young physician who was astute and competent." He had "admired his acumen" in annual medical meetings. Korcak thought many of the complaints at post about Dr. Lefton following Dr. Lefton's difficult divorce and remarriage came from persons at post who were sympathetic to Lefton's first wife. As a result of considerations such as these, it did not occur to Korcak or others in the Office of Medical Services to reprimand Dr. Lefton or to establish a plan for additional medical advice, support, and supervision in the event of a serious medical situation that might (and was more likely to) occur given Dr. Lefton's poor attitude and lack of availability.

## The injury

In September 1980, Linda Wheeler Tarpeh-Doe (then Linda Wheeler) became a certified public accountant (CPA). Her parents were also CPAs. She was then 23 years old. She applied for and was awarded a position as an accountant with AID. AID assigned her, for her first overseas station, to Monrovia, Liberia. On December 29, 1980, in preparation for her assignment, she began approximately 5 months of training in Washington, D.C.

On May 26, 1980, Linda Wheeler left the United States. She arrived in Monrovia on May 27. The next day, she began her first day of work at the Comptroller's Office of the AID mission there.

In July 1981, she developed gynecological problems. On the morning of July 7, 1981, she visited the health unit at the embassy. Either Dr. Lefton or Billie Clement, the State Department nurse stationed at the embassy health unit, told her that the embassy health unit did not treat gynecological conditions and referred her for treatment to Dr. Johnson, a local obstetrician and gynecologist. Clement called Dr. Johnson and arranged an appointment for Wheeler later that morning. Linda Wheeler visited Dr. Johnson on July 7 and 8, again on August 1 and 20, and on September 2, 1981. On September 9, 1981, she visited Dr. Kassas, another local doctor, to obtain a pregnancy test. The results were positive.

She had been referred to Dr. Kassas by Nyenpan (Ben) Tarpeh-Doe, an employee of the Liberian Ministry of Justice, whom she had met on her first day in Monrovia. She visited with Ben almost daily thereafter for several months. On July 12, Ben had asked her to marry him. On September 16 and 21, Ben and Linda visited the embassy health unit so that Ben could receive a physical examination and other tests required for their marriage. On January 16, 1982, Linda Wheeler and Ben Tarpeh-Doe were married. During one of the September visits to the embassy health clinic, Linda told Dr. Lefton that she was pregnant. Dr. Lefton normally referred patients to other doctors for prenatal care, but would also see a pregnant woman periodically to assure himself that things were well. However, he scheduled no such subsequent visit for Tarpeh-Doe and did not see her again until June 4, 1982, after she had delivered her baby.

Tarpeh-Doe visited Dr. Johnson for prenatal care throughout her pregnancy, which was easy and without complications. On May 18, 1982, Tarpeh-Doe delivered Nyenpan. Her delivery, attended by Dr. Johnson at

Cooper's Clinic (a local health facility unassociated with the embassy), was also complication free. On May 21, she was released from the clinic to return to her home in Monrovia.

She visited Dr. Johnson on May 23 when the baby's umbilical cord dropped and again on May 24 because the baby had thrush. On May 25, Dr. Johnson examined Tarpeh-Doe and found her to be well. On May 29, Dr. Johnson examined Nyenpan and found him to be well also. On the morning of Wednesday, June 2, Dr. Johnson again examined both mother and child. He found no sign of problems. That evening, however, according to Tarpeh-Doe's calendar notation, she became "sick with malaria."

The next day, Thursday, June 3, she still did not feel well. She was visited by Kate Jones Petrone. Petrone was a friend who lived in the same building. She was also employed by AID and had begun her first assignment overseas in May 1981, at the same time as Tarpeh-Doe. That evening, Petrone called the embassy health unit to ask that someone be sent to examine Tarpeh-Doe. In response, a Dr. Feir came to the Tarpeh-Does's apartment at approximately 10:00 p.m. He was the State Department psychiatrist assigned to the Liberian embassy (but did not live at the embassy). Nurse Billie Clement also came because Dr. Feir wanted a woman to be present. Dr. Lefton (who lived at the embassy) was unavailable; Clement could not recall why.

Clement found Linda in bed and Ben holding the child. Petrone recalled that Clement looked at the baby and said that she did not think the baby looked right. However, Clement did not recall examining the child. Dr. Feir gave Linda a limited examination without being able to examine, diagnose, and treat her fully. He suggested that she try to find Dr. Johnson that night and come to see Dr. Lefton at the embassy health unit the next morning. Ben located Dr. Johnson, who visited the apartment at about 1:00 a.m. on Friday, June 4. Dr. Johnson examined Linda and treated her for malaria, staphylococcal (staph) infection, and mastitis. He did not examine the baby, who was sleeping.

Later that Friday morning, Tarpeh-Doe visited the embassy health unit. There is a conflict of testimony as to whether she brought the baby with her. Dr. Lefton treated her with ampicillin for mastitis. Tarpeh-Doe had not been breast-feeding while she was ill. Nevertheless, Dr. Lefton advised her to resume breast-feeding. Dr. Lefton was not aware at that time that Feir and Clement had visited Tarpeh-Doe the night before, but had not examined the baby. There is no indication that he inquired into the condition of the baby or offered to see him.

Later that Friday, the baby was lethargic and was not feeding. At 5:00 p.m. that Friday evening, his parents took him to an emergency facility at Cooper's Clinic, where Dr. Tirad, a local physician, treated him with ampicillin for skin rash and fever. The baby did not improve, however. At 8:00 p.m. the same evening, his parents took him to the emergency room at the Catholic Hospital in Monrovia. There, two local doctors examined him and treated him with an electrolyte solution for dehydration. He was not admitted at either facility and returned home with his parents. He slept through the night, which he had never done before.

At 9:00 a.m. on Saturday morning, June 5, Tarpeh-Doe woke Nyenpan to try to feed him. The baby "became rigid" in her arms for 1 to 2 seconds, and the Tarpeh-Does left to take him to see Dr. Johnson in his office. On their way to Dr. Johnson's office, they passed Clement. Clement expressed surprise that Tarpeh-Doe was not home in bed due to her illness. When she heard that the baby was ill and that the parents were proceeding on their way to Dr. Johnson's office, Clement advised them to accompany her to the embassy health unit instead (testimony of Tarpeh-Doe). The four of them arrived at the embassy health unit at about 10:30 a.m. On the way, Nyenpan suffered a second period of rigidity or seizure.

Once there, Clement went to find Dr. Lefton. Within 5 minutes, Dr. Lefton arrived. He examined the baby, who experienced a third seizure at the clinic. Dr. Lefton administered gentamicin and procaine penicillin. He informed the parents that the child could be evacuated on a Pan Am flight scheduled to leave that evening at 11:00 p.m. Then, Dr. Lefton sent Mary Awantang, the State Department lab technician assigned to the Liberian embassy health unit, to find Dr. Van Reken, a pediatrician, and bring him to the clinic to examine the baby. Dr. Lefton had never referred a patient to Dr. Van Reken previously. A pediatrician to whom he had referred patients in the past was out of town on June 5.

When Awantang located Dr. Van Reken, he was lecturing to medical students. He left the lecture and came to the embassy, arriving at approximately 11:30 a.m. Dr. Van Reken, Dr. Lefton, and the other medical personnel took Nyenpan into an examining room. After examining the baby, the doctors informed the Tarpeh-Does that their son had spinal meningitis. Dr. Van Reken said that he could "make the baby well." The Tarpeh-Does expressed their preference for evacuation to the United States.

In an attempt to dissuade them, Dr. Van Reken told them of an Indian family whose child had contracted spinal meningitis. That family had flown to India for treatment. However, on returning, they informed Van Reken of the treatment given there. It was the same treatment Van Reken would have provided in Liberia had they stayed. The Tarpeh-Does still preferred evacuation. There is no indication that Drs. Lefton and Van Reken determined that evacuation would have been more risky than treatment in Monrovia.

Nonetheless, Dr. Lefton decided not to permit the parents to evacuate. Instead, he transferred the care of the child to Dr. Van Reken. Dr. Van Reken was the head of the pediatric ward at John F. Kennedy (JFK) Hospital in Monrovia and told the Tarpeh-Does that he wanted to admit the child there. Dr. Lefton had never sent a patient to JFK Hospital and was not familiar with its facilities or conditions. However, Ben Tarpeh-Doe, in his reporting work for a newspaper issued by the Liberian Ministry of Justice, had researched conditions at various Monrovian hospitals. The Tarpeh-Does informed the doctors that Ben had found that the conditions at JFK Hospital were appalling. The Tarpeh-Does vehemently opposed placement of their child in JFK Hospital, noting to the doctors that the hospital was known popularly as "Just for Killing."

Over the parents' objections, and with the knowledge and concurrence of Dr. Lefton, the baby was taken to JFK Hospital by the parents, accompanied by Dr. Van Reken and Clement. They arrived at about 12:00 noon. The hospital did not place him in a room until 1:30 p.m. During that hour and a half, the parents continued to express to Dr. Van Reken their objections to admitting their child to JFK Hospital. Once the baby was given a room, Dr. Van Reken left the hospital to deliver a speech. Clement also left after the baby was admitted to a room.

On Dr. Van Reken's instructions, Ben Tarpeh-Doe went to a local pharmacy to purchase certain prescriptions not available at the hospital. At 4:00 p.m., Dr. Van Reken returned and left instructions for administration of care during the night, such as when to administer various medications. Tarpeh-Doe stayed through the night accompanied by several friends, including Petrone; Charlene Fergusen, a nurse; and Welma Witten, a doctor. The spouses of Fergusen and Dr. Witten were on contract with or employed by AID.

The conditions at JFK Hospital were unsanitary. There were small cockroaches inside the baby's incubator that came out in large numbers when the heating unit in the incubator was turned on. There were also large cockroaches in the room and rats present both inside and outside the room (testimony of Tarpeh-Doe).

During the night of June 5–6, neither Dr. Van Reken nor Dr. Lefton visited the baby at JFK Hospital. Moreover, no hospital doctor could be located at crucial times during the night. Medical records from JFK Hospital indicate that the infant was treated by a Dr. Waiwaiku at 7:30 p.m., 9:00 p.m., and 6:30 a.m. Dr. Lefton did not know Dr. Waiwaiku or whether he was a resident or an intern. When the times came during the night to administer medicine as specified earlier by Dr. Van Reken, Tarpeh-Doe and her friends could not find any doctor in the hospital or any other person authorized to administer the medicines.

During the night, Nyenpan developed a fever and suffered more seizures. Dr. Witten felt that he should be on oxygen. Tarpeh-Doe and her friends asked the hospital employees for oxygen, but they were informed that the hospital had only one unit, and that unit was in use. They called the embassy to ask to use an oxygen unit. Someone there informed them that the embassy had no oxygen unit. When Tarpeh-Doe and her friends were unable to locate any other doctor or a nurse during the night, Dr. Witten, concerned about a particularly bad seizure, administered Valium.

Late the next morning, Sunday, June 6, Dr. Van Reken arrived at JFK Hospital. Tarpeh-Doe and her friends told Dr. Van Reken that they wanted Nyenpan transferred to another hospital. Dr. Van Reken at first refused. However, at the insistence of Tarpeh-Doe and her friends, especially Dr. Witten and Fergusen, he ultimately relented. But, he asked the Tarpeh-Does not to put anything in writing about the conditions at JFK Hospital. He also requested that they leave at the hospital the prescriptions they had purchased the previous evening and not used. Early that afternoon, Nyenpan was transferred to the ELWA hospital.

The conditions at ELWA were better than those at JFK Hospital. The facilities were cleaner, and the nurses were more attentive. The hospital had access to more medications. A private nurse was hired to attend the baby every night from 10:00 p.m. to 6:00 a.m. While Nyenpan was a patient at ELWA, Dr. Van Reken visited him daily. In addition, Ben Tarpeh-Doe was acquainted with a doctor at ELWA who was able to help them at times when they could not find other doctors. Dr. Lefton finally visited Tarpeh-Doe and Nyenpan at ELWA, but only once. He examined the mother, but not the baby. Ambassador Swing also visited them.

Nyenpan did not improve at ELWA. He continued to suffer periodically from seizures. His temperature did not remain constant. The doctors altered the dosage and mix of medications several times. The Tarpeh-Does discussed Nyenpan's condition with Dr. Van Reken, only to be informed that he did not know what was wrong or what was causing the meningitis. The Tarpeh-Does continually asserted their preference for evacuation and offered to pay the cost of evacuation if necessary. After a few days at ELWA, Dr. Van Reken agreed that the child should be evacuated and offered to accompany the child if necessary. Nonetheless, the evacuation was not authorized until June 17. On June 17, Nyenpan, the Tarpeh-Does, and Clement flew from Liberia to Colorado, by way of Dakar and New York. On arrival in Colorado, Nyenpan was admitted into the University of Colorado hospital.

Nyenpan was treated at the University of Colorado hospital for approximately 2 weeks. Doctors informed the Tarpeh-Does that their child had suffered severe brain damage. Toward the end of Nyenpan's stay at the University of Colorado hospital, the doctors asked the Tarpeh-Does whether they wanted the hospital to remove life support systems. The doctors believed that the child would die within 24 hours without life support. Nyenpan's parents agreed to the removal of life support, and feeding and other tubes were removed. Defying the doctors' predictions, Nyenpan survived. Three or four days later, on July 3, 1982, the Tarpeh-Does took Nyenpan to Marilyn Wheeler's home.

On July 25, 1982, AID assigned Tarpeh-Doe to work in its Washington, D.C., office. Nyenpan lived with her in Washington. He received daily therapy at the Hospital for Sick Children and was admitted at times to Children's Hospital. He continued to suffer from seizures. Dr. Adrian Smith, a neurologist who treated Nyenpan at Children's Hospital during that time, described his condition as spastic and noncommunicative. She also stated that he was incapable of meaningful motor movements and unable to feed himself. She believed that he was blind, but that there was some brain stem activity with respect to hearing. She testified that the damage was permanent, and that she was doubtful that there would be any improvement.

After Tarpeh-Doe had worked in Washington for more than a year, AID informed her that she would have to take another overseas assignment. To work overseas, an employee and dependents must be granted medical clearance (i.e., examined and found medically qualified) for a post. Nyenpan was not granted medical clearance. The family made arrangements for him to be admitted in December 1983 to the Wheat Ridge Regional Center in Colorado. To provide assistance for Nyenpan, the state of Colorado required that he have a resident guardian. Just before he was admitted to Wheat Ridge, Marilyn Wheeler became his legal guardian. On April 1, 1984, Linda Wheeler Tarpeh-Doe accepted an assignment with AID in Jamaica.

At Wheat Ridge, where Nyenpan remains and will remain for the foreseeable future, Nyenpan receives extensive care. He has no independent skills. He has no functional control over his arms and legs, although he can move them. He is blind. He continues to have 10 to 12 seizures a year. Care providers feed and dress him. They also turn him every hour or two to prevent skin breakdown. In addition, they sometimes give him baths or massages, read him stories, or take him outside in a wheelchair. He does not communicate in any meaningful way, but responds positively to the care providers who are familiar to him.

## *The treatment*

Plaintiffs allege that Drs. Lefton and Van Reken misdiagnosed and mistreated Nyenpan's illness in Monrovia. Specifically, they claim that Dr. Lefton's administration of antibiotics at the embassy health clinic on June 5, prior to any testing, masked accurate results in subsequent tests. They also argue that Nyenpan could have been evacuated immediately, and that he should have been evacuated sooner than June 17. Defendants argue that the doctors' actions did not fall below the standard of care. At trial, the parties produced extensive evidence in support of their positions. This evidence, summarized below, is relevant only to the degree that it relates to the issue of whether there was a causal link between the State Department's acts and omissions in Washington, D.C., and Nyenpan's injuries.

The medical experts who testified at trial agreed that Nyenpan's brain damage was caused by spinal meningitis, an infection of the meninges covering the spinal cord and brain. They suspected bacterial, rather than viral, meningitis. Bacterial meningitis can have a devastating effect very quickly in neonates (as it apparently did in Nyenpan's case). To identify the bacterial agent, the cerebrospinal fluid (CSF) of a patient, obtained by spinal tap or lumbar puncture, is cultured. Cultures of other samples can also aid in diagnosis.

However, neither Nyenpan's doctors nor the expert witnesses could identify with certainty the bacterial agent causing his meningitis — despite three CSF cultures, cultures of blood and other body fluids, and examination of other indicators, such as white blood cells (WBCs); glucose, potassium, and sodium analyses; and temperature levels. Using the diagnoses of the various treating physicians and laboratory reports, the experts identified three possible agents: staph, streptococcus (strep), and salmonella, all of which are endemic to western Africa. Staph and strep are "Gram-positive" bacteria; that is, they react in a particular way to a Gram stain. Salmonella, on the other hand, is a Gram-negative bacterium. Gram-positive and Gram-negative bacteria are treated with different antibiotics.

On June 5, when Nyenpan was first brought to the embassy health unit, Drs. Lefton and Van Reken, assisted by Clement and Awantang, took blood and stool cultures and a culture of fluid from skin lesions. In addition, Dr. Van Reken performed a lumbar puncture to obtain a CSF sample for testing. A smear of the CSF performed that morning revealed WBCs and two rare Gram-positive cocci on the stain of the CSF sample. That result was unusual, and left the medical personnel uncomfortable since, if the baby had meningitis, the stain should have evidenced numerous bacteria. However, the presence of WBCs indicated meningitis even without strong evidence of a bacterial agent. A Gram stain of the skin fluid showed "few gram positive cocci and many WBCs."

After overnight culture, the CSF sample taken at the embassy health clinic on June 5 was sterile, although it had revealed two rare Gram-positive cocci on smear the day before. In contrast, fluid taken from the skin lesions, after culture overnight, demonstrated heavy growth of Gram-positive cocci, which was later revealed to be staph. Stool cultures revealed a similar form of staph. No malarial parasites were found. Dr. Van Reken diagnosed and treated Nyenpan for "Group B" strep, a Gram-positive meningitis.

On June 10, blood and CSF tests were repeated at ELWA. Cultures of those tests were also sterile. Dr. Van Reken requested that Mary Awantang send a portion of the CSF sample obtained on June 10 to the State Department Office of Medical Services to obtain a counter immunoelectrophoresis (CIE) test. This test reveals specific antibodies and could have aided the doctors in detecting salmonella if present. However, instead of conducting a CIE test, the State Department in error sent the sample to a laboratory in Washington, D.C., accompanied by a request for an immunoelectrophoresis test, which is used to detect multiple sclerosis. When Nyenpan reached the University of Colorado hospital, blood, urine, and CSF cultures were repeated for a third time. The blood tests revealed salmonella. The other cultures were sterile. Accordingly, Nyenpan was treated in Colorado for salmonella sepsis, a blood infection.

Dr. Adrian Smith and Dr. Edward Gross, plaintiffs' experts, expressed the opinion that Nyenpan suffered from salmonella meningitis that Drs. Lefton and Van Reken failed to diagnose and treat. In support, they noted that a bacterial agent causing sepsis can cross the "blood/brain barrier" and lead to meningitis more readily than a bacterial agent causing a skin infection. Drs. Raoul L. Wientzen and Marianne Schuelein, defendants' experts, believed that Nyenpan's meningitis was caused by Gram-positive bacteria. Like Dr. Van Reken, Drs. Wientzen and Schuelein believed that the causative bacteria were Group B strep, even though strep was never cultured from any sample, and skin and stool cultures had revealed staph.

Defendants contend that Dr. Lefton was not responsible for Nyenpan's injuries because the child was already devastated and beyond hope of recovery when his parents brought him to the embassy health unit on June 5. Dr. Lefton had believed that when the child was brought to the embassy health unit on June 5, he was neurologically and physiologically intact. The experts offered conflicting views on the question of when Nyenpan was beyond hope of recovery.

Dr. Wientzen, whose expert testimony overall was highly persuasive, offered two answers to this question. When first asked whether Nyenpan was beyond hope of recovery at the embassy health clinic, Dr. Wientzen testified that he was beyond hope some time during the middle of the first hospital day (i.e., June 6). When asked again, though, he changed his opinion and stated that he believed the baby was beyond hope on June 5. However, he also testified that many people with the symptoms Nyenpan had on June 5 recover to lead a normal life. Dr. Gross believed that when Nyenpan was brought to the clinic, there was no permanent structural damage to the brain. He testified that, more likely than not, had the baby been treated aggressively for Gram-negative meningitis, he would have recovered. He believed the baby became devastated some time between June 5 and June 17, and he was not sure when. Dr. Schuelein believed that Nyenpan was devastated by the time he arrived at the embassy health unit.

The experts' conflicting opinions on this point suggest that it is very difficult, if not impossible, to pinpoint with certainty the earliest time at which Nyenpan was beyond hope of recovery. Nevertheless, appraisal of the testimony indicates that it is more likely that Nyenpan was beyond hope of recovery at least by the time of or shortly after his transfer to ELWA on June 6. Therefore, the critical time period for administering proper care was between June 3 and June 6.

On June 5, 1982, when Dr. Lefton first examined Nyenpan and before Dr. Van Reken arrived, Lefton promptly administered procaine penicillin and gentamicin before taking any samples for culture, such as from the blood, skin pustule, urine, or stool. Dr. Lefton also did not record any pulse or respiratory readings prior to administering antibiotics. Plaintiffs contend that the antibiotics took effect so quickly that the samples obtained by Dr. Van Reken 1 hour later were sterile.

The experts agreed that it would be below the standard of care not to obtain body fluid and other samples when possible prior to the administration of antibiotics. Nonetheless, treatment of Gram-positive bacteria leads almost immediately to sterilization of CSF cultures, while treatment of Gram-negative bacteria does not cause sterilization of CSF cultures for 1 to 11 days. Thus, it is unlikely that the medications administered by Dr. Lefton masked detection of Gram-negative bacteria in the CSF smear obtained on June 5 in the hour or so that elapsed between administration and the lumbar puncture. On the other hand, it is probable that the June 4 administration of ampicillin by Dr. Tirad at Cooper's Clinic along with Dr. Lefton's administration of procaine penicillin and gentamicin on June 5 masked detection of strep, staph, or other Gram-positive bacteria on June 5. Dr. Van Reken diagnosed Gram-positive meningitis and treated Nyenpan accordingly;

therefore, any masking effect of Gram-positive bacteria had little or no impact on the diagnosis and treatment.

Plaintiffs further argue that the decision not to evacuate Nyenpan on June 5 was below the standard of care. Dr. Lefton stated that he did not want to evacuate the baby because of the risk of lack of oxygen on the plane while the baby was having a seizure. He clarified that intubation (insertion of a tracheal tube) during a seizure would be more difficult in a plane. However, he also stated that he was not aware that there would be no oxygen available at JFK Hospital.

Dr. Gross testified that the technology and procedures that would have been required for evacuation on June 5 were no different from those that were in fact employed or available on June 17, namely, intubation, suction, intravenous feeding, and oxygen. Dr. Wientzen testified that intubation is easier in a hospital, that lighting is better, and that shock and respiratory failure could have caused problems on an airplane. However, he did not state that it would have been dangerous to move Nyenpan on June 5. He testified that, within a 48- to 72-hour period from when the parents presented Nyenpan at the embassy health clinic, there was no reason not to evacuate the baby. Dr. Schuelein testified that the baby should not have been evacuated due to the risk of continued seizures and status epilepticus, which might require administration of anticonvulsants. Nyenpan continued to suffer from seizures up to and following June 17.

Plaintiffs also contend that if Dr. Lefton felt that commercial evacuation was too dangerous, he could have requested the services of a Military Airlift Command (MAC) plane. MAC planes are specially equipped with medical equipment and personnel for transportation of severely ill or injured patients. State Department policies permit a regional medical officer to request MAC services when there is (1) an immediate threat to life, (2) no adequate local facility, and (3) no other available suitable transportation. The Air Force retains the discretion whether to grant a request for an MAC plane. According to Goff, if Dr. Lefton had requested MAC services to evacuate Nyenpan, that request would have been supported by the State Department. Dr. Lefton made no such request.

In addition, plaintiffs contend that Nyenpan could have been evacuated sooner than June 17. The Tarpeh-Does continually requested evacuation and offered to pay for it. Within a few days of Nyenpan's admission into ELWA, Dr. Van Reken advocated evacuation and offered to accompany the child. However, Dr. Lefton retained the final authority to approve evacuation, despite his withdrawal from decisions about Nyenpan's medical care. Defendants produced no evidence explaining or otherwise giving any reason why Dr. Lefton waited until June 17 to approve evacuation. It is more likely than not that, even if Nyenpan could not have been evacuated on June 5, he could have been evacuated much earlier than June 17. However, because he was probably beyond hope of recovery earlier than June 17, and perhaps as early as June 6, the failure of defendants to evacuate him between June 6 and June 17 did not cause his injuries.

## Make a list of the major problems presented in this case

- 
- 
- 
- 

## Hypothesis and mechanism

For the problems in your list above, give a cause or a reason for them to happen:

- 
- 
- 
- 

## Learning issues

Make a list of learning issues in the form of questions. Remember, your goal is to gather the medical, social, and all other relevant facts that may apply to the case.

The primary function of medicine for seriously ill neonates is sustaining life without prolonging the dying process. Providing life-sustaining treatment should be automatic unless what?
1. There is irreversible progression to imminent death.
2. The treatment is clearly ineffective or harmful.
3. Treatment causes more harm than good.
4. Their lives will be certainly filled with pain and suffering.

What should the child receive if the nontreatment option is selected?
1. The child should receive the best care, compassion, and support possible.
2. This care should include warmth, physical and social comfort, enteric feeding, hydration, and pain control.
3. The use of analgesics and sedatives to induce death or speed the dying process is unacceptable.

What should be considered in decisions promoting the well-being of the infant?
1. The infant must be protected from harm and well-being promoted.
2. Fairness must be used in terms of respecting the patient's or the family's values and their treatment decisions for the infant.

What are the different appraoches that different countries take in the face of uncertainty regarding end-of-life treatment decisions for seriously ill neonates?

1.  Statistical approach (Sweden): when statistical data suggest a grim prognosis, treatment of the neonate is withheld.
2.  Individualized approach (England): treatment is begun, but is withdrawn in the face of a deteriorating clinical situation.
3.  Waiting for near certainty (United States): treatment is initiated and continued until it is virtually certain the infant will die.

Ultimately, parents of the seriously ill neonate are morally and legally responsible for treatment decisions, with the best interests of the child in mind. This is considered true unless what?

1.  The parents are incompetent and cannot make decisions for themselves.
2.  The parents cannot resolve their differences.
3.  The parents do not claim responsibility for the child.
4.  The legal guardian is responsible if the parents are separated.

When the physician believes the treatment is in the best interest of the child, the physician must ensure the parents of the seriously ill neonate understand this. What if the parents disagree with the physician?

It is recommended that an ethics advisory committee get involved when there is a disagreement between parents and physicians or between health care professionals regarding treatment decisions.

What are the suggested guidelines for ethical decision making regarding the treatment of seriously ill neonates?

1.  Identify the decision makers. Do the parents have the capacity to make a decision? Who are the involved clinicians?
2.  Gather the relevant medical facts. What is the diagnosis? Prognosis? Are any further tests necessary? Is there necessary information from other clinicians?
3.  Solicit value data from all involved parties. Are there conflicts among values? Has the basis for the conflicts been identified?
4.  Define the available treatment options. For each option, what is the likelihood of cure or amelioration? What are the risks of an adverse effect? What is the minimum level of professionally acceptable treatment?
5.  Evaluate the possible treatment options and make a recommendation. The choice needs to be justified according to the values of various parties.
6.  Achieve a consensus resolution. Have all parties articulated their viewpoints? Would more factual information help resolve any disputes? Would a mediator (ethics consultant or ethics committee) be helpful?

## Literature review

To help you get ready to answer certain questions you anticipate being asked during the second part of the case, look in the local medical library and on the World Wide Web for helpful information. Please indicate in the spaces below (1) several helpful articles or books you found and (2) several helpful Web sites you found.

- **Helpful articles/books:**
  Catlin, A.J. and Carter, B.S., Resuscitation of marginally viable neonates, *Cambridge Q. Healthc. Ethics*, 9, 400–403, 2000.
  Glover, J.J. and Caniano, D.A., Ethical issues in treating infants with very low birth weight, *Semin. Pediatr. Surg.*, 9, 56–62, 2000.
  Hefferman, P. and Heilig, S., Giving "moral distress" a voice: ethical concerns among neonatal intensive care unit personnel, *Cambridge Q. Healthc. Ethics*, 8, 173–178, 2000.
  Jain, R. and Thomasma, D.C., Discontinuing life support in an infant of a drug-addicted mother: whose decision is it? *Cambridge Q. Healthc. Ethics*, 6, 48–54, 1997.
  Jain, R., Thomasma, D.C., and Ragas, R., Points of variance, *Cambridge Q. Healthc. Ethics*, 7, 94–96, 1998.
  Jain, R., Thomasma, D.C., and Ragas, R., Ethical challenges on the treatment of infants of drug-abusing mother, *Cambridge Q. Healthc. Ethics*, 8, 179–188, 1999.
  Muraskas, J. et al., Neonatal viability in the 1990's: held hostage by technology, *Cambridge Q. Healthc. Ethics*, 8, 160–172, 1999.
  Oberman, M., Response to ethics and drug infants by Renu Jain and David C. Thomasma (*CQ* Vol. 6, No. 1), *Cambridge Q. Healthc. Ethics*, 6, 235–239, 1997.
  Schneiderman, L.J. and Manning, S., The baby K case: a search for the elusive standard of medical care, *Cambridge Q. Healthc. Ethics*, 6, 9–18, 1997.

- **Helpful Web sites:**
  Canadian Pediatric Society: www.cps.ca
  University of Alberta — John Dossetor Health Ethics Center: www.ualberta.ca/BIOETHICS

## *Identify all relevant values that play a role in the case and determine which values, if any, conflict*

Nonmaleficence:

Beneficence:

Respect for persons:

Loyalty:

Distributive justice:

## Learning issues for next student-centered problem-based learning session

- List the options open to you. That is, answer the question, "What could you do?"
- Choose the best solution from an ethical point of view, justify it, and respond to possible criticisms. That is, answer the question, "What should you do, and why?"
- What are the different ways of thinking about the problem? Which conflict management techniques can be used in the situation?

## Part two

### The State Department's role

#### State Department policy

Plaintiffs allege that the Department of State in Washington, D.C., failed to provide the level of medical care promised in its policy manuals. The Uniform State/AID/USIA Regulations establish medical policies, benefits, and procedures for both employees and regional medical officers such as Dr. Lefton in the field as well as in the Office of Medical Services (also referred to as M/MED) and other organizations in the United States. As noted, the Uniform State/AID/USIA Regulations provide that the State Department's general policy is "to assist all American employees and their dependents in obtaining the best possible medical care . . . so that no employee need hesitate to accept an assignment to a post where health conditions are hazardous, medical service poor, or transportation facilities limited" (3 FAM § 681.2.; plaintiffs' Exhibit 59). The medical director of the Office of Medical Services in Washington is responsible for directing, managing, and supervising the medical and health program and operations, see 3 FAM § 681.6(j), plaintiffs' Exhibit 35, (effective June 16, 1972); § 681.6(k) (effective March 11, 1985), plaintiffs' Exhibit 59.

The State Department provides regional medical officers as a benefit of employment in locations where local medical services are poor because it would be difficult to find people to serve in many areas of the world without medical support. In 1982, the department employed 39 regional medical officers (not including psychiatrists). In addition to their responsibility for the provision of "medical care, counsel and examinations for American employees and their dependents" [§ 682.2–2(a)(1)], medical officers must "maintain liaison with Post Medical Advisors, local physicians, hospitals, laboratories, and public health officials on matters pertinent to the Department of State medical program" [§ 682.2–2(a)(3)].

Officials of the Office of Medical Services claim that it is impractical, if not impossible, for the office in Washington, D.C., to supervise the daily activities of regional medical officers in the field (testimony of Korcak, Goff). Nonetheless, regional medical officers normally consult the Office of Medical Services for cases involving serious medical problems. Indeed, the Uniform State/AID/USIA Regulations require such consultation: "The Department of State principal officer, medical officer, or nurse, will report telegraphically by 'MED CHANNEL' . . . to the Deputy Assistant Secretary for Medical Services (M/MED) each serious illness or injury of employees or their dependents" (3 FAM § 682.2–682.8). The regulations further provide: "The advice of a Department of State medical officer or the Office of Medical Services (M/MED) may be requested at any time. It should be obtained in all cases where there is doubt as to the need for the treatment recommended by another physician."

Moreover, regional medical officers generally obtain approval from the Office of Medical Services for evacuations. Thus, the Uniform State/AID/USIA Regulations provide:

> *Eligible American employees or dependents who are unable to obtain suitable medical care abroad for an overseas-incurred illness or injury may be authorized by the post to receive medical care in U.S. facilities. . . . In such cases, the post shall telegraph in advance via "MED CHANNEL" . . . to give the diagnosis and to request instructions from the Deputy Assistant Secretary for Medical Services (O/MED). In emergency situations where the well-being of the employee precludes prior consultation with O/MED, the delegated officer at post . . . may authorize travel to Washington, D.C.,*

*but shall immediately inform O/MED the reason for the*
*evacuation, give the date and mode of arrival, and request*
*that arrangements for hospitalization be made.*

(id. at § 685.4–2). Finally, the regulations provide that:

*any American Foreign Service employee or any of his de-*
*pendents . . . who require medical care for illness or injury*
*. . . while located or stationed abroad and there is no qualified*
*person or facility to provide such care . . . shall be eligible*
*to travel at Government expense to the nearest facility where*
*suitable care can be obtained, whether or not the medical*
*care is at Government expense.*

(3 FAM § 686.1). The Regulations thus demonstrate that, [**50] even though
the Office of Medical Services is unable practically to supervise the
day-to-day decisions of regional medical officers in the field, the office
strongly requires, or at least recommends and strongly supports, close communications during medical emergencies.


### State Department actions

Despite the regulations described above, the Office of Medical Services had
very little contact between June 5 and June 17, 1982, with Dr. Lefton or
anyone else in Monrovia regarding Nyenpan Tarpeh-Doe's illness. On June
5, when the Tarpeh-Does first brought Nyenpan to the embassy health unit
and Dr. Van Reken discussed evacuation with them, Tarpeh-Doe requested
that Petrone contact Tarpeh-Doe's mother, Marilyn Wheeler, to attempt to
arrange a receiving physician for the evacuation. On the afternoon of June
5, Petrone phoned Wheeler, informed her that Nyenpan was seriously ill,
and asked her to find a receiving physician in Colorado for Nyenpan's
evacuation.

On June 5 or 6, Wheeler located a neonatologist at the University of
Colorado, Dr. Gerhardt Schroeter, who agreed to serve as receiving physician. Dr. Schroeter told Wheeler that he thought it was essential that he speak
to the attending physician in Liberia as soon as possible. Wheeler was unable
to phone Liberia directly, so on Saturday or Sunday, June 5 or 6, she contacted
the State Department in Washington, using a list of telephone numbers given
to her by her daughter. She first called a medical emergency number. The
person who answered that call referred her to the Liberian desk. She
informed a person there that she had received a call about the evacuation
and been asked to locate a receiving doctor and hospital. She identified the
doctor and hospital and relayed the message that Dr. Schroeter thought it
was imperative that he speak with the attending physician. She was told
that they were not aware of the planned evacuation. At some point, she was
told they had sent a cable, but that the telephone was not working. Wheeler

did not receive a copy of the cable and did not hear again from the State Department until she received notice of the June 17 evacuation. Then, she again contacted Dr. Schroeter and arranged for an ambulance to meet the arriving family at the Denver airport.

In response to Marilyn Wheeler's June 5 or 6 telephone message to the State Department that she had arranged for a receiving physician in preparation for evacuation, the State Department sent a cable over "MED CHANNEL" to Liberia. That cable, dated June 7, stated:

> *1. M/MED INFORMED VIA TELEPHONE CALL FROM SUBJECT'S MOTHER THAT THE NEONATAL CENTER AT UNIVERSITY OF COLORADO WILL ACCEPT MRS. WHEELER AND INFANT. POINT OF CONTACT IS DR. GERHARDT SCHROTER [sic], TELEPHONE (303) 199–1211.*
>
> *2. TODATE [sic] M/MED UNAWARE OF THE ABOVE NEED. PLEASE ADVISE ASAP.*

(See plaintiffs' Exhibit 39). In response, on June 8, a cable from the embassy in Liberia stated:

> *1. SUBJECT BECAME ILL 3 JUNE 1982 PRESENTING WITH POOR SUCK, TEMPERATURE ELEVATION, LETHARGY, IRRITABILITY, STAPH LESSIONS [sic] OVER PERINEUM AND BUTTOCKS. MOTHER WHO HAD BEEN BREAST FEEDING WAS BEING TREATED BY LOCAL PHYSICIAN FOR BREAST ABSCESS.*
>
> *2. SPINAL FLUID POS FOR STAPH LIKE ORGANISM. SUBJECT IN ELWA HOSPITAL ON PENICILLIN AND CHLORAMPHENICOL. SEIZURE [sic] HAVE SUBSIDED. SUBJECT RECEIVING ANTICONVULSIVE MEDS.*
>
> *3. CONDITION STABILIZING. WOULD PLAN TO MOVE SUBJECT AT TIME WHEN PARENTERAL THERAPY COMPLETED. EARLIEST WOULD BE 13 JUNE.*
>
> *4. SUBJECT HAS CONTACTED HER PARENTS IN DENVER AREA REGARDING ACCEPTING FACILITY. SUBJECT WILL NEED CARE OF NEONATOLOGIST REGARDING CNS PROBLEMS. SPONSOR DESIRES TO COST CONSTRUCT DENVER IN LIEU OF FRANKFURT. PLS ADVISE.*

A return cable from the Department of State to the Liberian Embassy dated June 9 stated:

> 1. THE MEDICAL DIRECTOR AUTHORIZES MEDI-CAL TRAVEL OF SUBJECT TO DENVER, COLORADO ON COST CONSTRUCTION BASIS MONROVIA/FRANKFURT/MONROVIA.
>
> 2. MEDICAL CLEARANCE ANNULLED PENDING OUTCOME OF EVALUATION AND TREATMENT.
>
> 3. WILL SCHEDULE APPOINTMENTS WHEN DEFI-NITE ETA KNOWN.
>
> 4. CONTACT FOR REINSTATEMENT OF MEDICAL CLEARANCE AND ADMINISTRATIVE ASSISTANCE IS DR. HUNGERFORD OR DR. KEARY. 202–632–8122.

There is no evidence of further communication until June 16, when the Liberian embassy cabled the State Department that:

> 1. SUBJECT NOW STABLE ENOUGH TO TRAVEL TO NEONATAL INTENSIVE CARE UNIT AT U. OF COL-ORADO. . . .
>
> 4. AS YET HAVE NOT RECEIVED RESULTS OF CIE ON SUBJECT'S SPINAL FLUID OR BLOOD THAT WAS HAND CARRIED TO M/MED LAST WEEK. WOULD APPRECIATE KNOWING ORGANISM.

Dr. Lefton recalled communicating with the Department of State by telephone during this time. However, he could not remember with whom he spoke or what he discussed. There was no evidence of any contact regarding Nyenpan's illness between the Office of Medical Services in Washington, D.C., and any person in Liberia beyond that described in the cables above.

## Tarpeh-Doe's benefits

Plaintiffs claim that the State Department never informed Tarpeh-Doe that her medical benefits included the option to evacuate to deliver her child in Europe or the United States. Plaintiffs assert that, had she been informed, she would have taken advantage of that benefit and delivered her child in the United States, where bacterial infection is less prevalent, and medical care is more advanced. Tarpeh-Doe testified that she was never told and did not know of that right. However, defendants produced evidence to the contrary.

As part of employee training, Gertrude Slifkin presents a lecture on employee relations and insurance. She includes in her lecture information about the State Department policy regarding evacuation of pregnant women for delivery of their children (testimony of Slifkin). Tarpeh-Doe attended that lecture on December 30, 1980, the second day of her 9-week training course in Washington prior to traveling to Monrovia (see Tarpeh-Doe's lecture notes, plaintiffs' Exhibit 27 at 6). However, she does not recall mention of this benefit in the lecture and did not record such mention in her lecture notes. Slifkin did not recall the particular lecture attended by Tarpeh-Doe.

Alfreda Mitchell, a nurse assigned to the embassy health unit in Monrovia who was present when the Tarpeh-Does visited Dr. Lefton in September 1981 so that Ben could receive tests in preparation for their marriage, heard Tarpeh-Doe tell Dr. Lefton that she was pregnant. Mitchell recalled overhearing Dr. Lefton tell Tarpeh-Doe in response that she should evacuate for delivery (testimony of Mitchell). Tarpeh-Doe did not recall that Dr. Lefton so informed her. Moreover, Dr. Lefton did not testify that he so informed her. He stated that he was not aware of any other American mother who had delivered a child in Liberia. He also stated that a decision by a pregnant woman not to evacuate for delivery would have been reported on the woman's medical chart. No such decision was recorded on Tarpeh-Doe's chart. From 1969 to 1972, when Dr. Eben H. Dustin, director of medical services at the State Department in 1988, was regional medical officer in Monrovia, Liberia, no woman delivered her first child in Monrovia. When Dustin was regional medical officer in Monrovia, he discussed evacuation with every pregnant woman.

While the evidence described above is not conclusive, defendants produced additional evidence indicating that Tarpeh-Doe did not evacuate to deliver her child because she could not afford to forego pay during the time she would be required to be absent from her position to do so. The airlines and the State Department require pregnant women who want to deliver a child elsewhere to leave their overseas post 6 weeks prior to their scheduled delivery date and remain away for 6 weeks following delivery. Maternity benefits include reimbursement for travel and medical expenses for pregnant women who choose to evacuate to deliver their children, but do not include paid leave for the 12 weeks a woman must be away from her post. Thus, unless a woman has otherwise accumulated 12 weeks of paid leave, she must take leave without pay to take advantage of this "benefit." Petrone recalled asking Tarpeh-Doe why she did not go home to have the baby. Tarpeh-Doe responded that she could not afford to do so. However, Gertrude Slifkin testified that when Tarpeh-Doe visited her to discuss medical benefits on her return to the United States with Nyenpan, while the two walked across the street to the medical division, Slifkin asked Tarpeh-Doe why she had delivered her baby in Liberia. Tarpeh-Doe responded that she did not want to be away from post, and that she did not have enough accumulated leave to receive pay during her time away.

Therefore, the evidence does not clearly establish when and how defendants informed Tarpeh-Doe that her benefits included the right to evacuate for delivery, albeit without pay. But, Slifkin's recollection of Tarpeh-Doe's expressed reason for not evacuating to deliver her child indicates that it is more likely than unlikely that Tarpeh-Doe, although she may not have been aware of specific details of the options available to her for evacuation, was generally aware that evacuation was a possibility, but that she could not afford it. No evidence was adduced that any person informed her of the potential risks of delivery in Liberia, of the risks to neonates in Liberia, or of the prevalence of infectious diseases there.

This Court has jurisdiction over a claim against the United States for personal injury caused by the negligence of a governmental employee acting within the scope of employment. The Court's jurisdiction extends to "circumstances where the United States, if a private person, would be liable to the claimant in accordance with the law of the place where the act or omission occurred" [28 U.S.C. § 1346(b)]. The relevant acts and omissions, if any, took place in the District of Columbia. Therefore, District of Columbia tort law determines whether defendants are liable for plaintiffs' claims.

Defendants argue that the discretionary function exception to the Federal Tort Claims Act deprives the Court of jurisdiction here. The discretionary function exception exempts from the FTCA any claim "based upon the exercise or performance or the failure to exercise or perform a discretionary function or duty on the part of a federal agency or an employee of the Government, whether or not the discretion involved be abused" [28 U.S.C. § 2680(a)]. The Supreme Court has clarified the application of this provision as follows: First, whether an act or omission constitutes a discretionary function is determined by "the nature of the conduct, rather than the status of the actor" [*United States v. S.A. Empresa de Viacao Aerea Rio Grandense (Varig Airlines)*, 467 U.S. 797, 813, 81 L. Ed. 2d 660, 104 S. Ct. 2755 reh. denied, 468 U.S. 1226, 82 L. Ed. 2d 919, 105 S. Ct. 26 (1984)]. Second, the exception covers only actions that involve "an element of judgment or choice" [see *Berkovitz v. United States*, 486 U.S. 531, 536–537, 100 L. Ed. 2d 531, 108 S. Ct. 1954 (1988); *Dalehite v. United States*, 346 U.S. 15, 34, 97 L. Ed. 1427, 73 S. Ct. 956 (1953)]. Finally, the exception applies only to "government actions and decisions based on considerations of public policy" (*Berkovitz*, 486 U.S. at 537).

Thus, "where there is room for policy judgment and decision there is discretion" (*Dalehite*, 364 U.S. at 36). If regulations provide specific directions, therefore, an employee's failure to follow those directions is not protected by the discretionary function exception (*Berkovitz* at 542–543). For example, the Coast Guard's failure to ensure that a light bulb at a lighthouse was operational did not involve a permissible exercise of policy discretion [see id. at 538, discussing *Indian Towing Co. v. United States*, 350 U.S. 61, 100 L. Ed. 48, 76 S. Ct. 122 (1955)].

The Supreme Court has recently clarified the discretionary function exception [*United States v. Gaubert*, 113 L. Ed. 2d 335, 111 S. Ct. 1267 (1991)]. The plaintiff in *Gaubert* pursued a tort claim against the Federal Home Loan

Bank Board arising out of its supervision and day-to-day management of a thrift unit, the Independent American Savings Association. The Fifth Circuit, distinguishing between policy-making decisions and operational ones, determined that the discretionary function exception did not apply to the agency's intervention in day-to-day affairs. The Supreme Court disagreed and held that the discretionary function exception applies to operational decisions as well as policy and planning decisions (id. 111 S. Ct. at 1275). Describing the exception, the Court explained that

> *if a regulation mandates particular conduct, and the employee obeys the direction, the Government will be protected because the action will be deemed in furtherance of the policies which led to the promulgation of the regulation. If the employee violates the mandatory regulation, there will be no shelter from liability because there is no room for choice and the action will be contrary to policy. On the other hand, if a regulation allows the employee discretion, the very existence of the regulation creates a strong presumption that a discretionary act authorized by the regulation involves consideration of the same policies which led to the promulgation of the regulations.*
>
> *Not all agencies issue comprehensive regulations, however. Some establish policy on a case-by-case basis, whether through adjudicatory proceedings or through administration of agency programs. Others promulgate regulations on some topics, but not on others. In addition, an agency may rely on internal guidelines rather than on published regulations. In any event, it will most often be true that the general aims and policies of the controlling statute will be evident from its text.*
>
> *When established governmental policy, as expressed or implied by statute, regulation or agency guidelines, allows a Government agent to exercise discretion, it must be presumed that the agent's acts are grounded in policy when exercising that discretion.*

The Court further stated:

> *There are obviously discretionary acts performed by a Government agent that are within the scope of his employment but not within the discretionary function exception because these acts cannot be said to be based on the purposes that the regulatory regime seeks to accomplish.*

Therefore, defendants are protected by the discretionary function exception if their allegedly negligent acts or omissions involved an exercise of choice or judgment that conformed with the purposes of the State Department's medical policy. With respect to plaintiffs' claim that defendants failed to inform Tarpeh-Doe that her benefits included the option to deliver her child outside Liberia, any failure to inform was not based on a permissible exercise of discretion because the State Department's medical policy can in no way be furthered by a judgment that employees should not be informed about their benefits. Similarly, neither defendants' failure to transmit Marilyn Wheeler's message from Dr. Schroeter that he felt it was imperative that he speak with the treating physician nor defendants' failure to conduct the requested test on the sample of Nyenpan's spinal fluid sent to Washington, D.C., involved any permissible exercise of choice in conformance with the State Department's medical policy or any other public policy. That conduct more closely resembles an employee's failure to follow the directions specified in regulations in *Berkovitz* or the Coast Guard's failure to replace a light bulb in *Indian Towing* (see *Berkovitz*, 486 U.S. at 538 and 542–543).

In contrast, Korcak's participation in the decision to retain Dr. Lefton for part of the time it took to locate a replacement for him involved consideration of factors that conformed to the State Department's medical policy. The medical director is charged with providing medical officers in the field as well as removing medical officers who are unable to perform their responsibilities. Swing and Korcak jointly decided to curtail Dr. Lefton's assignment in Monrovia, but permit him to remain at post for several more months. One of the reasons for that decision — permitting Dr. Lefton to remain in Monrovia so that his daughter could proceed as planned to visit him in August 1982 — did not involve any permissible exercise of judgment related to the State Department's medical policy.

However, the decision was also based on an attempt to minimize the gap between Dr. Lefton's departure and the arrival of a replacement physician, taking into account the potential risks of leaving the post without an assigned physician. Consideration of those factors is protected by the discretionary function exemption. No evidence established the degree to which each reason affected the decision. But, the presence of protected considerations renders the entire decision immune. Accordingly, defendants are protected by the discretionary function exception from plaintiffs' claim that they negligently retained Dr. Lefton in Monrovia.

Nevertheless, defendants had a self-imposed responsibility under State Department regulations to supervise the provision of medical services by whomever they retained in Monrovia (see, e.g., 3 FAM §§ 681.2 and 685.4-1 and 4-2, defendants' Exhibit 1). Defendants' failure to supervise Dr. Lefton more closely even after the inspectors alerted defendants to Dr. Lefton's flagrant derelictions of his official and professional responsibilities was not a permissible exercise of choice or discretion; that failure involved no decision. When defendants permitted Dr. Lefton to remain at post for several months, they conspicuously failed to consider and to make any decision about enhanced supervision of Dr. Lefton in light of the manifestly increased risks to which they exposed State Department personnel in Monrovia by not replacing or reinforcing him. Thus, there is no evidence that defendants' lack of response was the result of any exercise of choice or judgment, much less a permissible choice or judgment based on State Department medical policy. The discretionary function exemption therefore does not apply to defendants' failure to supervise Dr. Lefton more closely.

To prove a tort claim under District of Columbia law, plaintiffs must show (1) a duty owed to plaintiffs by defendants, (2) a breach of that duty, and (3) an injury to plaintiffs proximately caused by defendants' breach of duty [see, e.g., *District of Columbia v. Fowler*, 497 A.2d 456, 462 (D.C. 1985); *Morrison v. MacNamara*, 407 A.2d 555, 560 (D.C. 1979)].

Plaintiffs contend that defendants had the duty to provide Tarpeh-Doe and her dependents with the best possible medical care as provided in Uniform State/USIA/AID Regulations (3 FAM § 681.2). Federal regulations do not establish a duty by the government in the absence of an analogous cause of action under local tort law [see, e.g., *Art Metal-U.S.A., Inc., v. United States*, 244 App. D.C. 1, 753 F.2d 1151, 1157 (D.C. Cir. 1985)]. Where an analogous duty is recognized under local law, however, federal regulations provide evidence that the government has assumed such a duty, as well as evidence of the standard of care assumed (id. at 1158). Plaintiffs argue that defendants voluntarily assumed the duty to provide Linda and Nyenpan with the best possible medical care.

Plaintiffs also contend that defendants assumed that duty as part of their special relationship with her. Plaintiffs further contend that defendants established that duty by publishing it in regulations and manuals. District of Columbia courts have found duties to exist in all of these circumstances. In this regard, see, for instance, *Arnold's Hofbrau, Inc., v. George Hyman Construction Company*, 156 App. D.C. 253, 480 F.2d 1145, 1148 (D.C. Cir. 1973) (voluntary assumption of duty); *Kline v. 1500 Massachusetts Avenue Apartment Corporation*, 141 App. D.C. 370, 439 F.2d 477, 482–483 (D.C. Cir. 970) (special relationship, including employer–employee relationship); *Lucy Webb Hayes Nat. Training School v. Perotti*, 136 App. D.C. 122, 419 F.2d 704, 710 (D.C. Cir. 1969) (duty based on normal practices as well as internal procedures or manuals).

Courts have also found that an employer's employment manuals are relevant to determining the terms of the employment contract [see, e.g., *Washington Welfare Association v. Wheeler*, 496 A.2d 613, 615 (D.C. 1985)]. The terms of a contract between parties, in turn, may in some circumstances help to define whether a defendant owes a duty to a plaintiff [see, e.g., *Kline*, supra, 439 F.2d at 481–482]. The State Department not only defines its medical policy as assisting all employees in obtaining the best possible care, but also defines the reason for that policy: "so that no employee need hesitate to accept an assignment to a post where health conditions are hazardous, medical service poor, or transportation facilities limited" (3 FAM § 681.2).

This explanation, supported by Korcak's testimony that it would be difficult to find employees to serve in certain areas of the world without medical support, indicates that defendants viewed the provision of enhanced medical services as a part of the employment contract — in consideration for which employees accepted assignments at medically risky posts. Reliance on those services by employees who accept a position for overseas service is highly likely. Reliance by plaintiffs is one factor District of Columbia courts have considered in finding a duty to exist under tort law based on a special relationship [see, e.g., *Morgan v. District of Columbia*, 468 A.2d 1306, 1313–1314 (D.C. 1983) (en banc)].

In addition, actual or constructive notice of dangerous conditions is relevant to whether there is a duty [see, e.g., id. at 481 and 483; *District of Columbia v. Fowler*, 497 A.2d 456, 461 (D.C. 1985)]. Here, the State Department had actual notice of Dr. Lefton's lack of availability and of his refusal to respond to serious medical situations on several occasions in the past, as well as the diseases that lurked in Monrovia. Moreover, the Foreign Affairs Statute provides that an action against the United States under the FTCA is the exclusive remedy for a claim for damages for personal injury allegedly arising from the negligence of "supporting personnel of the Department of State in furnishing medical care or related services" [22 U.S.C. § 2702(a); see also *United States v. Smith*, 113 L. Ed. 2d 134, 111 S. Ct. 1180 (1991)]. That statute thus anticipates tort liability for any negligent acts by Department of State employees related to the provision of health care. For all of these reasons, the State Department owed a duty to plaintiff to provide her with a level of medical care higher than that available from local facilities in Liberia. Defendants promised Tarpeh-Doe the best possible medical care. Although federal regulations provide some evidence of the standard of care to be applied, District of Columbia law also provides that the standard of care in negligence cases is "reasonable care under the circumstances" [see, e.g., *Morrison v. MacNamara*, 407 A.2d 555, 560 (D.C. 1979)].

Plaintiffs' claim that the State Department failed to inform Tarpeh-Doe of her right to evacuate to deliver her child must fail. As described above, the facts do not support Tarpeh-Doe's contention that she was not informed. Accordingly, even if defendants had a duty to inform her, plaintiffs fail to show a breach of that duty. Plaintiffs' claim that the Office of Medical Services failed to conduct the correct laboratory test on the CSF sample sent to Washington, D.C., on June 10, 1982, also must fail. To the extent that the Office of Medical Services offered to perform tests on samples sent to Washington, D.C., it had a duty to plaintiff to perform those tests competently. However, since Nyenpan's injuries were more likely than not irreversible by June 10 when a CSF sample was sent for a CIE test to the Office of Medical Services in Washington, D.C., any negligence by the Office of Medical Services in conducting the wrong test is unlikely to have caused Nyenpan's injuries.

Plaintiffs also claim that defendants negligently failed to relay a message from Dr. Schroeter indicating he felt it was imperative to speak with the treating physicians as soon as possible. By assuming responsibility for the provision of medical care and by accepting Wheeler's message, defendants had a duty to relay that message accurately. Defendants did not refute whether the message was relayed; thus, they breached that duty.

The more difficult question is whether that breach was the cause of Nyenpan's injuries. A defendant's conduct must be a "substantial factor" in causing a plaintiff's harm to support a finding of proximate cause [see, e.g., *Lacy v. District of Columbia*, 424 A.2d 317, 319–321 (D.C. 1980)]. Had Dr. Lefton or Dr. Van Reken received Dr. Schroeter's message and called him — and had Dr. Schroeter offered advice on which they could have more effectively treated the baby, all prior to the point at which the baby was beyond hope of recovery, perhaps the infant would have recovered.

However, this chain of causation is too attenuated to support a finding that defendants' failure to relay the message was a substantial factor in bringing about the injuries. The facts and inferences to be drawn from them indicate that the State Department in Washington delayed transmission of the first telegram (absent the message that Dr. Schroeter wanted to speak with the treating physicians) for approximately 2 days, until June 7. But because Nyenpan was likely beyond hope of recovery by June 6, it is unlikely that communication after that date could have served to help him. Furthermore, telephone communication between Liberia and the United States was not always possible. Moreover, no expert testified that if Dr. Schroeter had spoken with Dr. Lefton or Dr. Van Reken he could have offered advice that would have led to Nyenpan's recovery. As a result, plaintiffs' claim that defendants' failure to relay Dr. Schroeter's message caused the infant's injuries cannot succeed.

Plaintiffs allege that defendants negligently failed to supervise Dr. Lefton. District of Columbia courts recognize such a claim of negligent supervision [see *International Distributing Corp. v. American District Telegraph Co.*, 186 App. D.C. 305, 569 F.2d 136, 139 (D.C. Cir. 1977); *Kendall v. Gore Properties, Inc.*, 98 App. D.C. 378, 236 F.2d 673 (D.C. Cir. 1956); *Anderson v. Hall*, 755 F. Supp. 2, 5 (D.D.C. 1991); *Murphy v. Army Distaff Foundation, Inc.*, 458 A.2d 61 (D.C. 1983)]. A finding of negligent supervision does not require a finding that the tort was committed in the principal's interest, as does a finding of negligence on a theory of respondeat superior in the District of Columbia [see *International Distributing*, 569 F.2d at 139; *Lyon v. Carey*, 174 App. D.C. 422, 533 F.2d 649, 651 (D.C. Cir. 1976)]. Instead, to define negligent supervision claims, District of Columbia courts cite with approval the criteria listed in § 213 of the Restatement (Second) of Agency (1957):

> *A person conducting an activity through servants or other agents is subject to liability for harm resulting from his conduct if he is negligent or reckless:*
>
> 1. *in giving improper or ambiguous orders or in failing to make proper regulations; or*
> 2. *in the employment of improper persons or instrumentalities in work involving risk or harm to others; or*

3. *in the supervision of the activity; or*
4. *in permitting, or failing to prevent, negligent or other tortious conduct by persons, whether or not his services or agents, upon premises or with instrumentalities under his control.*

[see, e.g., *International Distributing Corp.*, 569 F.2d at 139; *Anderson*, 755 F. Supp. at 5; *Murphy*, 458 A.2d at 63–64]. Foreseeability is one factor considered by District of Columbia courts in imposing liability for negligent supervision (see, e.g., *Kline v. 1500 Massachusetts Ave. Apartment Corp.*, 439 F.2d at 483). But, foreseeability is not required — a defendant may be liable unless the "chain of events appears 'highly extraordinary' in retrospect" [*Lacy v. District of Columbia*, 424 A.2d 317, 319–320 (D.C. 1980)].

The facts and circumstances here support a finding of negligent supervision. First, defendants were on notice of Dr. Lefton's unavailability. Defendants knew that Dr. Lefton's unavailability was not the result of other commitments or responsibilities, but instead was the result of Dr. Lefton's unwillingness to provide medical care. The complaints from employees, relayed directly to both Beahler and Korcak from the inspectors, indicate that Dr. Lefton's reluctance to perform his duties went beyond the specific incidents described and extended to his patients' daily problems locating him, getting messages to him, and receiving any medical care after daytime weekday hours. Furthermore, defendants knew that Dr. Lefton had left the post repeatedly for personal travel, had refused to make house calls, and had refused to travel to administer medical care. Once Dr. Lefton's assignment had been curtailed, his supervisors should have recognized that his commitment to his responsibilities was unlikely to increase and was, if anything, likely to dwindle yet further.

Ambassador Swing may have realized this when he expressed to Korcak his concern for adding the provision of medical services to Dakar to Dr. Lefton's responsibilities during the summer. Korcak, however, dismissed these concerns. Unwilling to be dissuaded from his positive impression of Dr. Lefton, Korcak discouraged Swing from his attempts to curtail Dr. Lefton's assignment in Monrovia and encouraged Dr. Lefton to seek further extensions of his stay in Monrovia. The situation was rife with the potential for a serious mishap resulting directly from Dr. Lefton's inaction. A doctor's inaction, in addition to a doctor's actions, can constitute malpractice — a doctor who fails to provide needed medical services to a patient with whom that doctor has a professional relationship may be liable for abandonment unless the doctor is replaced by an equally qualified physician [see *Ascher v. Gutierrez*, 175 App. D.C. 100, 533 F.2d 1235, 1236 (D.C. Cir. 1976)]. The evidence indicates that Dr. Lefton's supervisors at the Office of Medical Services failed to appreciate, or even to consider, the risk of serious medical problems likely to arise from Dr. Lefton's reluctance to provide care. Accordingly, defendants breached their duty to Tarpeh-Doe.

Dr. Lefton's negligent actions and omissions proximately caused Nyenpan's injuries. Dr. Lefton did not administer or in any way supervise or check on any gynecological, prenatal, or obstetrical care to Linda Wheeler Tarpeh-Doe despite her manifest need for such care. Instead, he referred her to a local gynecologist and obstetrician for care for a period of over 9 months without advising her that she should or could call him if she needed advice, without arranging to see her even once to determine whether she was receiving adequate local care, and without inquiring about her care by her treating physicians. He did not inform her of the known risks of delivery and postnatal care of a child, particularly a first child, in disease-ridden Monrovia. He never alerted her to the conditions of the various clinics and hospitals in Monrovia, some of which were evidently notorious. He did not visit her on or after her delivery.

When she became sick on Thursday, June 3, and needed prompt attention at 10:00 p.m., he was unavailable for unexplained reasons — the likely inference being that he refused to make a house call as he had refused several times in the past. When Tarpeh-Doe visited Dr. Lefton for treatment for mastitis on Friday, June 4, Dr. Lefton did not examine, or even ask about, the child. He advised her at that time to resume breast-feeding. That advice, if followed, could have caused or increased the child's exposure to infectious bacteria. When the Tarpeh-Does came to Dr. Lefton on June 5, he did not administer any tests. Dr. Lefton considered, but decided against, attempting to evacuate the child by commercial airplane. He did not request the services of an MAC flight for evacuation.

He handed over all care to Dr. Van Reken, a physician to whom he had never referred a patient. Against the baby's parents' vehement objections, he permitted Dr. Van Reken to admit Nyenpan, at a critical point in the baby's care, to a local hospital that had deplorable conditions. He was not familiar with the conditions at JFK Hospital, despite his duty to be aware of conditions at local health facilities to advise State Department and AID employees where to safely obtain services.

He did not visit or inquire about his American charges at JFK Hospital during the initial afternoon of June 5, and he did not visit or inquire that night or the next morning. He never evaluated its facilities to determine whether the parents' pronounced fears were justified. He did not check to see whether medications, oxygen, or 24-hour care by doctors or other trained medical attendants would be available there.

He did not contact the Office of Medical Services immediately to request advice or support in the United States from a neonatologist or an expert in bacterial spinal meningitis. Moreover, he did not cable the Office of Medical Services until he received a brief request for information from them. When he did cable the office, he did not inform persons there that he had not examined the child since June 5, or that he had turned over care to Dr. Van Reken; he did not request assistance or advice. He did not visit Tarpeh-Doe until June 12. After the June 5 visit to him at the embassy health clinic, he did not examine the baby. He did not authorize evacuation either on the parents' repeated requests or on Dr. Van Reken's approval of evacuation.

In short, Dr. Lefton washed his hands of Linda Wheeler Tarpeh-Doe and her baby and turned his back on them, doing as little as possible to attend to Tarpeh-Doe's care during pregnancy or to plan for the close medical supervision of mother and child after delivery. He was supposed to be the family doctor. Had Dr. Lefton provided Tarpeh-Doe with gyneco-logical or prenatal care or taken any interest at all in her condition by anticipating and preparing himself and herself for the risks awaiting the mother and child after delivery, he would have visited her or otherwise made himself available so that she would have automatically called or visited him with the child on Friday, or even Thursday, when she first noticed signs of illness. Had she felt that he would willingly, rather than reluctantly, attend to her medical needs, she would have sought him out instead of waiting until Nyenpan required emergency care and seeking that care from local, inadequate, facilities.

On June 5, had Billie Clement not directed the Tarpeh-Does to the embassy health unit, it is even possible that Nyenpan would have received better care from Dr. Johnson at Cooper's Clinic than he received from Dr. Lefton, who permitted Dr. Van Reken to place him in a hospital with roaches and rats and with no medications, no medical attendants during the night, and no oxygen. From Tarpeh-Doe's arrival in Monrovia throughout her pregnancy and delivery and, most important, from the onset of the postnatal illness of mother and child, Dr. Lefton took none of the initiatives required of him by the State Department directives or by any conceivable standard of care by a physician in his circumstances.

Dr. Lefton's acts and omissions render it difficult to determine with any degree of certainty the true cause of the infant's failure to recover. District of Columbia courts have established that when a defendant's acts or omis-sions create uncertainty as to whether, had the defendant acted otherwise, the outcome would have been more favorable to the plaintiff, that uncer-tainty does not provide a defense against the plaintiff's showing of proximate cause [see, e.g., *Daniels v. Hadley Memorial Hospital*, 185 App. D.C. 84, 566 F.2d 749, 757 (D.C. Cir. 1977); *Ascher v. Gutierrez*, 175 App. D.C. 100, 533 F.2d 1235, 1238 (D.C. Cir. 1976)]. It is more likely than unlikely that improved prenatal and postnatal care for Linda Wheeler Tarpeh-Doe and Nyenpan, advice for sanitary precautions, or earlier treatment for Nyenpan would have averted this tragedy or resulted in the child's full recovery. Dr. Lefton was responsible for failing to provide that earlier advice and treatment. Therefore, plaintiffs have shown by a preponderance of the evidence that Dr. Lefton's conduct, in particular his omissions, were a substantial factor in causing Nyenpan's injuries.

The ultimate question remains whether defendants are liable for "per-mitting, or failing to prevent" Dr. Lefton's negligence [Restatement (Second) of Agency § 213]. Defendants argue that it would have been impossible for the Office of Medical Services to participate in decisions regarding

Nyenpan's care. This contention is controverted by defendants' own regulations. The Uniform State/AID/USIA Regulations require the Office of Medical Services to support regional medical officers in serious medical emergencies that take place in foreign countries, to receive notification of medical emergencies, and to authorize evacuations. Dr. Lefton could and should have instantly communicated with Washington. In addition, while 3 FAM § 681.2 provides that post officers "are cautioned to be alert to any medical and health problems of employees and their dependents and to take appropriate action promptly," only medical officers at the Office of Medical Services in Washington had the medical expertise required to predict the risk of medical emergencies stemming from Dr. Lefton's failure to provide services. Therefore, Dr. Lefton's negligent acts and opinions were under defendants' control [see Restatement (Second) of Agency § 213(d)].

Moreover, Dr. Lefton's lack of care could have and should have been foreseen by the U.S. defendants. Dr. Lefton's supervisors at the Office of Medical Services could and should have anticipated and taken several steps to decrease the likelihood of the medical disaster that occurred here. Defendants could and should have directed Dr. Lefton to focus more attention on his responsibilities and to make himself available in the evenings and on weekends. Furthermore, defendants could and should have imposed additional reporting requirements.

For example, they could have advised or ordered Dr. Lefton to report any serious illness immediately by telephone or telegram. Medical officers in Washington (the only responsible persons competent to fully assess the medical risks of Dr. Lefton's poor attitude and lack of availability in a tropical climate like that of Monrovia) also could have warned Ambassador Swing and Deputy Chief of Mission Perkins, as well as supporting medical personnel, including Nurse Clement and Dr. Feir, to alert the Office of Medical Services immediately of any potential need for medical advice or treatment — such as the first pregnancy of a woman planning to deliver in Monrovia. They could have required Dr. Lefton to put in place plans for the care of the mother and child in the event of a pregnancy of and birth to an AID employee during the time remaining to Dr. Lefton in Monrovia.

Had defendants done so, it is more likely than unlikely that Dr. Lefton or someone else in Monrovia would have informed the Office of Medical Services of Tarpeh-Doe's pregnancy and delivery and Nyenpan's illness. Had defendants been advised of the pregnancy and delivery, they could have taken steps to ensure that Tarpeh-Doe was fully informed of risks to neonates in Monrovia and advised as to safety precautions and that Dr. Lefton was prepared for the event. Had they been advised of Nyenpan's illness on June 3 or 4, or even on being alerted of the illness by Marilyn Wheeler, presumably on June 5, defendants could have acted promptly to ensure, by promptly phoning and telegraphing Liberia to find out what the situation was and offering support and advice, that Dr. Lefton was not again declining to provide medical services as he had in the past.

Defendants could have arranged for a neonatologist familiar with meningitis to discuss Nyenpan's care directly with Drs. Lefton and Van Reken. Defendants could have advised Dr. Lefton whether evacuation was possible or advisable. In that next 24 hours, very likely a crucial period, defendants could have supported and supervised many of Dr. Lefton's decisions. Again, defendants' failure to supervise Dr. Lefton more closely creates uncertainty whether, had they acted otherwise, Nyenpan would have recovered (see *Daniels*, 566 F.2d at 757; *Ascher*, 533 F.2d at 1238). Defendants thus "[permitted] or [failed] to prevent negligence or other tortious conduct by persons... under [their] control" [Restatement (Second) of Agency § 213]. In the unusual circumstances here, having been alerted to Dr. Lefton's deficiencies and knowing the severe risks of tropical diseases such as those confronting a newborn and its mother in Monrovia, defendants had a self-imposed duty to see to it that Dr. Lefton was informed, readily available, and in charge with a previously approved plan for treatment if necessary and hospitalization or evacuation in just such an emergency as occurred.

Defendants urge the Court to find that Tarpeh-Doe was contributorily negligent by failing to seek Dr. Lefton's services earlier than June 5. This contention is not supportable. Tarpeh-Doe was a 24-year-old woman with little experience living and obtaining medical care overseas. She had just experienced her first pregnancy and delivery. She was learning for the first time how to care for an infant, without the support of family or friends from years past, in a country with poor local health facilities. She received virtually no support or medical care from Dr. Lefton. She was sick with malaria, staph infection, and mastitis when her infant became critically ill; in that condition, she took him to two emergency rooms and the embassy health unit and stayed up overnight in his hospital room, attended only by friends and not by the professionals responsible for her care or the care of her child. Tarpeh-Doe's actions and omissions in this case were reasonable under the circumstances. Therefore, for the reasons stated, defendants are liable to plaintiffs for any damages they suffered.

*List the options open to you. That is, answer the question, "What could you do?"*

- 
- 
- 
- 

*Choose the best solution from an ethical point of view, justify it, and respond to possible criticisms. That is, answer the question, "What should you do, and why?"*

- 
- 
- 
- 

*Select one member of your PBL group to role-play as Dr. Lefton and have another member of your PBL group role-play as Linda Wheeler Tarpeh-Doe. How might the two converse about different ways of thinking and techniques for conflict management?*

- 
- 
- 
- 

*Again, please select one member of your PBL group to role-play as Dr. Lefton and have another member of your PBL group role-play as Linda Wheeler Tarpeh-Doe. How might Dr. Lefton use what is known about stages of change and about motivational interviewing to solve what you consider the major problem presented in the case?*

- 
- 
- 
- 

## Part three

Plaintiffs' damages include amounts paid for past care for the child as well as future payments for care and lost income Nyenpan would have earned as an adult. The parties agree on the appropriate method of computing the expected rate of increase in the cost of future medical care offset by the present value of future payment for that care. However, as discussed below, the parties dispute Nyenpan's life expectancy and the amount of future lost wages.

Plaintiffs claim damages of $322,443.57 for Nyenpan's institutionalization at Wheat Ridge Regional Center to date, $4,969.18 for unreimbursed expenses paid by Tarpeh-Doe on his behalf, $4,657,400 for the present value of the cost of future medical and personal care at Wheat Ridge, and $1,008,434 in income and benefits Nyenpan could have received over his lifetime, less expenses and taxes. These claims total $5,993,246.75. Plaintiffs also seek damages for emotional suffering, pain, and disfigurement. Defendants argue that if plaintiffs are entitled to recover, the damage award should total $1,281,563, consisting of $4,969 for unreimbursed expenses by Tarpeh-Doe, $702,844 for the present value of future expenses, and lost income of $573,750. Defendants argue that damages should not include the past costs of hospitalization at Wheat Ridge because those costs were paid by Medicare. However, plaintiffs filed on the record in this case an assignment agreement between the Department of Social Services of the State of Colorado and plaintiffs' attorneys (see Notice of Filing [filed November 26, 1990]). That agreement states that the state of Colorado has the legal right to recover the amount of Medicaid payments made by it from any third party liable for the recipient's injuries (id.). In that agreement, plaintiffs agree to pay to Colorado the amount the state has paid in expenses from any recovery up to the amount of 50% of that recovery. Accordingly, damages awarded to plaintiffs by the terms of the agreement will be payable to the state of Colorado to the extent indicated.

Plaintiffs' expert economist Dr. Herman Miller calculated Nyenpan's lost income to be $1,008,434, using the census tables to determine the present value of the income of an American male college graduate with a work life of 38 years, less taxes and plus benefits (Miller dep. at 15). Defendants, in contrast, argue that the expected earnings should be reduced significantly (see defendants' Exhibit 41; [testimony of Schiller]). In support, defendants' expert economist Dr. Bradley Robert Schiller argues that, since Nyenpan's father was Liberian and his mother worked in Liberia when he was born, he could not be expected to spend his entire working life in the United States. (Plaintiffs noted on cross-examination of Dr. Schiller that Ben Tarpeh-Doe was now an American citizen and worked in the United States.) Aside from the reduced wages he could be expected to receive in Liberia, Dr. Schiller argued that his work life would be shorter by several years. He also believed that, once part of his work life had been spent in Liberia, he would receive less income in the United States. Moreover, Dr. Schiller argued that the appropriate measure of future earnings in the United States for Nyenpan (whose mother is white and whose father is black) is the average earnings of black men, not those of all men (defendants' Exhibit 41 [testimony of Schiller]).

Defendants' argument that Nyenpan's projected earnings should be reduced because he might spend part of his working life in Liberia is not convincing. Insufficient evidence exists to support such a reduction. Furthermore, defendants' argument that average black male earnings are an appropriate measure of Nyenpan's future earnings cannot be accepted since Nyenpan is half black and half white. Moreover, it would be inappropriate to incorporate current discrimination resulting in wage differences between the sexes or races or the potential for any future such discrimination into a calculation for damages resulting from lost wages. The parties did not cite any precedent on this question.

Accordingly, on request by the Court, Schiller submitted a calculation of the average earnings of all college graduates in the United States without regard to sex or race (defendants' Exhibit 44). Adjusted for changes in work life expectancy, this calculation resulted in lost wages of $882,692. Dr. Schiller further adjusted this amount to reduce the income amount to earnings, to include payroll taxes in the tax deduction, and to make certain adjustments in the net discount rate, resulting in total lost wages of $573,750.

These adjustments appear to be reasonable and were not contested by plaintiffs. The average wages for all persons are lower than average black male wages; thus, the incorporation of women's expected earnings lowers the estimate even further than defendants' estimate. Nevertheless, estimating Nyenpan's future earnings based on the average earnings of all persons appears to be the most accurate means available of eliminating any discriminatory factors. Accordingly, the accompanying order grants plaintiffs $573,750 in lost earnings.

In calculating the cost of future care, plaintiffs rely on the opinion expressed by their expert Dr. Harold Stevens, a neurologist, that Nyenpan's life expectancy is 10% less than the life expectancy of an average person (see Stevens dep. at 12). Dr. Stevens based this estimate not on any statistical evidence, but on his personal experience of encounters with hundreds of children he followed through adulthood who had severe nervous system damage (id. at 21–22). He also noted that there is tremendous variability of longevity in persons suffering from postmeningitic syndromes.

Plaintiffs' expert economist Dr. Miller testified that the average 8-year-old male has a life expectancy of 72 years (i.e., 64.3 additional years) (Miller dep. at 10–11). Thus, plaintiffs assumed that Nyenpan would live 55 more years, 10% less than average. Although costs at Wheat Ridge, which were $232 a day or $84,680 a year in 1990, had increased at the rate of 18% a year during the past 5 years, Miller estimated the growth rate of medical costs over Nyenpan's life would average 7% a year. In arriving at that figure, he explained that medical costs had increased by an average of 8% a year for the past 20 years, and that he could not conceive of the costs increasing at the rate of 18% a year for the next 55 years. To determine the present value of those costs, Miller used a discount rate of 7%, which he derived from the rate of return on long-term, insured, tax-free municipal bonds (id. at 17 and 20). On the assumption that the increase in cost would equal the discount rate, Miller calculated future medical costs by multiplying the number of years Nyenpan was expected to live (55) by the annual cost of care ($84,680), arriving at $4,657,400.

Defendants' expert Dr. Marianne Schuelein testified in contrast that she believed that Nyenpan's life expectancy was an additional 8.3 years, not 55 years. She based that figure on an article in the *New England Journal of Medicine*, "The Life Expectancy of Profoundly Handicapped People with Mental Retardation" (defendants' Exhibit 33). A study of 4513 profoundly mentally retarded persons who were immobile and were fed by others found an average life expectancy for children aged 5–9 to be an additional 8.3 years (defendants' Exhibit 33 at 588, Table 4). The average life expectancy of persons who survived to the age of 20 years rose, rather than fell. Dr. Schuelein also testified that most children with Nyenpan's difficulties die in the first 9 years, and that in her 23 years of experience, she had not seen persons with Nyenpan's injuries survive beyond the age of 20 years. One of the problems she noted was the difficulty diagnosing diseases in such persons (testimony of Dr. Schuelein). Like Dr. Miller, defendants' expert economist Dr. Schiller believed that the increase in medical costs over the years would be offset by the discount rate. Accordingly, defendants estimated Nyenpan's future medical costs to be $702,844.

This conflict of expert opinion as to Nyenpan's life expectancy creates an issue that is difficult to resolve equitably. A lump sum award of damages may be too crude an instrument. If the 8.3-year estimate is too low, the plaintiffs will lose relief to which they are plainly entitled. If the 55-year estimate is too high, they will realize a gross windfall at great expense to the taxpayers. There should be a way to minimize the guesswork. It can be determined with reasonable certainty what it will cost to maintain Nyenpan per year (i.e., $ 84,680.00), adjusted in future years for inflation (or deflation).

A solution may be available through one of several alternative mechanisms. First, defendants could undertake to pay an annual amount (adjusted for inflation) for the benefit of Nyenpan during his lifetime. Second, defendants could be required to contribute to a trust a discounted principal sum measured originally by the 55-year life expectancy anticipated by plaintiffs' experts, with distributions by the trustee from income and, if necessary, from principal, in amounts appropriate to maintain Nyenpan during his lifetime, with the remainder reverting to defendants at his death. For instance, see *Friends for All Children v. Lockheed Aircraft Corporation*, 563 F. Supp. 552 (D.D.C. 1983); 587 F. Supp. 180, 202 (D.D.C. 1983). Finally, it is conceivable that commercial insurance companies would be willing to bid on a commercial annuity, the cost of which would be measured by Nyenpan's life expectancy as determined by the insurance carrier on the basis of actuarial experience generally adjusted to reflect Nyenpan's unique condition [see, e.g., *Nemmers v. United States*, 795 F.2d 628, 635 (7th Cir. 1986); but see *Friends for All Children*, 563 F. Supp. at 553]. Accordingly, the accompanying order will require counsel for both parties to investigate these alternatives and to file on or before September 9, 1991, either a joint proposal or separate ones for payment by defendant of the cost of maintaining Nyenpan during his remaining years.

Finally, it is found and ruled that, in addition to a sum (to be determined) for future maintenance of Nyenpan, plaintiffs are entitled to (1) $322,443.53 for the cost of his maintenance incurred through October 1990, (2) $4,969.18 for unreimbursed expenses incurred on behalf of Nyenpan by his mother Linda Tarpeh-Doe, and (3) $573,750, the present value of Nyenpan's prospective lost earnings. The accompanying order will enter judgment for the resulting total of $901,162.71 and schedule further pleadings with respect to reimbursement for the cost of future maintenance for life.

Plaintiffs' request for damages for Nyenpan's emotional distress and pain and suffering must be denied. It is highly likely that Nyenpan has suffered and will suffer extreme emotional distress as a result of his condition. However, Nyenpan now receives excellent and caring attention from those who attend to his needs. It is not clear that a monetary award would serve to compensate him for his suffering or otherwise benefit him in any way. Furthermore, such an award may be barred under the FTCA as punitive damages. In this regard, see, for instance, *Molzof v. United States*, 911 F.2d 18 (7th Cir. 1990), cert. granted, 113 L. Ed. 2d 239, 111 S. Ct. 1305 (1991); see also *Flannery v. United States*, 718 F.2d 108, 111 (4th Cir. 1983), cert. denied, 467 U.S. 1226, 81 L. Ed. 2d 874, 104 S. Ct. 2679 (1984); but see *Rufino v. United States*, 829 F.2d 354, 362 (2d Cir. 1987); *Shaw v. United States*, 741 F.2d 1202, 1208 (9th Cir. 1984); *Kalavity v. United States*, 584 F.2d 809, 811 (6th Cir. 1978). Should the Supreme Court resolve the split in the circuits on this issue by determining that an award of damages for loss of enjoyment of life to a comatose or similarly incapacitated plaintiff is appropriate under the FTCA, the Court will consider an application from plaintiffs for modification of judgment with respect to damages for pain and suffering.

Plaintiffs request leave to amend their complaint to request a total of $8,000,000 in damages [filed December 3, 1990]. That motion is moot. For all of the reasons explained above, an accompanying order grants judgment for plaintiffs, grants judgment of $901,162.71, and requests further briefing on the discount rate and rate of increase in costs to apply to a calculation of future medical costs.

## Conclusion

The medical field tries to find treatment options for seriously ill neonates. These include therapy to sustain life while not prolonging the dying process. The best interest of the child should be taken into consideration at all times. If the treatment option will not be beneficial overall , it should not be used. The best care, support, and comfort should be provided to the child. When considering treatment options, the values of the family need to be taken into consideration.

Ultimately, the parents have moral and legal responsibility to the child and have the right to make the decision regarding the treatment. If the parents cannot make the decision due to incompetence or if the parents are separated, the legal guardian makes the decision. Also, if the physician finds a treatment option, the physician must ensure the parents know and understand fully what needs to be done. The suggested guidelines for decision making are not mandatory, but they provide a tool for parents to use when making decisions regarding their child.

Modern medicine and technology have the ability to prolong life and are so advanced that there is a real danger that the prolongation of life becomes the sole end. These decisions to use life-sustaining or life-prolonging medical treatment must be made with the best interest of the child in mind. The child's best interest must take priority over family stability or well-being or the well-being of the caretakers. However, the burdens that are placed on the family must be included in making a decision. All outcomes must be examined in the decision of treatment or nontreatment to ensure the best possible care for seriously ill neonates.

## case ten

# Distributive justice

This problem-based learning session is based on the following: *Connecticut v. Physicians Health Services of Connecticut, Inc.*, Docket No. 00-7986, U.S. Court of Appeals for the Second Circuit, 287 F.3d 110; 2002 U.S. App. Lexis 5357; 27 E.B.C. 2496. May 1, 2001, Argued. March 27, 2002, Decided. As Amended April 10, 2002. Writ of certiorari denied: *Connecticut v. Physicians Health Services of Connecticut, Inc.*, 2002 U.S. Lexis 6430 (U.S. Oct. 7, 2002). It is reprinted here with permission of LexisNexis.

## Objectives

The objectives of this problem-based learning case are to understand issues of access barriers to health care associated with:

- Health care delivery systems
- Managed care
- Impact of technology
- Individual rights and public health

## Introduction

Although distributive justice implies that everyone gets equal access to quality care in our health care delivery system, intensity and quality of care have always been impacted by different issues of access barriers.

## Part one

On December 14, 1999, the state of Connecticut brought this suit for equitable relief in the U.S. District Court for the District of Connecticut against Physicians Health Services of Connecticut, Inc. ("PHS"), an insurance company offering managed care plans to Connecticut residents. The State seeks an order pursuant to Section 502(a)(3) of the Employment Retirement Income Security Act of 1974 ("ERISA"), 29 U.S.C. § 1132 (a)(3), enjoining the defendant PHS from using a drug "formulary" — a list of drugs preapproved by

PHS for reimbursement — that allegedly prevents plan enrollees from receiving drugs prescribed for them by their physicians that are medically necessary or preferable to a comparable listed drug. Under § 1132(a)(3), "a participant, beneficiary, or fiduciary" may bring a civil action for equitable relief to redress violations of ERISA or the terms of an ERISA-regulated plan. The State asserts standing to sue in its capacity as *parens patriae,* and as the assignee of eight individual participants in PHS plans who have purportedly assigned the State their right to seek "appropriate equitable relief" with respect to "any cause of action" they may have as plan participants or beneficiaries (Compl., Exs. 1–8 P 2). The district court (Stefan R. Underhill, Judge) granted the defendant's motion to dismiss the State's complaint for lack of standing [*Connecticut v. Physicians Health Services of Connecticut, Inc.,* 103 F. Supp. 2d 495 (D. Conn. 2000) (*PHS*). The court, in a thorough and careful opinion, held that the State did not meet the requirements for standing under § 1132(a)(3) (id. at 511). The State filed a timely appeal.

We conclude that the State as assignee of the plan participants' rights to bring equitable actions against the defendant lacks standing under Article III of the Constitution. We further hold that the State cannot bring this suit in a *parens patriae* capacity. Because Congress "carefully drafted" § 1132, parties other than those explicitly named therein — plan participants, beneficiaries, and fiduciaries — may not bring suit [*Pressroom Unions–Printers League Income Sec. Fund v. Continental Assurance Co.,* 700 F.2d 889, 893 (2d Cir.), cert. denied, 464 U.S. 845, 78 L. Ed. 2d 138, 104 S. Ct. 148 (1983)]. The State in its *parens patriae* capacity is not one of these enumerated parties. We therefore affirm the district court's grant of the defendant's motion to dismiss all the State's claims for lack of standing.

## Background

In its complaint filed on December 14, 1999, the State alleges that the PHS drug formulary system violates provisions of ERISA that impose on PHS: (1) a fiduciary duty to administer its health care plans solely in the interests of the plan participants; (2) a duty to disclose the full details of its plans to plan participants; and (3) a duty to provide plan participants with adequate notice of reasons for denials of claims for reimbursement. The State asserts that PHS's drug formulary system injures plan participants by denying them "access to safe, effective, and medically necessary" drugs prescribed by their doctors. The details of the State's allegations are set forth in the district court's opinion. Because we do not reach the merits of the claims, we need describe them no further here.

Relying on 29 U.S.C. § 1132 (a)(3), which allows a participant, beneficiary, or fiduciary of an ERISA-regulated plan to bring a civil action for injunctive and other equitable relief, the State seeks an order:

> 1. *requiring the defendant to provide its enrollees with the prescription medications ordered by the attending physician unless the defendant submits to the Court, and the*

> *Court approves, a plan for substituting the defendant's preferred medications for those prescribed while insuring [sic] that (I) the substitution is approved by the attending physician, and (ii) the enrollee experiences no unreasonable delay before receiving an appropriate medication; and*

> 2. *requiring the defendant to comply with the dictates of ERISA and disclose to enrollees information sufficient to inform them fully and accurately, prior to their enrollment or re-enrollment in the plan, concerning the true nature of the prescription drug benefit to which they are entitled; and*

> 3. *requiring that whenever an enrollee requests coverage of a prescription drug by presenting a completed prescription form to a participating pharmacy and coverage is denied, the defendant shall give the enrollee a written denial notice setting forth the specific reason for the denial, and the steps necessary to file an appeal.*

The complaint also requests "such other and further relief as the Court may deem necessary and proper."

The State advances two theories of standing. First, it asserts standing as the assignee of the rights of eight plan participants as individuals and as representatives of a class consisting of all Connecticut residents enrolled in PHS's managed care plans. Second, it asserts standing in its *parens patriae* capacity to protect its interest in the health and well-being of its citizens. Each of these plan participants executed a document purporting to assign to the State his or her right to sue for injunctive or other equitable relief pursuant to 29 U.S.C. § 1132 (a)(3). The right to sue for money damages was not assigned and remains with the plan participants. Attached to the complaint are copies of these assignments. Each states:

> *I hereby assign to the State of Connecticut any cause of action I may have arising from my status as a participant in or beneficiary of an employee welfare benefit plan established pursuant to the Federal Employee Retirement Income Security Act of 1974 ("ERISA"), upon the following conditions:*

> 1. *I believe my managed care organization has improperly and illegally obstructed my access to safe and effective prescription medications. I believe many other Connecticut residents have been injured in a similar way. I cannot afford to hire private attorneys to protect my rights under ERISA.*

2. *By this assignment I intend to empower the State of Connecticut, by and through the Attorney General, to take action to protect me, and people like me, pursuant to 29 U.S.C. 1132 (a)(3), which provides that I, or my assignee, may bring an action to enjoin any act or practice which violates the terms of my health care plan, or to obtain other appropriate equitable relief to redress such violations or to enforce provisions of ERISA or the plan. I agree to cooperate with the Attorney General's Office in any such action, and I agree that the facts of my case should be made public. I am willing, if necessary, to testify under oath.*

3. *Any positive result the Attorney General is able to obtain will help me, and other people in my position, to receive the medically necessary prescription medications to which we are entitled and which are essential to our health and well-being.*

In exchange for this assignment, the State neither promised to prosecute the assignors' claims nor provided other consideration.

On January 24, 2000, PHS filed a motion to dismiss the complaint pursuant to Rules 12(b)(1) and 12(b)(6) of the Federal Rules of Civil Procedure on the grounds that: (1) the State lacked standing to bring this action, (2) the assignor–plan participants had not suffered any injuries compensable under ERISA, and (3) the State failed to state a cause of action under ERISA. On July 13, 2000, the district court granted the defendant's motion to dismiss, holding that the State lacked standing to pursue its claims either as *parens patriae* or as the assignee of the named participants — either individually or as representatives of a class (*PHS*, 103 F. Supp. 2d at 497). The district court concluded that "Congress carefully limited the persons authorized to" sue under § 1132(a)(3) to "either 'a participant, beneficiary, or fiduciary'" and that "the State does not meet any of these statutory requirements of standing, and cannot overcome its omission from section [1132(a)(3)] either through the doctrine of *parens patriae* or through the assignment of rights from persons who would have standing" (*PHS*, 103 F. Supp. 2d 495). The district court did not address PHS's other asserted grounds for dismissal.

This appeal followed. The sole issue before us is whether the State has standing in either of the two capacities it asserted in the district court.

*Make a list of the major problems presented in this case*

- 
- 
- 
-

## Hypothesis and mechanism

For the problems in your list above, give a cause or a reason for them to happen:

- 
- 
- 
- 

## Learning issues

Make a list of learning issues in the form of questions. Remember, your goal is to gather the medical, social, and all other relevant facts that may apply to the case.

Although distributive justice implies that everyone gets an equal access to quality care in our health care delivery system, intensity and quality of care have always been impacted by different issues of access barriers.

What are the three basic types of health care systems in the United States?
   Fee for service — physician treats and bills you for a particular service
   Managed care — health maintenance organizations (HMOs), PPOs, POSs
   Public Health — public health clinics
   Important notes: One of the basic types of health care systems is fee for service. Although this is the most common system, the care it provides is limited to what the doctor determines and what the patient can afford. The doctor often recommends a hospital for certain care. Managed care (HMOs) is a fairly new system in which physicians, hospitals, and other providers treat patients that are enrolled. However, this system also has its own barriers to quality care. The managed care company, to keep costs down, can limit services, surgery, or hospitalization. People who work for a small company of fewer than 25 employees may not have access to care through HMO enrollment. In addition, cost sharing (co-pay) reduces drug utilization by 25%. This is a barrier to quality care if the patient does not have resources for the co-pay. Other barriers may include nonformulary drugs that are too expensive for patients to afford, formulary drugs that are based on cost containment, and the fact that doctors may be required to change treatment choices to conform to present formulary. Public health services such as MCH services and general ambulatory care are designed for low-income families, and services are funded by federal, state, or local government. However, most of public services, especially communicable disease control (for sexually transmitted diseases, STDs) and chronic diseases (cancer detection

clinics) are preventive services. This means that patients with low incomes may not have access to other care services that they need and that are not provided by public health services.

Managed care organizations (HMOs) have access barriers. Explain.
  In 1973, the approval of the Health Maintenance Organization Act required that employers of 25 or more employees provide an HMO enrollment as an alternative to indemnity insurance.
  Cost sharing requires that the patient share the burden of drug cost utilization. This reduces drug utilization by 25%.
  Of HMOs, 95% have formularies. Most of them are closed formularies, which means that drugs, particularly expensive innovator drugs, outside the formulary are usually not covered.
  Drugs selected for formularies are based on cost containment, not necessarily on the patient's best interest.
  Of HMOs, 18% use capitation in regard to drug prescriptions.
  The physician is placed at a financial liability for drug utilization.

Does every citizen have an individual right to health care?
  These rights, by contemporary U.S. society, are guaranteed fundamentally in the U.S. Constitution (such as the right of free speech, the right of the press, etc.).
  There is no law that states that a patient has a right to health care, but rather there is a moral obligation that is reinforced by laws.
  Public health is services provided by federal, state, or local government. Examples include services for communicable disease control, MCH, chronic diseases, and general ambulatory care.
  Important notes: Today, patients believe that they have the right to health care and expect that clinicians will employ their knowledge and experience in caring for them. At first glance, our American health care system seems fundamentally based on ensuring the rights of patients, such as the right to choose their physician, pharmacy, hospital, and treatment. This is not true with the newly passed HMOs, which limit these individual rights.

What has been the impact of technology on health care?
  Patients have access to on-line pharmacies and other health care services.
  Doctors have access to on-line telemedicine to improve the quality of care for the patients.
  Medical devices are available for patients at their convenience.
  Patients, especially those in rural areas, may not have access to the Internet (computers), may not have the knowledge to use this technology, or may consider needed medical devices too expensive. These are the barriers.
  Important notes: Technology today has impacted access to quality care greatly. Medical devices help patients monitor their glucose levels

and increase self-care, which shortens hospital stays and reduces costs. Internet or telemedicine helps reduce medical and medication errors, provides patients with on-line pharmacy and videoconferencing consultation with their doctors without having to leave the comfort of their office or home, and so on. Barriers to care arise when patients do not have access to technology, when they do not have the knowledge to use it, or maybe when the medical devices are too expensive.

## Literature review

To help you get ready to answer certain questions you anticipate being asked during the second part of the case, look in the local medical library and on the World Wide Web for helpful information. Please indicate in the spaces below (1) several helpful articles or books you found and (2) several helpful Web sites you found.

- **Helpful articles/books:**
  Bailey, T. C., Real time notification errors, *Health Manage. Technol.*, 21, 24–26, 2000.
  CibaGeneva Pharmaceutical, *CibaGeneva Pharmacy Benefit Report*, Summit, NJ, 1996.
  Leitner, P.J., The world and I, *Washington Times Corporation*, 15,140–147, 2000.
  Manning, W.G. et al. Health insurance and the demand for medical care, *Am. Econ. Rev.*, 77, 251–277, 1987.
  McCarthy, R.L., *Introduction to Health Care Delivery: a Primer for Pharmacists*, Aspen Publishers, Gaithersburg, MD, 1998.

- **Helpful Web sites:**
  American Association of Retired Persons: www.aarp.org/programs/health/hdiwhat.html
  Benton Foundation: www.benton.org/Library/health/two.htm
  Cornell Law School, U.S. Code Collection, requirement of health maintenance organizations: www4.law.cornell.edu/uscode/42/300e.html

## *Identify all relevant values that play a role in the case and determine which values, if any, conflict*

Nonmaleficence:

Beneficence:

Respect for persons:

Loyalty:

Distributive justice:

## Learning issues for next student-centered problem-based learning session

- List the options open to you. That is, answer the question, "What could you do?"
- Choose the best solution from an ethical point of view, justify it, and respond to possible criticisms. That is, answer the question, "What should you do, and why?"
- What are the different ways of thinking about the problem? Which conflict management techniques can be used in the situation?

# Part two

## Standard of review

Because "standing is challenged on the basis of the pleadings, we 'accept as true all material allegations of the complaint, and must construe the complaint in favor of the complaining party'" [*United States v. Vazquez*, 145 F.3d 74, 81 (2d Cir. 1998), quoting *Warth v. Seldin*, 422 U.S. 490, 501, 45 L. Ed. 2d 343, 95 S. Ct. 2197 (1975)]. This appeal depends solely on questions of law, which we review *de novo*.

## The State's standing as assignee

We reach the same conclusion as that of the district court, that the State lacks standing to pursue this action as an assignee of the eight plan participants' right to bring an action in equity, although our reasoning differs from the district court's. The court concluded that the State lacks standing as an assignee because "the civil enforcement provisions of ERISA are exclusive and provide standing only to . . . specifically enumerated" parties, who include plan participants and beneficiaries, but not their assignees (*PHS*, 103 F. Supp. 2d at 510). We do not reach this issue. Rather, we conclude that the State, in its capacity as an assignee of the right to bring suit for equitable relief, did not suffer an injury of a nature that would confer standing on it under Article III of the Constitution.

The assignments purport to transfer to the State any right of action for equitable relief possessed by the plan participants by virtue of their status as plan participants or beneficiaries. They do not, the State acknowledges, confer "actual" rights or benefits under ERISA on the State (Pl.'s Br. at 15–17). The right to recover benefits or to seek money damages remains with the assignors. Moreover, the assignments divorce the equitable cause of action aimed at an alleged breach of fiduciary duty from the duty itself because they do not create a fiduciary duty running from PHS to the State. And, the assignments do not shift the loss suffered by individual enrollees from the alleged breach of such duty from the individuals to the State. "Whether a party has a sufficient stake in an otherwise justiciable controversy to obtain judicial resolution of that controversy is what has traditionally been referred to as the question of standing to sue" [*Sierra Club v. Morton*, 405 U.S. 727, 731–732, 31 L. Ed. 2d 636, 92 S. Ct. 1361 (1972)].

Article III, § 2 of the U.S. Constitution restricts federal courts to deciding "Cases" and "Controversies." From this has emerged the doctrine of constitutional standing. Federal courts must determine [standing] at the threshold of every case. . . . "It would violate principles of separation of powers for us to hear a matter that was not a case or controversy and therefore not delegated to the [federal] judiciary under Article III" [*Vermont Right to Life Comm., Inc., v. Sorrell*, 221 F.3d 376, 381–382 (2d Cir. 2000), quoting *United States v. Cambio Exacto, S. A.*, 166 F.3d 522, 527 (2d Cir. 1999)].

At an "irreducible constitutional minimum," Article III standing requires that the plaintiff "have suffered an injury in fact — an invasion of a legally protected interest which is (a) concrete and particularized; and (b) actual or imminent, not conjectural or hypothetical" [*Lujan v. Defenders of Wildlife*, 504 U.S. 555, 560, 119 L. Ed. 2d 351, 112 S. Ct. 2130 (1992); accord *Vermont Agency of Natural Resources v. United States ex. rel. Stevens*, 529 U.S. 765, 771, 120 S. Ct. 1858, 146 L. Ed. 2d 836 (2000); *St. Pierre v. Dyer*, 208 F.3d 394, 401 (2d Cir. 2000); *Vazquez*, 145 F.3d at 80; cf. *Valley Forge Christian College v. Americans United for Separation of Church and State, Inc.*, 454 U.S. 464, 472, 70 L. Ed. 2d 700, 102 S. Ct. 752 (1982) ("At an irreducible minimum, Art. III requires the party who invokes the court's authority to show that he personally has suffered some actual or threatened injury as a result of the putatively illegal conduct of the defendant")]. The Supreme Court has noted, as a "prudential principle. . . that the plaintiff generally must assert his own legal rights and interests, and cannot rest his claim to relief on the legal rights or interests of third parties" (*Valley Forge Christian College*, 454 U.S. at 474).

The State does not bring suit here as a party injured itself, but as an assignee of others who assert injury. The Supreme Court has held that, in at least some cases, an "assignee of a claim [does have] standing to assert the injury in fact suffered by the assignor" (*Vermont Agency*, 529 U.S. at 773). Typically, the assignee, obtaining the assignment in exchange for some consideration running from it to the assignor, replaces the assignor with respect to the claim or the portion of the claim assigned and thus stands in the assignor's stead with respect to both injury and remedy.

For example, we have held that a health care provider that spends money on behalf of a patient for drugs and in return receives an assignment of the patient's rights to reimbursement under the health care plan has standing as assignee in a lawsuit under ERISA against the plan that refused the reimbursement [See *I.V. Servs. of Am., Inc. v. Trs. of Am. Consulting Eng'rs Council Ins. Trust Fund*, 136 F.3d 114, 117 n.2 (2d Cir. 1998)]. In *I.V. Services*, the injury — the unreimbursed cost of drugs prescribed for the assignor — was assumed by the assignee, and in return the right to seek redress for it passed from the patient to the provider under the assignment. We noted our agreement "with our sister circuits that, under federal common law, the assignees of beneficiaries to an ERISA-governed insurance plan have standing to sue under ERISA" (id. [citations omitted]). By sustaining the plaintiff's standing as a matter of federal common law, we implicitly held that health care providers under these circumstances have constitutional standing.

There are also situations for which, even though an assignee incurs no injury, expense, or loss in exchange for the assignment, a valid and binding assignment of a claim (or a portion thereof) — not only the right or ability to bring suit — may confer standing on the assignee. In *Vermont Agency*, the Supreme Court held that the plaintiff had standing under Article III to bring a qui tam civil action pursuant to the False Claims Act, which allows a private person (the relator) to bring suit on behalf of the U.S. government and in return recover a share of the proceeds from the action (529 U.S. at 769, 771–778). The Court concluded that "the United States' injury in fact suffices to confer standing on [the relator]" (id. at 774). The Court explained that an "adequate basis for the relator's suit for his bounty is to be found in the doctrine that the assignee of a claim has standing to assert the injury in fact suffered by the assignor. The [False Claims Act] can reasonably be regarded as effecting a partial assignment of the Government's damages claim."

The case before us differs critically from *Vermont Agency* and *I.V. Services*. The qui tam relator in the former and the health care provider in the latter each had a "'concrete private interest in the outcome of [its] suit'" (see *Vermont Agency*, 529 U.S. at 772 [quoting *Lujan*, 504 U.S. at 573]). That is, the outcome had the potential to affect the qui tam relator and health care provider in a "personal and individual way": they both stood, personally and individually, to recover a monetary award (see *Lujan*, 504 U.S. at 560 and [noting that an "injury in fact" must be "particularized" and defining "particularized" as affecting "the plaintiff in a personal and individual way"]). Furthermore, their interest in the suit was directly related to the assignors' original injuries (see *Vermont Agency,* 529 U.S. at 772 ["An interest unrelated to injury in fact is insufficient to give a plaintiff standing"]). The money damages they sought to recover would be awarded in recompense for the property interest allegedly injured by the defendants.

As assignee in the present case, however, the State fails to meet the injury requirement because it does not have a "concrete private interest in the outcome of the suit" (see id. [citation and internal quotation marks omitted]). In other words, it has failed to allege that it suffered an injury in fact that is particularized. The actions of the defendant, as alleged, do not "affect the plaintiff in a personal and individual way." Through the assignments, the State has acquired only the right to control the equitable portion of a lawsuit seeking redress of the assignor–participants' rights under ERISA. None of the remedies being sought would flow to the State as assignee. As the State puts it, "this case is brought solely for the benefit of the assignors and those similarly situated" (Pl.'s Br. at 11). Even if the assignments are valid as a contractual matter, they thus merely give the State the right to act as a nominal party. Compare *New York ex rel Abrams v. Cornwell Co.,* 695 F.2d 34, 38 (2d Cir. 1982), holding that a quasi-sovereign interest that will support *parens patriae* standing must be distinguished "from [*inter alia*] . . . private parties' interests where the State serves merely as a nominal party," vacated in part on other grounds, 718 F.2d 22 (2d Cir. 1983). The State as an assignee therefore lacks standing under Article III of the Constitution.

"We have no doubt about the sincerity of [the State's] stated objectives and the depth of [its] commitment to them. But the essence of standing is not a question of motivation but of possession of the requisite . . . interest that is, or is threatened to be, injured by the unconstitutional conduct" (*Valley Forge Christian College,* 454 U.S. at 486). We hold that the State as purported assignee of the right to seek equitable relief for the assignors' alleged injury lacks Article III standing because it does not, through that assignment, possess the requisite interest that is or is threatened to be injured by PHS's conduct.

## The State's standing as parens patriae

### Article III standing

As an alternative basis for jurisdiction, the State asserts the right to institute this action in its capacity as *parens patriae.* The doctrine of *parens patriae* allows states to bring suit on behalf of their citizens in certain circumstances by asserting a "quasi-sovereign interest" [*Alfred L. Snapp & Son, Inc. v. Puerto Rico ex rel. Barez,* 458 U.S. 592, 601, 73 L. Ed. 2d 995, 102 S. Ct. 3260 (1982)]. The doctrine of *parens patriae* derives from the common-law principle that a sovereign, as "parent of the country," may step in on behalf of its citizens to prevent "injury to those who cannot protect themselves."

The district court, in concluding that the State had no Article III standing to bring this litigation, reviewed various factors that the Supreme

Court, this Court, and others have viewed as prerequisites for *parens patriae* standing (*PHS*, 103 F. Supp. 2d at 504–509). The court concluded that the State had "articulated an interest apart from the interests of the particular private parties referenced in the complaint," and that it had met the requirement that the injury asserted be to "a sufficiently substantial segment of its population." The court held, however, that ERISA's broad preemption clause removed from the State its "quasi-sovereign interest in the specific relief sought by this lawsuit," and, in "a very close call," that there were "adequate alternative means of civil enforcement by which individual plaintiffs may obtain complete relief." Based on its last two holdings, the district court concluded that the State lacked *parens patriae* standing under Article III.

We might be inclined to disagree with the district court were it necessary to address the issue of Article III *parens patriae* standing. We do not think, however, that it is.

*List the options open to you. That is, answer the question, "What could you do?"*

- 
- 
- 
- 

*Choose the best solution from an ethical point of view, justify it, and respond to possible criticisms. That is, answer the question, "What should you do, and why?"*

- 
- 
- 
- 

*Select one member of your PBL group to role-play as a representative of the PHS and have another member of your PBL group role-play as a representative of the State of Connecticut. How might the two converse about different ways of thinking and techniques for conflict management?*

- 
- 
- 
-

*Again, please select one member of your PBL group to role-play as a representative of the PHS and have another member of your PBL group role-play as a representative of the State of Connecticut. How might the representative of the PHS use what is known about stages of change and about motivational interviewing to solve what you consider the major problem presented in the case?*

- 
- 
- 
- 

# Part three

## Statutory standing

Whether the State has *parens patriae* standing under Article III, we conclude that it lacks statutory standing under ERISA's § 1132(a)(3). When determining whether a state has *parens patriae* standing under a federal statute, we ask if Congress intended to allow for such standing. See *Hawaii v. Standard Oil Co. of California*, 405 U.S. 251, 260–266, 31 L. Ed. 2d 184, 92 S. Ct. 885 (1972), parsing statutory language and examining legislative history before deciding that states cannot bring *parens patriae* actions for damages under § 4 of the Clayton Act because Congress did not intend to allow such suits; *Illinois v. Life of Mid-American Insurance Co.*, 805 F.2d 763, 766 (7th Cir. 1986), concluding that *parens patriae* standing was absent because "even if the complaint did sufficiently allege an injury to the state in its quasi-sovereign capacity, it [was] not clear to [the court] that Congress, in enacting the RICO statute, intended to permit such a *parens patriae* proceeding"; see also *New York ex rel Vacco v. Reebok International Ltd.*, 96 F.3d 44, 46 (2d Cir. 1996), noting that the Hart–Scott–Rodino Antitrust Improvement Act of 1976 explicitly provides for *parens patriae* standing.

Section 1132(a)(3) allows a participant, beneficiary, or fiduciary of an ERISA-regulated plan to bring a civil action for injunctive and equitable relief. Other subparts of § 1132 allow the Secretary of Labor to bring specified actions [id. §§ 1132(a)(2), (4), (5), (8), (9)]. Section 1132(a)(7) authorizes states "to enforce compliance with a qualified medical child support order," and § 1169(b) of the same title authorizes states to acquire the rights of third parties through assignment for the limited purpose of recouping payments made under state plans for medical assistance. Nowhere else in § 1132 are states authorized to bring suit.

Courts have consistently read § 1132(a)(3) as strictly limiting "the universe of plaintiffs who may bring certain civil actions" [*Harris Trust and*

*Savings Bank v. Salomon Smith Barney, Inc.*, 530 U.S. 238, 247, 147 L. Ed. 2d 187, 120 S. Ct. 2180 (2000) (emphasis deleted)]. Absent a valid assignment of a claim, at least, non-enumerated parties lack statutory standing to bring suit under § 1132(a)(3) even if they have a direct stake in the outcome of the litigation. In this regard, see *Franchise Tax Board v. Construction Laborers Vacation Trust*, 463 U.S. 1, 27, 77 L. Ed. 2d 420, 103 S. Ct. 2841 (1983) ("ERISA carefully enumerates the parties entitled to seek relief under [§ 1132]; it does not provide anyone other than participants, beneficiaries, or fiduciaries with an express cause of action"); *Pressroom Unions*, 700 F.2d at 892 [concluding that § 1132(e)(1), which states that pension plan participants, beneficiaries, and fiduciaries may sue for certain violations of ERISA, "should be viewed as an exclusive jurisdictional grant" of standing to the parties specified]; see also *Great-West Life and Annuity Insurance Co. v. Knudson*, 534 U.S. 204, 122 S. Ct. 708, 712, 151 L. Ed. 2d 635 (2002) ("ERISA's carefully crafted and detailed enforcement scheme provides strong evidence that Congress did not intend to authorize other remedies that it simply forgot to incorporate expressly").

Because states are not mentioned in § 1132(a)(3), Congress — which "carefully drafted [the] provisions" of § 1132 — did not intend for them to have the ability to bring suit pursuant to § 1132(a)(3) (see *Pressroom Unions*, 700 F.2d at 893). Furthermore, as the district court explained, "the inference that Congress intentionally omitted states from section [1132(a)(3)] finds strong support in the fact that states are expressly empowered by section [1132(a)(7)] to bring only a very limited class of cases" to enforce qualified medical child-support orders [*PHS*, 103 F. Supp. 2d at 502; see also 29 U.S.C. § 1169 (b), allowing states to use assignments in certain circumstances not present in this case].

By holding that the State lacks *parens patriae* standing because § 1132(a)(3) does not expressly provide for such standing, we do not, of course, intend to imply that states may only sue in their *parens patriae* capacity when a statute specifically provides for suits by states. There is considerable authority for the proposition that "states have frequently been allowed to sue in *parens patriae* to . . . enforce federal statutes that . . . do not specifically provide standing for state attorney generals" [*New York ex rel Vacco v. Mid Hudson Medical Group, P.C.*, 877 F. Supp. 143, 146 (S. D.N.Y. 1995) (collecting cases), but, compare *Standard Oil Co.*, 405 U.S. at 264 (rejecting *parens patriae* standing in a suit for damages in the absence of a "clear expression of congressional purpose" allowing such standing because of the concern of double recovery)]. As the district court correctly pointed out, however, "the federal statutes under which states have been granted *parens patriae* standing all contain broad civil enforcement provisions" that "permit suit by any 'person' who is 'injured' or aggrieved'" (*PHS*, 103 F. Supp. 2d at 509–510 [collecting federal statutes with broad enforcement provisions]). Section 1132 of ERISA, by contrast, carefully limits the parties who may seek relief.

By our holding, we reject the State's argument that Congress cannot limit states' power to sue as *parens patriae*. Specifically, the State argues that "the ability of states to act in the interest of their citizens in a *parens patriae* capacity is an essential attribute of the inherent sovereignty of states that may not be diminished in light of the principles of our federalism that are reflected in the Constitution and the Tenth Amendment" (Pl.'s Ltr. Br. of June 12, 2001, at 14).

The Tenth Amendment provides that "the powers not delegated to the United States by the Constitution, nor prohibited by it to the States, are reserved to the States respectively, or to the people." Federal statutes validly enacted under one of Congress's enumerated powers — here, the Commerce Clause — cannot violate the Tenth Amendment unless they commandeer the states' executive officials [see *Printz v. United States*, 521 U.S. 898, 933, 138 L. Ed. 2d 914, 117 S. Ct. 2365 (1997)] or legislative processes, see *New York v. United States*, 505 U.S. 144, 161–166, 120 L. Ed. 2d 120, 112 S. Ct. 2408 (1992); see also *Cellular Phone Taskforce v. Federal Communications Commission*, 205 F.3d 82, 96 (2d Cir. 2000), holding that a federal telecommunications law preempting states' ability to regulate the health and safety issues with respect to certain personal wireless service facilities does not violate the Tenth Amendment because the "statute does not commandeer local authorities to administer a federal program", cert. denied, 531 U.S. 1070, 148 L. Ed. 2d 661, 121 S. Ct. 758 (2001); *City of New York v. United States*, 179 F.3d 29, 35 (2d Cir. 1999), holding that the Tenth Amendment is a "shield against the federal government's using state and local governments to enact and administer federal programs" not a "sword allowing states and localities to engage in passive resistance that frustrates federal programs", cert. denied, 528 U.S. 1115 (2000); *United States v. Sage*, 92 F.3d 101, 107 (2d Cir. 1996), concluding that the Child Support Recovery Act does not violate the Tenth Amendment because it does not "compel a State to enact and enforce a federal family program", cert. denied, 519 U.S. 1099, 136 L. Ed. 2d 727, 117 S. Ct. 784 (1997); *United States v. Bostic*, 168 F.3d 718, 724 (4th Cir.), holding that a federal gun statute does not violate the Tenth Amendment because it was validly passed under the Commerce Clause and imposes no "affirmative obligation" on the states, cert. denied, 527 U.S. 1029, 144 L. Ed. 2d 785, 119 S. Ct. 2383 (1999). Section 1132 does not commandeer any branch of state government because it imposes no affirmative duty of any kind on any of them. It therefore does not violate the Tenth Amendment.

For the foregoing reasons, the judgment of the district court is affirmed.

## Conclusion

The barriers to health care are basically accessibility, availability, and acceptability. People such as African Americans, Native Americans, and Native Alaskans who live in rural areas may lack accessibility and availability. Others may not accept or be aware of health and social services that are available in the community. Other factors that many people may face are communication difficulties, discrimination, the lack of education and promotion. Access to health care has for a while been one of the big issues that the United States has faced and has been trying to improve through reform. Presidential candidates often use this issue as one of their campaign tools.

---

# Unethical experimentation

This problem-based learning session is based on the following: *Bibeau v. Pacific Northwest Research Foundation.*, No. 97-35825, U.S. Court of Appeals for the Ninth Circuit, 1999 U.S. App. Lexis 38092. September 15, 1998, Argued. September 16, 1998, Submission Deferred. September 28, 1998, Submitted, Portland, Oregon. August 19, 1999, Filed. As Amended on Denial of Rehearing April 12, 2000, Reported at: 2000 U.S. App. Lexis 6639. It is reprinted here with permission of LexisNexis.

## Objectives

The objectives for this problem-based learning case are:

- To study the history of experiments and the ethical issues behind the procedures performed by researchers
- To find the role of informed consent in these cases
- To present appropriate research methods

## Introduction

Looking at research in the 20th century, you will find ethical issues regarding the use of human subjects. Human subjects were sometimes misinformed or forced to participate in studies without their consent. Here we will examine five well-known studies involving ethical issues. Experiments in Nazi Germany involved forced participation in numerous detrimental or fatal studies. Human subjects unknowingly participated in the Tuskegee syphilis experiment, Willowbrook, Jewish Chronic Disease Hospital study, and various human radiation studies.

## Part one

In the 1960s, Harold Bibeau was an inmate at the Oregon State Penitentiary (OSP). During that time, Dr. Carl Heller of the Pacific Northwest Research

Foundation (PNRF) conducted a series of experiments under the auspices of the Atomic Energy Commission to determine the human body's responses to various experimental regimens, among them the effect of radiation on human testicular function. Inmates were paid for participating and proselytized other inmates to sign up for the experiments. As a result of this encouragement, Bibeau volunteered for the testicular irradiation experiments.

Bibeau's involvement with the Heller experiments consisted of four steps: First, a biopsy was taken of his testicles before he underwent irradiation. Next, his testicles were exposed to approximately 18.5 rads of radiation. Biopsies were then periodically taken from his testicles to monitor the effects of the radiation. Finally, prior to his departure from the OSP, and in accordance with a consent form he signed prior to his participation in the experiments, he underwent a vasectomy to prevent contamination of the genetic pool by mutated chromosomes.

Following his release from the OSP, Bibeau became a self-described drifter, moving from place to place and spending many years as a long-haul truck driver. After marrying and settling near Portland, Bibeau lived a relatively peaceful life, not thinking about his time in the OSP. One day in 1993, he came across a news report of a speech by Energy Secretary Hazel O'Leary, which contained an apology from the U.S. government for its use of human subjects during the Cold War era. Bibeau thought the events she described sounded suspiciously similar to the program in which he had been involved, so he began an "obsessive" search for the truth about the Heller experiments. Just short of 2 years after the O'Leary speech, Bibeau filed this action in the District of Oregon as the putative representative of a class of persons similarly situated. After Bibeau's claims were narrowed on a motion to dismiss, the court found that all of his claims were barred by the statute of limitations and granted the defendants' motions for summary judgment.

Bibeau claims he was the victim of a conspiracy to fraudulently induce him to participate in the experiments, and that he was lied to about the possible side effects of the radiation and about the nature and purpose of the experiments. He also brings related state law claims for fraud, battery, breach of fiduciary duty, strict liability for ultrahazardous activity, and intentional infliction of emotional distress. These claims have their roots in the events of over three decades ago, and the parties agree that the statute of limitations applicable to both the federal and the state claims is 2 years. The question remains, two years from when?

Because it is inequitable to bar someone who has no idea he has been harmed from seeking redress, the statute of limitations has generally been tolled by the "discovery rule." Under this rule, the statute only begins to run once a plaintiff has knowledge of the "critical facts" of his injury, which are "that he has been hurt and who has inflicted the injury." In addition to being a rule of Oregon law, the discovery rule has been observed as a matter of federal law.

There is a twist to the discovery rule: the plaintiff must be diligent in discovering the critical facts. As a result, a plaintiff who did not actually know that his rights were violated will be barred from bringing his claim after the running of the statute of limitations if he should have known in the exercise of due diligence. But "what [a plaintiff] knew and when [he] knew it are questions of fact." The district court held that Bibeau had failed to investigate his symptoms diligently; as a result, he had run out of time to file suit. Notably, however, the district court did not specify *when* Bibeau was, or should have been, aware of the fact that he had been injured by the Heller experiments. This is a telling point, for it highlights the fact-intensive nature of the issue the district court resolved in granting summary judgment.

In support of the district court's ruling, defendants contend that Bibeau's claims accrued when the pain he experienced during his biopsies was much more severe than he had been told to expect, which should have alerted him that Dr. Heller was lying. Although a jury might find that someone who experienced much greater pain than he had been told to expect should have begun to question the bona fides of the experiments, we cannot hold as a matter of law that a reasonable person would be put on notice of his claims by such an event. Pain is subjective and cannot be described in precise terms. Bibeau may well have believed that he was experiencing the degree of pain he had been told to expect, but had misunderstood how much that would be. It also is not clear why pain during the biopsies should have alerted him to the long-term effects of the radiation, especially since the biopsies and the irradiation were distinct operations performed during the experiments.

Alternatively, defendants point to certain physical symptoms, which may have had their roots in the Heller experiments, that Bibeau experienced over the course of the many years since he left the OSP. These ailments consisted of recurrent, severe testicular pain, which Bibeau experienced since the 1970s; a periodic groin rash he suffered from the early 1970s; a wart on the inside of his left upper leg, which he discovered in 1979; and certain lymph node lumps that appeared on his arm and back in 1979. Despite suffering from these symptoms over the course of decades, Bibeau never consulted a doctor, and it did not cross his mind that they could be associated with the Heller experiments. He claims that he believed some of these symptoms were common male complaints. The district court held, however, that a reasonable person "would have associated the pain with the experiments, accurately or not, or at least would have made inquiries regarding a possible connection."

We cannot agree with the district court. A trier of fact could find that a reasonable person would not necessarily have connected Bibeau's symptoms to the Heller experiments. It is a closer question whether the symptoms created a duty to consult a doctor. Under both federal and Oregon law, the question of diligence in cases like this is twofold. Initially, we must ask "'whether the plaintiff could reasonably have been expected to [consult a doctor] in the first place.'" If we answer this question in the affirmative, we must next determine whether a medical examination would have disclosed the nature and cause of plaintiff's injury to put him on notice of his claim.

While we have held that the plaintiff has a duty of inquiry, none of our cases deals with a situation in which a plaintiff fails to seek medical attention that might have led him to discover his claim. In *Schiele*, however, the Oregon Supreme Court did deal with such a situation and held that while "not everyone goes to a doctor with the same degree of alacrity," there is a point beyond which "delay in seeking medical attention is no longer reasonable," in which case plaintiff will be charged with "any knowledge which a medical examination would otherwise have disclosed" (*Schiele*, 587 P.2d at 1014).

Under *Schiele*, Bibeau may have hesitated too long in seeking medical attention, in which case he would be charged with whatever he would have learned from consulting a doctor. But, it makes no difference in this case because the record fails to demonstrate irrefutably that, had Bibeau consulted a doctor, he would have discovered his claims. In holding Bibeau's claim barred by the statute of limitations, the district court explained: "Given the plethora of information in the public domain regarding the risks of radiation exposure, generally, and the Heller experiments, specifically, *had Bibeau explained his participation in the Experiments to a medical doctor*, to the extent there is merit to his case, presumably he would have learned that there was a possibility that his symptoms were related to the Experiments" (*Bibeau*, 980 F. Supp. at 355. The district court's ruling presupposes that Bibeau not only would have seen a doctor about his symptoms, but also that he would have "explained [to him] his participation in the [Heller] Experiments" (id.) But, for Bibeau to have done so, he would have had to suspect a connection between the experiments and the symptoms, and we have already held that this is not necessarily the case (see p. 9434 supra).

The question the district court *should* have addressed is whether, had Bibeau seen a doctor about his symptoms, the doctor would have discovered Bibeau's participation in the experiments and then made a connection between the two. The defendants did not submit any expert testimony or other evidence demonstrating that a normally competent doctor would have put Bibeau on the right track. With all that was in the public domain, it is possible that a competent doctor would have done so. But, while we may determine what a "reasonable person" would do, we cannot, without any evidence in the record, say what a normally competent doctor would do in this situation. This genuine issue of material fact precluded summary judgment.

As a second justification for their insistence that Bibeau must have known he had been injured by the Heller experiments, the defendants advance a litany of news reports and other public revelations regarding the OSP and the Heller experiments. Indeed, the results of the experiments themselves were published in scientific journals, just as the inmates who participated in them were told they would be. Surely, the defendants contend, given the volume of public attention the experiments received, Bibeau cannot plausibly claim to have been unaware of the torts that he now alleges.

It is true that many news articles were published regarding the experiments, most notably around the time they ended and in the mid-1980s when the names of those involved were released. However, that does not mean that Bibeau must be lying about his ignorance, or that a reasonable man would necessarily have discovered the truth. The fact that Bibeau was employed as a long-haul trucker, and thus was often traveling around the country during the time that a rash of lawsuits over the Heller experiments were filed in Oregon, would help explain why he did not hear of the suits. He claims not to have been worried about the possible deleterious effects of radiation because his military experience led him to believe that radiation was safe. And, given his modest educational background, it is not entirely surprising that he would not have come across any articles published in scientific journals. All of these factors and the inferences that can be drawn from them present questions of fact for a jury to resolve (cf. *Swine Flu*, 764 F.2d at 641 regarding additional fact finding necessary to determine if general community awareness was sufficient to indicate that a plaintiff reasonably should have known of the cause of his wife's death).

We also reject the argument that Bibeau must be presumed to have known that he was injured as of 1987, when the Oregon legislature passed a bill providing for payment of medical expenses of inmates who participated in the Heller experiments. Defendants rely on the adage that everyone is presumed to know the law, but that is actually a misstatement of the rule. What the law presumes is that everyone is aware of the obligations the law imposes on them. When a piece of legislation — usually of a criminal nature — adjusts the legal responsibilities of citizens, they cannot escape the effect of that law by claiming ignorance. Were the rule otherwise, citizens could frustrate the legislature's exercise of authority by an ostrichlike effort not to learn their legal obligations. But, that is very different from saying that every citizen is presumed to know every word of every law passed by the legislature. The 1987 Oregon statute imposed no obligations on Bibeau. On the contrary, the law imposed obligations on others to provide Bibeau with certain benefits. It was their responsibility to notify him of his rights, a responsibility they undertook only halfheartedly.

For much the same reasons, we cannot hold that Bibeau should be presumed to be aware of a 1986 report issued by the U.S. House of Representatives. It would stretch the rule that individuals are presumed to know their legal obligations to the breaking point to presume that they are aware of every report, white paper, and floor statement delivered within the halls of the legislature. The legislative report, like the 1987 Oregon legislation, may have given Bibeau actual notice, in which case he would be barred. But, Bibeau claims that he was unaware of either, and therefore his state of awareness is a contested question of fact that cannot be resolved on summary judgment.

In sum, although we sympathize with the view that there is a time when stale claims must come to rest and a defendant's right to repose outweighs a plaintiff's right to redress, we are unable to say that the time has come to declare Bibeau's claims to be barred as a matter of law.

## Make a list of the major problems presented in this case

- 
- 
- 
- 

## Hypothesis and mechanism

For the problems in your list above, give a cause or a reason for them to happen:

- 
- 
- 
- 

## Learning issues

Make a list of learning issues in the form of questions. Remember, your goal is to gather the medical, social, and all other relevant facts that may apply to the case.

Describe the important features of the Jewish Chronic Disease Hospital Study.
- In 1963, the Jewish Chronic Disease Hospital in New York City performed studies regarding the transplant rejection process.
- The doctors injected chronically ill and debilitated patients with live cancer cells.
- It was known that healthy individuals injected with live cancer cells would soon after reject the transplant.
- The researcher failed to obtain a written consent form from the individuals undergoing the study.
- The patients did not know they were injected with live cancer cells. The doctors did not want to "frighten" the patients unnecessarily.
- The debilitated patients rejected the cancer cells eventually. The rejection took substantially longer than for those who were not ill.

Describe the important features of the Tuskegee Study of Untreated Syphilis (1932–1972).

African-American men (400) in rural Alabama thought they were being treated for syphilis; in reality, they were going untreated.

Penicillin was widely used to treat syphilis by 1946, but was withheld from these patients.

The U.S. Public Health Service (PHS) was actually studying the long-term effects of syphilis on black males.

The government doctors failed to obtain informed consent; however, they did offer incentives for participation.

Incentives included: free physical exams, free rides to and from the clinics, hot meals on examination days, and a guaranteed burial stipend.

This study was unethical and immoral and perhaps even racist because of the lack of informed consent and immoral experiments on human subjects.

The PHS believed the information the study would eventually provide would exceed the possible risk to the men.

Not until July 1972 did the story break, and lawsuits formed against the institutions and individuals involved in the study.

By this time, over 100 of the African-American men infected with the disease had died.

Living participants and the heirs of the deceased received settlements; however, no apologies were ever made by the PHS.

Not only did this study examine medical research, but it also examined ethical dilemmas such as the need for patient education in determining personal therapy.

Describe the important features of the Human Radiation Studies.

Irradiation of pregnant women, mentally retarded students, workers, soldiers, medical patients, and prison inmates at dose rates known to have harmful effects

Objective: To discover whether and under what conditions soldiers on an atomic battlefield would be cognitively impaired

Responsible organizations: Funded by Department of Defense, researched by University of Cincinnati, under leadership of Eugene Saenger

No "informed consent": Due to subjects' "low-educational level, low-functioning intelligence quotient, and strong evidence of cerebral organic deficit"

Researchers claim: Subjects "benefit" from radiation exposure, treatment not intended to have therapeutic effect, and an estimated eight deaths would be attributed to treatment

Chronology of significant events in history of this human radiation study:

1971: The *Washington Post* reveals study conducted by University of Cincinnati.

1972: Researchers quietly end experiment when evidence of harmful effects begins to mount.

1975: Senator Edward Kennedy chairs hearings on human experimentation funded by Department of Defense.

Early 1980s: Network of activist–researchers starts to compile full and extensive record of U.S radiation experiments on humans.

Mid-1980s: Network accumulates enough documentation on human experimentations to go public.

1985–1986: Labor council representing workers at the Department of Energy's Fernald, Ohio, plant, demands disclosure of all studies involving uranium and plutonium, toxic release to environment, use of atomic workers as experimental subjects, and the body-snatching program.

1992: Dotte Troxell holds a hunger strike to be continued until death unless the government releases all data on the experiments and provides care for all survivors.

1993: Emma Craft, who never knew that she had been fed radioactive iron in the 1940s, finds out her 11-year-old daughter died from cancer.

1994: Craft, along with many others who learned they have been experimental subjects, files a class action lawsuit against a long list of defendants, led by Vanderbilt University.

Describe the important features of the Willowbrook study.

The purpose was to study the etiology of the disease and attempt to create a protective vaccine against it.

These studies took place at the Willowbrook State School during the period 1963 through 1966.

The study was of the natural history of infectious hepatitis and subsequent testing of the effects of gamma globulin in preventing or ameliorating the disease.

Children were infected with the hepatitis virus.

Subjects were fed stools from an infected person, and later these subjects received injections of more purified virus preparation.

Defense for the study was that the majority of these children acquired the infection anyway and maybe it would be better for them to be infected under carefully controlled research conditions.

Willowbrook closed its doors during these studies.

What studies prompted the creation of the Nuremberg Code and the Declaration of Helsinki to protect the rights of human subjects?

Freezing/hypothermia

Genetics: twin experiments

Infectious diseases: facial fungus

Interrogation and torture

High altitude: compression chambers

Pharmacological: sulfanilamide
Sterilization: formalin injections, x-rays, and castration
Surgery
Traumatic injuries: wound, infection

## Literature review

To help you get ready to answer certain questions you anticipate being asked during the second part of the case, look in the local medical library and on the World Wide Web for helpful information. Please indicate in the spaces below (1) several helpful articles or books you found and (2) several helpful Web sites you found.

- **Helpful articles/books:**
  Bernstein, J.E., Ethical considerations in human experimentation, *J. Clin. Pharmacol.*, 15, 579–590, 1975.
  Lederer, S., *Subjected to Science: Human Experimentation in America before the Second World War*, John Hopkins University Press, Baltimore, 1998.
  Lock, S., Research ethics—a brief historical review to 1965, *J. Int. Med.*, 238(6), 513–520, 1995.
  Shevell, M.I., Neurosciences in the Third Reich: from Ivory Tower to death camps, *Can. J. Neur. Sci.*, 26(2), 132–138, 1999.

- **Helpful Web sites:**
  The University of Texas Medical Branch, Why research Became Regulated: http://www.utmb.edu/gcrc/INCLUDE/Training%20Class/1999-2000/Handouts/Vanderpool.htm
  National Cancer Institute. A Guide to Understanding Informed Consent: History http://www.cancer.gov/clinicaltrials/conducting/informed-consent-guide/page4

## *Identify all relevant values that play a role in the case and determine which values, if any, conflict*

Nonmaleficence:



Beneficence:

Respect for persons:


Loyalty:


Distributive justice:


## Learning issues for next student-centered problem-based learning session

- List the options open to you. That is, answer the question, "What could you do?"
- Choose the best solution from an ethical point of view, justify it, and respond to possible criticisms. That is, answer the question, "What should you do, and why?"
- What are the different ways of thinking about the problem? Which conflict management techniques can be used in the situation?


## Part two

Many of the defendants also assert that they are shielded from the federal claims by the doctrine of qualified immunity. We conclude that some of them are.

Both the PNRF and Mavis Rowley (who was Dr. Heller's assistant) contend that, as government contractors that did not violate any clearly established constitutional rights, they are entitled to qualified immunity. According to them, recent Supreme Court decisions, such as *Richardson v. McKnight* [521 U.S. 399, 138 L. Ed. 2d 540, 117 S. Ct. 2100 (1997)] and *Wyatt v. Cole* [504 U.S. 158, 118 L. Ed. 2d 504, 112 S. Ct. 1827 (1992)], "strongly imply" that private entities briefly associated with the government are entitled to share in governmental qualified immunity. It is true that, in *Richardson*, the Supreme Court, although refusing to grant the defendant prison contractors qualified immunity, "answered the immunity question narrowly, in the context in which it arose" (*Richardson*, 521 U.S. at 413) and also refused to rule on whether the defendants might assert "a special 'good faith' defense" (id.). However, circuit precedent suggests that the private defendants are not entitled to qualified immunity here; see *Halvorsen v. Baird*, 146

F.3d 680, 686 (9th Cir. 1998), (determining that "a firm systematically organized to assume a major lengthy administrative task" was not entitled to
share in governmental qualified immunity).

Our situation is little different from those in past cases that found qualified immunity absent. This is not a firm that was "briefly associated with a
government body" (*Richardson*, 521 U.S. at 413), but rather a firm that conducted research at the OSP for a decade, from 1963 to 1973. We can find no
principled distinction between private researchers such as the PNRF, the
private prison guards involved in *Richardson*, and the private detoxification
facility in *Halvorsen*. Accordingly, PNRF and Rowley are not entitled to
qualified immunity.

DiIaconi, who was the chief medical officer at the OSP during the time
in question, claims he is entitled to qualified immunity as a state employee
who acted in good faith and did not violate any clearly established rights.
Bibeau counters that DiIaconi violated his "clearly established constitutional
right to be free from the non-consensual, non-therapeutic invasion of [his]
bodily integrity." He claims to have met his burden of pointing to clearly
established law existing at the time of the events by citing decisions such as
*Rochin v. California* [342 U.S. 165, 96 L. Ed. 183, 72 S. Ct. 205 (1952)] and
*Skinner v. Oklahoma* [316 U.S. 535, 86 L. Ed. 1655, 62 S. Ct. 1110 (1942)].

This claim is problematic because those cases refer to the right at a high
level of generality, and the Supreme Court has instructed that "the contours
of the right must be sufficiently clear that a reasonable official would understand that what he is doing violates that right" [*Anderson v. Creighton*, 483
U.S. 635, 640, 97 L. Ed. 2d 523, 107 S. Ct. 3034 (1987)]. A right to bodily
integrity defined only by these cases could leave a reasonable governmental
official in doubt whether any battery would lead to a constitutional violation.
But, we need not decide whether these cases clearly establish a right to bodily
integrity as we hold that DiIaconi's actions here did not violate any such
right, even if it was clearly established.

Once the relevant right is identified, the question becomes whether a
reasonable officer could have believed that his actions affecting that right
were lawful [see *Sinaloa Lake Owners Association v. City of Simi Valley*, 70 F.3d
1095, 1099 (9th Cir. 1995)]. "An official is entitled to qualified immunity even
where reasonable officers could disagree as to the lawfulness of the official's
conduct, so long as that conclusion is objectively reasonable" (id.). Even
assuming that Bibeau had a clearly established right to bodily integrity
requiring that he be fully informed of all known risks of the experiments he
had agreed to undergo, DiIaconi denies he was involved in the allegedly
flawed process of obtaining consent. Instead of coming forward with evidence to suggest otherwise, Bibeau points to DiIaconi's position as chief
medical officer at the prison and the fact that he performed biopsies and
vasectomies on inmates, including Bibeau.

But, DiIaconi performed those operations pursuant to signed consent
forms obtained by the experimenters, which he could have reasonably taken
to indicate that the inmates had been informed of all the risks of the

experiments. Bibeau has alleged that DiIaconi was convinced of "the worth of the program" (according to a report he coauthored after the experiments were conducted), but a belief that the program was worthwhile implies nothing about his knowledge of the adequacy of the notice given the inmates. Indeed, Bibeau admitted in his deposition that the reason he included DiIaconi in this suit was because he "assumed" and "believed" that DiIaconi was involved with Dr. Heller and attended many of Dr. Heller's meetings, and that there was no other reason that he was named in this litigation. A reasonable doctor could have believed that he was respecting the inmates' clearly established rights when he operated on them pursuant to seemingly valid consent forms.

Bibeau also complains that DiIaconi failed to advise former inmates that they should receive follow-up examinations as a result of the experiments, even though he considered his duty to his patients a continuing one. Assuming such a failure would be actionable under state tort law — and we express no view on the subject — a violation of a tort duty certainly is not enough to show that DiIaconi violated clearly established constitutional rights. As the Supreme Court has said, qualified immunity protects "all but the plainly incompetent or those who knowingly violate the law" [*Malley v. Briggs*, 475 U.S. 335, 341, 89 L. Ed. 2d 271, 106 S. Ct. 1092 (1986)]. A reasonable doctor could have believed that operating on seemingly consenting patients and allowing the experiments to be conducted in the prison in which he worked was consistent with clearly established constitutional rights; therefore, we hold that DiIaconi is entitled to qualified immunity.

To resolve the question of the Division of Biology and Medicine heads Totter and Liverman's entitlement to qualified immunity, we enter into a murky area on the border between qualified immunity and liability under Section 1983. Generally, the key question to be answered for purposes of qualified immunity is whether the law was clearly established at the time of the alleged acts. Claims, such as Totter and Liverman's, that a defendant was not involved in the events giving rise to liability are cut from a different cloth because they present factual disputes rather than distinct legal questions [see, e.g., *Velasquez v. Senko*, 813 F.2d 1509, 1511 (9th Cir. 1987)]. Although an officer not present at the scene of a beating obviously could not have violated any clearly established rights, such factual defenses are treated differently from claims based on the state of the law. As an example, an interlocutory appeal will not lie for such claims if the district court determines that there are genuine issues of fact involved [see *Johnson v. Jones*, 515 U.S. 304, 319–320, 132 L. Ed. 2d 238, 115 S. Ct. 2151 (1995)]. We need not worry about such jurisdictional considerations in evaluating these claims, however, as this is an appeal from a final judgment, not an interlocutory appeal. Therefore, we apply normal summary judgment principles to determine whether defendants are entitled to qualified immunity.

Like DiIaconi, Totter and Liverman do not dispute Bibeau's claim to a clearly established right to bodily integrity; rather, they argue that their actions did not violate Bibeau's rights. This resembles a claim that "a reasonable officer [could] have believed [his] conduct was lawful" in light of clearly established law, which is the second prong of our test for qualified immunity [*Act Up!/Portland v. Bagley,* 988 F.2d 868, 871 (9th Cir. 1993)]. At the same time, Totter and Liverman's defense also looks like they claim that Section 1983 liability will not lie for the actions performed as a matter of Section 1983 doctrine. Thus, it could very well be that what we have here are not claims to qualified immunity so much as claims that Section 1983 supplies no remedy for the acts alleged. We see these as flip sides of the same coin. Whether we denominate these assertions as claims of qualified immunity or claims that they are not subject to liability under Section 1983 for their actions, the result is the same: Totter and Liverman were entitled to summary judgment on this point.

Aside from the fact that Totter and Liverman headed the Division of Biology and Medicine (Totter from 1967 to 1972 and Liverman from 1972 to 1979), Bibeau adduced no substantial connection between them and the Heller experiments. Indeed, he forthrightly admitted that Totter and Liverman relied on the reports of their staff that the experiments were being conducted satisfactorily, although in doing so he added the legal conclusion that "Totter and Liverman as Directors were ultimately responsible for the Heller Experiments." Another way of phrasing Bibeau's "ultimate responsibility" theory is "respondeat superior," and such liability does not lie in either *Bivens* or Section 1983 actions [see, e.g., *Terrell v. Brewer,* 935 F.2d 1015, 1018 (9th Cir. 1991) (*Bivens*); *Taylor v. List,* 880 F.2d 1040, 1045 (9th Cir. 1989) (Section 1983)].

Bibeau attempts to avoid this bar by alleging that Totter and Liverman had sufficient involvement in the Heller experiments to render them liable because they attended various meetings and reviewed certain proposals, but failed to take any steps to ensure that the inmates were properly informed. Even setting aside the fact that Liverman became head of the Division of Biology and Medicine after Bibeau had been released from the OSP, Bibeau has not adduced enough evidence to raise a genuine issue of material fact as to whether Totter and Liverman were more than peripherally connected with the Heller experiments due to their alleged awareness of the project. This is further pointed up by the fact that Bibeau complains not about their actions, but about their inaction. Without more involvement in the experiments, they did not violate any of Bibeau's clearly established rights and therefore are entitled to qualified immunity.

The defendants assert various other defenses, but we decline to consider their arguments because the discovery schedule indicates that the summary judgment motions were set only for questions relating to the statute of limitations and qualified immunity. Therefore, we will allow the district court to rule on these other contentions in the first instance.

*List the options open to you. That is, answer the question, "What could you do?"*

- 
- 
- 
- 

*Choose the best solution from an ethical point of view, justify it, and respond to possible criticisms. That is, answer the question, "What should you do, and why?"*

- 
- 
- 
- 

*Select one member of your PBL group to role-play as Dr. Heller and have another member of your PBL group role-play as Mr. Bibeau. How might the two converse about different ways of thinking and techniques for conflict management?*

- 
- 
- 
- 

*Again, please select one member of your PBL group to role-play as Dr. Heller and have another member of your PBL group role-play as Mr. Bibeau. How might Dr. Heller use what is known about stages of change and about motivational interviewing to solve what you consider the major problem presented in the case?*

- 
- 
- 
-

## Part three

More than 30 years ago, plaintiff Harold Bibeau suffered the unkindest cut of all. Today, he seeks to bring suit against those he claims are responsible for injuring him. The defendants parry by raising the statute of limitations. The district court agreed and entered summary judgment in favor of all defendants. We must decide whether Bibeau was or should have been aware of his injuries and is therefore barred from bringing suit as a matter of law.

The judgment of the district court is reversed, and this case is remanded for further proceedings consistent with this opinion.

## Conclusion

The results of these studies uniformly demonstrated a lack of informed consent. The researchers denied the participants their human rights. The lack of informed consent among human patients is not in accordance to the Belmont Report. The researchers in these studies failed to:

1. Inform patients of the procedures, purpose, and risks of the study
2. Present information in a manner that the patient would understand
3. Allow patients to make their own decision without feeling pressured into participating in the study

The Belmont Report identified three basic ethical principles that also need to be followed. They are:

1. *Respect for persons (autonomy):* This principle acknowledges the dignity and freedom of every person. It requires obtaining informed consent from all potential research subjects (or their legally authorized representatives).
2. *Beneficence:* This principle requires that researchers maximize benefits and minimize harms or risks associated with research. Research-related risks must be reasonable in light of expected benefits.
3. *Justice:* This principle requires the equitable selection and recruitment and fair treatment of research subjects.

*case twelve*

# Research principles

This problem-based learning session is based on the following: *Warner-Lambert Company v. Heckler*, Nos. 85-3371, 85-3377, 85-3383, U.S. Court of Appeals for the Third Circuit, 787 F.2d 147; 1986 U.S. App. Lexis 23635, January 6, 1986, Argued, April 1, 1986. It is reprinted here with permission of LexisNexis.

## Objective

The objectives of this problem-based learning case are:

- To be familiar with the major codes, statements of ethical principles, and laws/regulations that prescribe responsible conduct in research, including the Nuremberg Code, the Declaration of Helsinki, the Belmont Report, and governmental and institutional regulations

## Introduction

Human torture, prolonged disease states, humans coerced into harmful situations, discrimination, and abuse of privileges by medical professionals — these are just some of the things that can result from the lack of principles, standards, and regulations regarding human research.

The Nuremberg Code, Declaration of Helsinki, and Belmont Report are portrayed through government and institutional regulations. These are some of the major codes and regulations that are required to be followed by parties involved in human research to avoid tragic results.

## Part one

The petitioners, who manufacture and market oral proteolytic enzymes (OPEs), are Warner-Lambert (Warner), who produces the OPE Papase, and Armour Pharmaceutical Company, William H. Rorer, Inc., and Wallace Laboratories (collectively ARW), who presented their case jointly before the Food and Drug Administration (FDA) and before this court and who produce, respectively, the OPEs Chymoral, Ananase, and Avazyme.

The OPEs are prescription medications that the manufacturers claim are effective for use as adjunctive relief of swelling and inflammation associated with accidental trauma; surgical, obstetrical, and dental procedures; and infections and allergic reactions. Some of the drug companies claim that their OPEs will ease pain and accelerate tissue repair.

The manufacturers obtained FDA approval for the OPEs prior to 1962. At the time approval was granted, the Food, Drug, and Cosmetic Act required the FDA to determine only that a drug was safe for human use. In 1962, Congress amended the act to require drug manufacturers to prove to the FDA that drugs they wished to market were effective as well as safe. The 1962 amendments also required the FDA to reevaluate drugs that it had previously been approved.

The Supreme Court opinion in *Weinberger v. Hynson, Westcott, and Dunning, Inc.* [412 U.S. 609, 37 L. Ed. 2d 207, 93 S. Ct. 2469 (1973)] reviews the legislative history leading to the 1962 amendments, the major provisions enacted, and the subsequent administrative actions to enforce the new statutory requirements. As the Court pointed out, substantial numbers of drugs were being marketed for which efficacy could not be shown. The panels evaluating 16,500 claims made on behalf of 4000 drugs found that 70% of the claims were not supported by substantial evidence of effectiveness.

Pursuant to the statutory mandate, the FDA requested the OPE manufacturers to submit documentation showing the effectiveness of their drugs. Manufacturers of nine OPEs submitted data for evaluation. Based on these initial submissions, the commissioner of the FDA found in 1970 that the OPEs were "possibly effective" for "diagnostic gastric lavage" and for relieving symptoms associated with the obstetrical procedure episiotomy, and that the OPEs lacked substantial evidence of effectiveness for all other claims.

In the same notice, the OPE manufacturers were required to delete from their labeling the indications for which the drug had been classified as lacking substantial evidence. They were also required to provide additional data that would constitute substantial evidence of the effectiveness of OPEs for those indications for which the drugs had been classified as possibly effective. Five years later, the FDA published an extensive review of the additional data submitted in which the agency concluded that the manufacturers had not supported any of their claims of effectiveness for any indication. Therefore, the FDA announced that it proposed to withdraw approval for the OPEs. Seven OPE manufacturers were granted a formal hearing on the question of whether the OPEs were effective, the other manufacturers having withdrawn or having failed to submit data. Before the hearing, two more OPE manufacturers withdrew.

After prehearing conferences in February and March 1980, a hearing before an administrative law judge was held in July and August of that year. Warner and ARW submitted a total of 31 studies, 13 on behalf of Warner and 18 on behalf of ARW, to demonstrate the effectiveness of their OPEs. In addition, the manufacturers presented the testimony of many of the investigators who conducted the studies. The manufacturers sought to bolster this evidence by the testimony of experts, who testified that, based on their review of the submitted studies, the drugs had been shown to be effective. In opposition, the FDA produced the testimony of several employees of the agency's Bureau of Drugs and several outside experts.

In April 1981, the ALJ (administrative law judge) issued his initial decision in the matter. In a lengthy opinion that reviewed each of the studies submitted by the sponsoring manufacturer, the ALJ concluded that each study failed to meet the requirements for adequate and well-controlled clinical investigations. The ALJ thus found that the drug manufacturers had not met their statutory burden of producing evidence demonstrating that the OPEs were effective. The ALJ therefore ordered withdrawal of approval for the drugs.

The parties filed extensive exceptions to the ALJ's decision with the commissioner. Four years later, the commissioner issued his decision withdrawing approval for the OPEs. The commissioner rejected all the manufacturers' challenges to the conduct of the hearing. In a detailed opinion, the commissioner reviewed each of the studies submitted by the manufacturers in support of the efficacy of the OPEs and found each methodologically inadequate, although in some cases for reasons different from those on which the ALJ had relied. The commissioner also found that there was a lack of substantial evidence that the five OPEs had the effects represented, and, accordingly, he withdrew approval. The commissioner stayed this decision pending judicial review.

## The statutory and regulatory framework

Under the Federal Food, Drug, and Cosmetic Act, 21 U.S.C. §§ 301–392, a drug manufacturer or sponsor cannot market a new drug unless the FDA first approves the drug. To obtain approval, a drug's sponsor must submit to the FDA full reports of investigations that have been made to show whether such drug is safe for use and whether such drug is effective in use.

The act requires drug manufacturers not only to show that the drug is safe, but also to show by "substantial evidence" that the submitted drug "will have the effect it purports or is represented to have under the conditions of use prescribed, recommended, or suggested." Substantial evidence is defined in the act as follows:

> *evidence consisting of adequate and well-controlled investigations, including clinical investigations, by experts qualified by scientific training and experience to evaluate the effectiveness of the drug involved, on the basis of which it could fairly and responsibly be concluded by such experts that the drug will have the effect it purports or is represented to have under the conditions of use prescribed.*

The statute mandates the same standard when the commissioner is deciding whether to withdraw approval for a drug that previously received FDA approval.

Because the act uses the plural "investigations," the FDA requires drug manufacturers to submit at least two "adequate and well-controlled" studies showing the effectiveness of the drug. The FDA has issued regulations defining adequate and well-controlled by several substantive criteria: (1) the study must select subjects in a way that ensures that they are suitable for the study, that assigns subjects to test groups in a way designed to minimize bias, and that reduces the effect of other individual factors, such as the subjects' age, sex, or use of other drugs; (2) the study must explain its methodology, including the steps taken to minimize investigator and subject bias; (3) the study must use a method of control that permits "quantitative evaluation"; and (4) the drug tested must be standardized for identity, strength, purity, quality, and dosage form. The regulations also require that a study provide a clear statement of its objectives, a summary of the methods of analysis, and an evaluation of the data derived from the study. Uncontrolled studies alone are not sufficient to show effectiveness, but the FDA will consider them as corroborative support. A failure to meet any of these criteria renders the study unacceptable for meeting the statutory requirement of substantial evidence.

Judicial review of the commissioner's decision is pursuant to 21 U.S.C. § 355(h), which provides that the secretary's findings of fact "if supported by substantial evidence, shall be conclusive." In addition, under the Administrative Procedure Act, a reviewing court shall "set aside agency action, findings, and conclusions found to be . . . arbitrary, capricious, an abuse of discretion, or otherwise not in accordance with law." Although our review of the commissioner's legal decision is plenary, it is clear that, to the extent the commissioner's decision involves interpretation of the Food, Drug, and Cosmetic Act, we must give "considerable weight" to his construction.

## Make a list of the major problems presented in this case

- 
- 
- 
- 

## Hypothesis and mechanism

For the problems in your list above, give a cause or a reason for them to happen:

- 
-

- •
- •

## Learning issues

Make a list of learning issues in the form of questions. Remember, your goal is to gather the medical, social, and all other relevant facts that may apply to the case.

What is the Hippocratic oath? The writings of Hippocrates, a Greek physician, had an impact on the ethics of medical practice. The Hippocratic oath represents the traditional Hippocratic doctor–patient relationship, in which the patient was silent and obedient to the physician and trusted that the physician would act in their interest and do no harm.

> I *swear by Apollo the physician, the Aesculapius, and Health, and All-heal, and all the gods and goddesses, that, according to my ability the judgement, I will keep this Oath and this stipulation to reckon him who taught me this Art equally dear to me as my parents, to share my substance with him, and relieve his necessities if required; to look upon his offspring in the same footing as my own brothers, and to teach them this art, if they shall wish to learn it, without fee or stipulation; and that by precept, lecture, and every other mode of instruction, I will impart a knowledge of the Art to my own sons, and those of my teachers, and to disciples bound by a stipulation and oath according to the law of medicine, but to none others. I will follow that system of regimen which, according to my ability and judgement, I consider for the benefit of my patients, and abstain from whatever is deleterious and mischievous. I will give no dead-ly medicine to any one if asked, nor suggest any such coun-sel; and in like manner I will not give a woman pessary to produce abortion. With purity and with holiness I will pass my life and practice my Art. I will not cut persons laboring under the stone, but will leave this to be done by men who are practitioners of this work. Into whatever houses I enter, I will go into them for the benefit of the sick, and will abstain from every voluntary mischief and corruption; and further from the connection with it, I see or hear, in the life of men, which ought not to be spoken of abroad, I will not divulge, as reckoning that all such should be kept secret. While I continue to keep this Oath unviolated, may it be granted to me to enjoy life and practice of the Art, respected by all men, in all times. But should I trespass and violate this Oath, may the reverse be my lot.*

What is the Nuremberg Code?

The Nuremberg Code of 1947 is generally regarded as the first document to set ethical regulations in human experimentation based on informed consent. It was a response to the horrors of Nazi experimentation in the death camps. The legacy of Nuremberg and the trial, in which physicians were found to have special obligations to use their power to protect human rights, has changed 'the way physicians conduct medical research on human subjects since 1947. A set of regulations was established by American judges that must be followed each time an experiment is conducted. Two of the regulations are designed to protect the rights of the subjects of human experimentation, and eight are to protect their welfare.

The two American physicians who helped prosecute the Nazi doctors at Nuremberg, Leo Alexander and Andrew Ivy, are the code's authors.

In this ten-point statement, humane experimentation is justified only if the results benefit society, and the experimentation is carried out in accordance with basic principles that satisfy moral, ethical, and legal concepts.

The code served as a blueprint for today's principles that ensure the rights of human subjects in medical research.

It has not been officially adopted in its entirety as law by any nation or as ethics by any major medical association. It has been universally accepted and is articulated in international law in Article 7 of the United Nations International Covenant on Civil and Political Rights (1966).

Physicians and researchers in medicine failed to see that the code applied to them because it was linked to the Nazi atrocities, thus it was only relevant to the Nazi doctors. Doctors felt the code was too stringent and legalistic to be applied to modern research. As soon as the code was written, there were attempts to marginalize it.

Directives for Human Experimentation

1. Voluntary informed consent is essential.
2. Experiment results should be for the good of society and not obtained by other methods or means of study.
3. Experiment should be based on prior animal studies and knowledge of the disease or other problem being studied.
4. Avoid all unnecessary physical and mental suffering and injury.
5. There should be no expectation that death or disabling injury will occur from the experiment.
6. Degree of risk should never exceed the benefits of the experiment.
7. Adequate preparations and facilities should be provided to protect human subjects from injury, disability, or death.
8. Only scientifically qualified individuals should conduct the experiment.

9. The human subjects should be at liberty to terminate their involvement in the experiment at any time.
10. Scientist in charge of the experiment must be prepared to terminate the experiment at any stage if there is probable cause of injury to the human subject.

What is the Declaration of Helsinki?

The Declaration of Helsinki was developed by the World Medical Association in 1964 and later amended in 1975, 1983, 1989, 1996, and most recently in 2000. The declaration serves as an ethical guideline to physicians and other participants in biomedical research involving human subjects. It emphasizes the obligations of the physician–investigators to protect the welfare of the subjects.

History

Original text brought to the World Medical Association by various national medical associations.

Declaration of Helsinki was officially adopted by the 18th World Medical Assembly in Helsinki, Finland, in 1964.

During World War II, the World Medical Association was established and tried to substitute informed consent with peer review in its Declaration of Helsinki.

The Declaration of Helsinki reestablished physician-centered guidelines, thereby continuing the Hippocratic tradition.

Purpose

The declaration serves as the ethical principles to provide guidance to physicians or investigators in biomedical research involving humans.

Basic principles for all medical research (research combined with clinical care and nontherapeutic research)

Biomedical research involving human subjects must be used to improve diagnostic, therapeutic, and prophylactic procedures and the understanding of the etiology and pathogenesis of disease.

The physicians' duty is to protect life, health, privacy, and dignity of human subjects.

Research with humans should be based on laboratory and animal experimentation.

The experimental protocol should be reviewed by an independent committee.

The research protocol should contain a statement that says ethical considerations involving research comply with the principles of the Declaration of Helsinki.

The research is conducted only by medically/scientifically qualified individuals.

Researchers should assess predictable risks in comparison with benefits to the subjects.

The subjects must be volunteers and informed participants.

Informed consent

Subjects who are minors or those with mental/physical incapacities should have informed consent from a lawful guardian.

Publications of research results should be accurate and present both positive and negative findings.

At the conclusion of the study, every patient should be ensured access to the best proven prophylactic, diagnostic, and therapeutic methods identified by the study.

What is the Belmont Report?

The Belmont Report, created in 1979 by the U.S. Department of Health, Education, and Welfare, provides the three basic principles: respect for persons, beneficence, and justice. Respect for persons dictates that informed consent, which consists of information, comprehension, and voluntariness, should be recognized. Beneficence states the assessment of risks, including the nature and scope of risks, and the benefits, and the systematic assessment of risks and benefits should be applied. Justice deals with the selection of subjects and making sure the process is fair. The report allows all parties involved to understand the correct procedures that must take place to conduct research that is as safe and beneficial as possible.

The Nuremberg Code was the prototype of the Belmont Report.

The report indicates a distinction between research and practice. It provides "the philosophical underpinnings for the current laws governing human subjects research."

Research that "relies on data from or about human subjects should be carried out in accordance with *Belmont Report* guidelines."

It contains three basic ethical principles that are relevant to research involving human subjects and the application of these principles: respect for persons, beneficence, and justice.

What are the boundaries between practice and research?

*Practice* refers to "interventions that are designed solely to enhance the well-being of an individual patient or client and that have a reasonable expectation of success." Medical or behavioral practice provides diagnosis, preventive treatment, or therapy to particular individuals.

*Research* refers to "an activity designed to test an hypothesis, permit conclusions to be drawn, and thereby to develop or contribute to generalizable knowledge." Research is described in a formal protocol and indicates an objective and the procedure to reach that objective.

What are the basic ethical principles?

*Respect for persons* states that "individuals should be treated as autonomous agents," which are individuals capable of making decisions about personal goals and living by those decisions. It also states "persons with diminished autonomy are entitled to protection."

These individuals are not capable of making self-determined decisions and need to have their personal rights protected. The extent of protection given depends on the "risk of harm and the likelihood of benefit."

*Beneficence* is described as covering "acts of kindness or charity that go beyond strict obligation." The Belmont Report has two expressions of beneficent action: "(1) do no harm and (2) maximize possible benefits and minimize possible harms." Beneficence affects individual investigators and society. Problems result in the determination of when it is acceptable to seek certain benefits despite the risks and when benefits should be avoided due to the risks.

*Justice*, in essence, is "'fairness in distribution' or 'what is deserved.'" It describes guidelines by which burdens and benefits should be distributed. These guidelines are: "(1) to each person an equal share, (2) to each person according to individual need, (3) to each person according to individual effort, (4) to each person according to societal contribution, and (5) to each person according to merit."

How have the basic ethical principles been applied?

*Informed consent* gives subjects the opportunity to decide what will or will not happen to them, to the degree that they are capable of deciding. The consent process contains three elements: information, comprehension, and voluntariness.

*Assessment of risks and benefits* provides both "an opportunity and a responsibility to gather systematic and comprehensive information about proposed research." It consists of "The Nature and Scope of Risks and Benefits" and "The Systematic Assessment of Risks and Benefits."

*Selection of subjects* describes the selection of subjects of research, which occurs at two levels: "the social and the individual." Social justice requires that "distinction be drawn between classes of subjects that ought, and ought not, to participate in any particular kind of research, based on the ability of members of that class to bear burdens and on the appropriateness of placing further burdens on the already burdened persons." Individual justice requires that subjects not be chosen because they are favorable for a particular research or they are "undesirable" individuals, such as prison inmates, subject to risky research.

Describe government and institutional regulations from 1980 to the present.

General requirements for informed consent

No investigator may involve a human being as a subject in research covered by these regulations unless the investigator has obtained the legally effective informed consent of the subject or the subject's legally authorized representation.

Elements of informed consent

A statement that the study involves research, an explanation of the purposes of the research, and the expected duration of the subject's participation

A description of any reasonably foreseeable risks and benefits to the subject

A disclosure of appropriate alternative procedures or courses of treatment, if any, that might be advantageous to the subject

A statement describing the extent, if any, to which confidentiality of records identifying the subject will be maintained and notes to the possibility that the FDA may inspect the records

An explanation as to whether there is any compensation and an explanation as to whether any medical treatments are available

A statement that participation is voluntary, that refusal to participate will involve no penalty or loss of benefits to which the subject is otherwise entitled, and that participation may be discontinued at any time

An explanation of whom to contact for answers to pertinent questions about the research and research subjects' rights and whom to contact in the event of a research-related injury to the subject

The approximate number of subjects involved in the study

A statement of significant new findings developed during the course of the research that may relate to the subject's willingness to continue participation

Documentation of informed consent

Informed consent shall be documented by a written consent form approved by the institutional review board (IRB) and signed by the subject or the subject's legally authorized representative.

The consent form can be either:

A written consent document that embodies the elements of informed consent

A short-form written consent document stating that the elements of informed consent have been presented orally to the subject or the subject's legally authorized representative. When this method is used, there shall be a witness.

Institutional review board

Intended to protect the rights and welfare of human subjects involved in such research

Shall have at least five members with varying backgrounds to promote complete and adequate review

Shall review and have authority to approve, require modifications to, or disapprove all research activities

Criteria for IRB approval of research:

Risks to subjects are minimized

Selection of subjects is equitable

Informed consent is obtained from each prospective subject or the subject's legally authorized representative

Appropriate documentation of informed consent

When appropriate, adequate provisions to protect the privacy of subjects and to maintain the confidentiality of data

Terminate ongoing studies subject to this part when doing so would not endanger the subjects

Suspension or termination of IRB approval of research:

An IRB shall have authority to suspend or terminate approval of research that is not being conducted in accordance with the IRB's requirements or that has been associated with unexpected serious harm to subjects. Any suspension or termination of approval shall include a statement of the reasons for the IRB's action and shall be reported promptly to the investigator, appropriate institutional officials, and the FDA.

Disqualification of an IRB or an institution:

The commissioner may disqualify an IRB or the parent institution if the commissioner determines that:

The IRB has refused or repeatedly failed to comply with any of the regulations.

The noncompliance adversely affects the rights or welfare of the human subjects in a clinical investigation.

If the commissioner determines that disqualification is appropriate, the commissioner will issue an order that explains the basis for the determination and prescribe any actions to be taken with regard to ongoing clinical research conducted under the review of the IRB.

The FDA will not approve an application for a research permit for a clinical investigation that is to be under the review of a disqualified IRB or that is to be conducted at a disqualified institution.

What are the roles of the FDA and IRBs in protecting the welfare of human subjects?

The government (FDA) and the institutional review board protect the welfare and rights of human subjects. The investigators must document all of the informed consent provided and follow the rules and regulations the government sets out to obtain approval and funding for the project.

How have these various codes been applied?

U.S. regulations governing federally supported research with human subjects derive in part from the Nuremberg Code and the Declaration of Helsinki: "Concern for the interests of the subject must always prevail over the interest of science and society."

Informed consent principle and minimal risks concept utilized by federal regulations to protect the rights and welfare of subjects in human research

To different viewpoints on placebo comparisons: Is it unethical and irrelevant?

Antidepressant studies in the United States

Clinical trials of AIDS vaccines in developed and developing countries

## Literature review

To help you get ready to answer certain questions you anticipate being asked during the second part of the case, look in the local medical library and on the World Wide Web for helpful information. Please indicate in the spaces below (1) several helpful articles or books you found and (2) several helpful Web sites you found.

- **Helpful articles:**
  Amdur, R.J. and Biddle, C., Institutional review board approval and publication of juman research products, *JAMA*, 277, 909–914, 1997.

  Bloom, B.R., The highest attainable standard: ethical issues in AIDS vaccines, *Science*, 279, 186, 1998.

  Grodin, M., *Science, Ethics and Law. Children as Research Subjects*, Oxford University Press, New York, 1994, pp. 15–16, 81–84, 103–140, 113–117, 218–219.

  Lasagna, L., The Helsinki Declaration: timeless guide or irrelevant anachronism? *J. Clin. Psychopharmacol.*, 15, 96–98, 1995.

  Pranulis, M.F., Protecting rights of human subjects, *West. J. Nurs. Res.*, 18, 474–478, 1996.

  Rothman, K.J. and Michels, K.B., Declaration of Helsinki should be strengthened, *BMJ*, 321, 442–445, 2000.

  Skolnick, B.E., Ethical and institutional review board issues, *Adv. Neurol.*, 76, 253–262, 1998.

  Vollmann, J. and Winau, R., Informed consent in human experimentation before the Nuremberg Code, *BMJ*, 313, 1445–1449, 1996.

  Woodward, B., Challenges to human subject protection in U.S. medical research, *JAMA*, 282, 1947–1952, 1999.

- **Helpful Web sites:**
  Nova online — Hippocratic oath — classical version: www.pbs.org/wgbh/nova/doctors/oath_classical.html

  National Institutes of Health — the Nuremberg Code: ohsr.od.nih.gov/nuremberg.php3

  The Food and Drug Administration — the Belmont Report: www.fda.gov/oc/ohrt/irbs/elmont.html

  World Medical Association Declaration of Helsinki: www.wma.net

  Informed consent checklist — basic and additional elements: ohrp.osophs.dhhs.gov/humansubjects/assurance/consentckls.htm

*Identify all relevant values that play a role in the case and determine*
*        which values, if any, conflict*

Nonmaleficence:

Beneficence:

Respect for persons:

Loyalty:

Distributive justice:

*Learning issues for next student-centered problem-based learning*
*        session*

- List the options open to you. That is, answer the question, "What could you do?"
- Choose the best solution from an ethical point of view, justify it, and respond to possible criticisms. That is, answer the question, "What should you do, and why?"
- What are the different ways of thinking about the problem? Which conflict management techniques can be used in the situation?

## Part two

The drug companies have filed extensive challenges to the commissioner's decision. They attack the commissioner's determination that each of the 31 investigations they submitted failed to meet the regulatory criteria for an adequate and well-controlled investigation. The commissioner filed an exhaustive opinion of 585 pages, in which he painstakingly reviewed each investigation and gave at least two reasons why each was rejected. We do not discuss each investigation, but refer to particular studies when appropriate or as illustrative.

In addition to challenging the commissioner's rejection of the individual studies, the drug companies present certain general challenges to the commissioner's decision. All argue that the commissioner gave inadequate weight to the testimony and opinions of their expert witnesses, ARW argues that the commissioner improperly required that the clinical investigations show therapeutically significant evidence of improvement, and all claim that the commissioner erred by failing to find that they had established effectiveness under the statutory standard. Warner also raises two procedural issues relating to the ALJ's conduct of the proceedings specific to it. It contends that the ALJ impermissibly allowed the hearing to extend beyond the issues outlined in the prehearing stipulation and erred by excluding the direct testimony of three of Warner's experts.

We consider first petitioners' argument that the commissioner improperly substituted his view for that of the experts. If petitioners are correct, then of course the decision could not stand.

## Commissioner's authority to assess studies

Warner and ARW make the novel and potentially far-reaching argument that the opinions and conclusions of their experts, rather than the opinion of the commissioner, must determine whether studies submitted by the drug companies were adequate and well controlled and whether they proved the effectiveness of the drugs under consideration. Thus, Warner argues that the statutory language "obligates the Commissioner to base any decision on the adequate and well-controlled character of a clinical study, and on the determinations of a drug's effectiveness drawn there from, solely on the conclusion of qualified experts" (Warner's brief at 27). Warner stresses that the views of the experts on these issues were intended to "be paramount and controlling."

We believe that this argument and the comparable one made by ARW run counter not only to the statutory scheme and the legislative history, but also to the policy and rationale underlying use of administrative agencies. In establishing a regulatory scheme such as that administered by the FDA, Congress has chosen to place rule making, administrative control, and enforcement authority in an expert agency. Its chief officer, the Commissioner of Food and Drugs, to whom the Secretary of HHS has delegated the statutory responsibility [21 C.F.R. § 5.10 (1985)] has the obligation of effectuating the intent of Congress that drugs on the marketplace be both safe and effective. The commissioner's decision that studies submitted by drug manufacturers should be evaluated pursuant to "well-established principles of scientific investigations," as set forth in the regulations promulgated for that purpose, was approved by the Supreme Court in *Weinberger v. Hynson,*

*Westcott, and Dunning, Inc.* [412 U.S. 609, 37 L. Ed. 2d 207, 93 S. Ct. 2469 (1973)], but see also *Pharmaceutical Manufacturers Association v. Richardson* [318 F. Supp. 301, 306–310 (D. Del. 1970), approvingly cited in *Hynson*, 412 U.S. at 619 n. 13].

If, as Warner and ARW suggest, the commissioner were required to defer to the opinions of experts testifying with respect to the validity of the methodology used in particular studies and the ultimate question of effectiveness, the commissioner's statutory function would be significantly curtailed. Moreover, he would not even be able to ensure that his own regulations were interpreted uniformly and consistently. Patently, the drug companies' argument would undercut the traditional discretion such statutory schemes relegate to the administrator.

The drug companies argue, however, that the interpretation they proffer is compelled by the statutory definition of "substantial evidence," which refers to conclusions reached "by . . . experts." The language of the statutory definition of substantial evidence as consisting of "adequate and well-controlled investigations . . . on the basis of which it could fairly and responsibly be concluded by such experts that the drug will have the effect it purports . . . to have" [21 U.S.C. § 355(d)] hardly supports the drug companies' startling claim that the experts' view must be binding on the commissioner. The plain import of the reference to experts in the definition of substantial evidence is that the investigations submitted be of such quality that the investigating experts could responsibly rely on them for a conclusion. The definition does not suggest any allocation of responsibility for decision making between the commissioner and the experts, and it is unlikely that Congress would use a definition for that purpose. Elsewhere, the statute makes clear that withdrawal of new drug approval is the prerogative of the secretary "if the Secretary finds . . . that there is a lack of substantial evidence that the drug will have the effect it purports or is represented to have" [21 U.S.C. § 355(e)(3)].

The petitioners also claim that their interpretation is supported by the decision of Congress to permit the drug manufacturers to prove the effectiveness of their drugs by substantial evidence rather than the higher standard of preponderance of the evidence [see S. Rep. No. 1744, Pt. 2, 87th Cong., 2d Sess. 6 (1962)]. That fact, while relevant to the issue of the quantity of evidence, also does not go to the allocation of decision-making responsibility. The legislative history hardly suggests that Congress intended that the commissioner have no role in determining whether substantial evidence exists as to a particular drug. The Senate report, in its explanation of the statutory definition of substantial evidence, makes clear that the commissioner may reject the experts' conclusions. The report states:

> *[A] claim could be rejected if it were found (a) that the investigations were not "adequate;" (b) that they were not "well controlled;" (c) that they had been conducted by experts not qualified to evaluate the effectiveness of the drug*

*for which the application is made; or (d) that the conclusions drawn by such experts could not fairly and responsibly be derived from their investigations.*

Any doubt as to the intention of Congress to vest in the secretary, and not the drug company experts, the responsibility of making the ultimate decision called for in the statute is plainly dispelled by the unambiguous language of the Senate report:

*What the Secretary is required to do is evaluate the claims of effectiveness in the light of the information submitted to him in the new drug application and any other information before him with respect to such drug and to decide whether there is substantial evidence, as defined above, to support the claim. The question of whether the claim would or would not be allowed would be determined by his evaluation of whether the claim had been supported by substantial evidence as defined above. If on the basis of his evaluation the Secretary finds that the claim is not supported by substantial evidence, as defined above, it will not be allowed; if he finds that it is so supported, it will be allowed.*

It would defeat the clear purposes of the act to transfer the commissioner's authority to the manufacturers' experts as petitioners propose. We thus conclude that the concern of Congress with the quality of the expert submissions leads to the conclusion that it is the commissioner who must determine, after giving full consideration to all of the evidence that has been submitted, including expert opinions, if the studies meet the regulatory criteria and show effectiveness.

## Required showing of effectiveness

ARW contends that the commissioner erred in reviewing each study to determine if the results were therapeutically significant, interchangeably referred to as clinically significant. Therapeutic or clinical significance is contrasted for this purpose with statistical significance, which ARW accurately characterizes as based on a premise of the elimination of chance results (ARW reply brief at 6—7). ARW argues that the commissioner must look only to whether any of the submitted studies show statistically significant differences between the test groups given the OPE and the control groups. If so, the commissioner must find the drug effective, and any determination of therapeutic value must be left to the individual prescribing physician. In essence, ARW's claim is that "effectiveness" as used in the act means only that the drug will have the effect the manufacturer claims for it; the amount of the effect is irrelevant, except to the treating physician.

To support its view, ARW points to the statute that requires the FDA to find only that the submitted drug "will have the effect it purports or is represented to have under the conditions of use prescribed, recommended, or suggested in the labeling thereof" [21 U.S.C. § 355(e)(3)]. ARW also points to statements in the legislative history that indicate that Congress believed that effectiveness would be measured by the claims made for the drug by the manufacturer [see, e.g., S. Rep. No. 1744, 87th Cong., 2d Sess. reprinted in 1962 U.S. Code Cong. and Ad. News 2884, 2892; Drug Industry Antitrust Act, Hearings on H.R. 6245 before Subcommittee on Antitrust and Monopoly, 87th Cong., 2d Sess. 143 (1962)]. These isolated sentences, however, do not support ARW's inference, which is contrary to the policy behind the act.

The act does not define effectiveness, thus leaving the task of deciding how effective a new drug must be to the agency to which Congress delegated enforcement. It is important to note that the commissioner does not contend that the effectiveness shown must amount to a "medical breakthrough," as ARW complains, but contends in his brief that he would be satisfied with even a modest clinical or therapeutic effect (respondents' brief at 23).

The commissioner's interpretation of the statute as requiring a showing of clinical significance, rather than merely statistical significance, is persuasive for several reasons. First, in requiring evidence of therapeutic effectiveness, the FDA is interpreting the language of the Food, Drug, and Cosmetic Act, which Congress has entrusted to that agency's supervision. As the Supreme Court has frequently noted, "the construction of a statute by those charged with its administration is entitled to substantial deference" [*United States v. Rutherford*, 442 U.S. 544, 553, 61 L. Ed. 2d 68, 99 S. Ct. 2470 (1979); see *Chevron, U.S.A., Inc. v. Natural Resources Defense Council, Inc.*, 467 U.S. 837, 104 S. Ct. 2778, 2782, 81 L. Ed. 2d 694 (1984)]. We may not substitute ARW's interpretation of effectiveness for that of the FDA unless the commissioner's interpretation is arbitrary or irrational or unless it is established that Congress meant to foreclose the requirement of therapeutic effectiveness.

The fact that the drug, not chance, can be assumed to have contributed to the factor measured does not necessarily establish that patients will receive a benefit from the drug. The commissioner has consistently required a showing of some benefit as an element of the statutory requirement of effectiveness [see Benylin, Final Order, 44 Fed. Reg., 51512, 51521 (1979); Luxtrexin, Withdrawal of Approval of New Drug Application, 41 Fed. Reg., 14406, 14419 (1976)].

It is difficult to conceive of any good reason why the commissioner should be required to find a drug effective if there has been no showing of its therapeutic effect. For example, in the Soule, Wasserman, and Burstein study of the effect of the OPE Chymoral (marketed by Armour) on symptoms associated with episiotomy, the investigators made 240 comparisons between the study and control groups on factors such as edema (swelling), erythema (skin redness), bruising, and the subject's pain while resting, sitting, and walking. These were studied at different time periods after delivery. There were no statistically significant results in favor of Chymoral for reduction of swelling or bruising. Of the 240 tests, only 6 provided statistical results indicating that Chymoral had some effectiveness in the reduction of pain, but these results were shown only after stratification of the subjects into subgroups that the commissioner found had no scientific basis. For example, statistically significant results were reached showing effectiveness of Chymoral for reduction of pain "on sitting on day four in subjects with labors over eight hours"; for reduction of pain "on sitting, on post-partum days two and three, in the 20 subjects less than 21 years old"; and for reduction of pain in multipara subjects (those who had earlier pregnancies) "on ambulation on post-partum days three, four and five," but not in primiparas (first pregnancy subjects) as a group.

ARW argues that these positive results in 6 of 240 comparisons constitute the required statutory showing of effectiveness. The commissioner stated that the most reliable test of effectiveness is the comparison of the total drug group to the total placebo group, a comparison never made in this study. Since there was expert evidence to support the commissioner's conclusion that the *post hoc* stratification was inappropriate, the commissioner's conclusion that six statistically significant findings cannot support a finding of effectiveness was supported by substantial evidence.

Another illustration of the ARW position is afforded by the Lee, Larsen, and Posch Study No. 1, which was proffered to show Chymoral's effectiveness in reducing edema in subjects with hand surgery. The largest difference in measurements between the drug group and the placebo group in absolute figures (rather than percentages) was approximately a quarter inch. Although the percentage difference was statistically significant, the commissioner rejected the study, in part based on expert testimony that the difference in measurements was "therapeutically trivial."

The commissioner's construction that clinically significant evidence of effectiveness must be shown accords with the policies behind the 1962 amendments to the act. These amendments were passed to increase the protection accorded to the consuming public. In a somewhat related context, the Supreme Court recognized that the requirement of effectiveness added by these amendments necessarily entails a showing of some benefit to the patient. The Court stated, "in the treatment of any illness, terminal or otherwise, a drug is effective if it fulfills, by objective indices, its sponsor's claim of prolonged life, improved physical condition, or reduced pain. See 42 Fed. Reg., 39776–39786 (1977)" (*United States v. Rutherford*, 442 U.S. at 555).

Congress rejected the notion, asserted here by ARW, that individual physicians should be left to decide whether particular drugs were effective. For example, in separate concurring remarks accompanying the Senate report, Senator Kefauver, the leading figure behind the legislation, joined by four other members of the Senate Judiciary Committee, made the following observations:

*Leading physicians testified that it is impossible to keep currently informed of the state of medical knowledge to be found scattered in hundreds of medical journals on the 400 new drugs introduced each year. Moreover, they stressed that the marketing of a safe but ineffective drug may well be positively injurious to the public health. When an ineffective drug is prescribed, it is usually in place of an older but effective drug. The problem is compounded by the fact that usually a considerable period elapses between the time when a highly-advertised new drug is put on the market and when knowledge becomes widely disseminated among the medical profession that its performance falls seriously short of its claims.*

(S. Rep. No. 1744, 87th Cong., 2d Sess, 1962 U.S. Code Cong. and Ad. News 2902 [views of Senators Kefauver, Carroll, Hart, Dodd, and Long]).

Congress wanted to ensure that prescribing physicians received sufficient and accurate information concerning the effectiveness of FDA-approved drugs (see *Weinberger v. Hynson, Westcott & Dunning, Inc.*, 412 U.S. at 619), a task that had become impossible due to the sheer volume of new drugs and to the heavy and persistent drug company advertising. See 108 Cong. Rec. 21070 (1962) (remarks of Representative Fogarty), "medical practitioners cannot keep abreast [of new information] on each drug"; 108 Cong. Rec. 17382 (1962) (colloquy between Senators Kefauver and Hart), discussing drug company advertising; see also *Upjohn Company v. Finch*, 422 F.2d 944, 952–54 (6th Cir. 1970), rejecting contention that the public is protected because a physician must prescribe the drugs.

Given the strength of the congressional concern with the protection to the public underlying the Drug Amendments of 1962, it would be anomalous to hold that drug manufacturers may demonstrate effectiveness merely by showing statistical significance. Therefore, we hold that the commissioner did not err in requiring petitioners to show that OPEs are therapeutically effective. This interpretation accords with long-standing FDA policy and with the policies embodied in the Food, Drug, and Cosmetic Act.

## Substantial evidence

The pivotal issue on this appeal is whether there is any basis for us to overturn the commissioner's conclusion that petitioners had not produced substantial evidence that the OPEs will have the purported or represented effects. Central to this conclusion was the commissioner's determination that all of the investigations submitted by the petitioners did not meet the requirements of adequate and well-controlled studies.

As we commented, the commissioner's review of each of the submitted studies was extensive. For each study, the commissioner first reviewed the factual data of the investigation, including information concerning the subjects, the condition tested, the method of reporting results, and the claimed results. Second, the commissioner reviewed the administration of the OPE and stated whether the subjects had received concomitant medication. Finally, the commissioner reviewed the parties' exceptions to the ALJ's findings on each study, the information contained in each study, and the expert testimony supporting the study. Neither ARW nor Warner challenges the accuracy of the commissioner's descriptions of the studies.

Instead, petitioners challenge the commissioner's bases for the rejections. They argue that all of the studies they submitted demonstrate the effectiveness of the particular drug at issue, but Warner directs our attention particularly to the commissioner's rejection of four studies it submitted, and ARW focuses on the commissioner's rejection of six of its studies, two supporting each OPE.

Because the commissioner's findings in this case were made after a hearing, we review them under the substantial evidence test [see 21 U.S.C. § 355(h); see also *Weinberger v. Hynson, Westcott, and Dunning, Inc.*, 412 U.S. at 622]. That review standard does not require that we resolve scientific disputes over the evidence, even though some expert witnesses may have drawn conclusions different from those of the experts on whom the commissioner relied [see *Rhone-Poulenc, Inc., Hess and Clark Division v. FDA*, 205 U.S. App. D.C. 42, 636 F.2d 750, 753 (D.C. Cir. 1980)]. The requirement of substantial evidence also does not require a finding of preponderant or conclusive evidence [see *United States v. An Article of Drug Consisting of 4680 Pails*, 725 F.2d 976, 985 (5th Cir. 1984)]. Rather, we must determine if the commissioner's decision has a reasonable basis [see *Pfizer, Inc., v. Richardson*, 434 F.2d 536, 546–547 (2d Cir. 1970)].

Although courts frequently express reluctance to intrude into complex scientific or medical issues on which we have inadequate technical background, see, for instance, *Cooper Laboratories, Inc., v. Commissioner Federal FDA*, 163 U.S. App. D.C. 212, 501 F.2d 772, 788 (D.C. Cir. 1974) (Leventhal, J., dissenting), (understanding and applying "the drug law and regulations [require] technical knowledge that is not part of this court's working kit"), we cannot completely abdicate the review function imposed on us by Congress and inherent in a democratic society that looks to the judiciary to check excesses from other branches of the government. Fortunately, the issues in this case involve in the main those relating to scientific methodology cognizable even to laypeople (see *Pfizer, Inc., v. Richardson*, 434 F.2d at 546–547).

### Concomitant medication

The basis given by the commissioner most frequently in rejecting the submitted studies was that the investigators' use of concomitant medication was uncontrolled. In 16 studies, the commissioner found that the case report forms were missing information as to the dosage, frequency, or length of administration of the concomitant medication, and that the investigation could therefore not be used as evidence in support of the claims. It is unclear whether the petitioners are challenging the commissioner's position that accurate and complete details about the administration of concomitant medication is a *sine qua non* of an acceptable clinical investigation, or whether they are merely challenging the commissioner's requirement that dosage, frequency, and length of administration must have been contemporaneously recorded on the case report form.

In his opinion, the commissioner fully explained the importance of reviewing the use of concomitant medication and cited to the supporting expert opinion in that connection. He stated that the uncontrolled use of concomitant medication "violates several of the most basic scientific principles governing clinical explanations." These principles are embodied in the commissioner's regulations [see, e.g., 21 C.F.R. § 314.111(a)(5)(ii)(a)(b) and (c)]. Because many concomitant medications, such as analgesics and anti-inflammatory drugs, and concomitant treatments, such as ice packs, are active treatments for the symptoms that the OPEs purport to help alleviate, the use of concomitant medications in both the test and the control groups makes it difficult to state which results in the test group can be attributed to the OPE treatment. However, the commissioner rejected the position that a *per se* rule applies to the use of concomitant medication and instead opted for "the more flexible scientific approach" that entailed examination of the case report forms to determine if the actual effect of the concomitant medications can be determined. The commissioner concluded that, if the concomitant medication is uncontrolled, and the reports of the studies do not provide the details necessary to permit a scientific evaluation of the use of concomitant medication, then the study cannot be considered as part of the basis for approval of effectiveness claims.

Ample precedent supports the commissioner's insistence on "well-controlled investigations." In *Weinberger v. Hynson, Westcott, and Dunning*, the Court stated: "The standard of 'well-controlled investigations' particularized by the regulations is a protective measure designed to ferret out those drugs for which there is no affirmative, reliable evidence of effectiveness" (412 U.S. at 622). Moreover, the expert evidence in the record supports the commissioner's conclusion that use of concomitant medication flaws a clinical study unless it can be determined whether such use was controlled.

ARW raises three related challenges to the commissioner's analysis of concomitant medication. First, ARW argues that the commissioner in effect held that concomitant medication could never be used because of the stringent restrictions he required to constitute control of their use. According to ARW, to meet these requirements, clinical investigators would have had to administer the OPEs in isolation. Because OPEs are adjunctive therapy, not primarily intended to reduce pain or to be used alone, it would be unconscionable to withhold the concomitant medication to subjects suffering painful postsurgical trauma symptoms.

We recognize that clinical investigation of adjunctive therapy raises research difficulties that may not be presented when studying other types of drugs. However, the commissioner cited expert testimony in this record to show that means of controlling concomitant medication existed. Indeed, the adjunctive use of OPEs would seem to indicate that more, rather than less, control over concomitant medication would be necessary to demonstrate effectiveness (cf. *Cooper Laboratories v. Commissioner*, Federal FDA, 501 F.2d at 779, rejecting argument that controlled tests are impossible for drugs designed to relieve pain).

Furthermore, the petitioners would be in a more sympathetic posture to complain about the difficulties of showing effectiveness of adjunctive therapy if their studies had reported the use of concomitant medication in accordance with settled scientific research principles. As the commissioner commented, "In no OPE study criticized by the ALJ because of the use of concomitant medication did all subjects receive the same type and amount of concomitant medication or receive it in a blinded manner." A holding that the commissioner cannot require clinical investigations to be strictly controlled would undermine the intent of Congress to have effectiveness proven by a "strict and demanding" test (see *Weinberger v. Hynson, Westcott, and Dunning, Inc.*, 412 U.S. at 619). Moreover, we find it significant that Congress has not accepted proposals to delete the statutory requirement of a showing of effectiveness [see, e.g., H.R. 12573, 94 Cong., 2d Sess. (1976)].

ARW's second argument is that "so long as patients in control groups and test groups receive at random, concomitant medications, the groups should be roughly equal." The commissioner rejected this argument because it would essentially require him to disregard the use of concomitant medication. He concluded he could not be assured, as the drug companies argued, that randomization balanced out the amounts of concomitant medications used in the studies. In addition, based on expert testimony, the commissioner concluded that, while random assignment of subjects could help minimize the effects of unknown and uncontrollable factors, it should not be used to minimize the effect of factors that are known and can be otherwise controlled.

Finally, ARW argues that the FDA has approved two other drugs that were supported by studies in which concomitant medication was used. This argument is irrelevant. We have already held that the commissioner may insist on strict controls on the use of concomitant medication. That he approved other drugs that were tested with concomitant medications does not bear on the decision in this case, especially when no showing has been made that the studies supporting the other drugs lacked sufficient controls. We decline to overturn the commissioner's decision in this case on the basis of unsupported allegations about the decision in another.

### Other bases for rejection of individual studies

ARW and Warner object to the commissioner's other reasons for rejecting numerous studies. We have reviewed the commissioner's decision and the studies and testimony on which he relied, and we are unable to agree with petitioners. The commissioner fully met the requirement set forth in *Cotter v. Harris* [642 F.2d 700, 706 (3d Cir. 1981)], cited by Warner, regarding the need for an adequate discussion of the evidence in an adjudicatory decision. The commissioner painstakingly reviewed the petitioners' submissions, devoting 370 pages to analysis of the evidence submitted in support of petitioners' OPEs. Each study was rejected for at least two violations of the regulatory criteria, and of the studies petitioners particularly focus on in this court, six were rejected for three or more reasons. It would serve little purpose here to review each of these reasons. Illustrative of the reasons given by the commissioner for finding particular studies were not adequate and well controlled were the failure to show that adequate steps were taken to minimize bias and that blinding was maintained (JA at 150), the failure to record the investigator's initial expectations in studies using the "comparison with expectations" method of analysis, the absence of assurance that the drug and placebo groups were comparable for severity of disease, and the use of an inappropriate statistical method to evaluate data. Our review convinces us that the commissioner disqualified each study "in light of the pertinent regulations" (*Weinberger v. Hynson, Westcott, and Dunning, Inc.*, 412 U.S. at 622).

We emphasize that it is not the court's role to substitute its judgment for that of the commissioner. Warner argues that there is a facial implausibility to the commissioner's rejection of 31 studies, but we cannot find that he did not have a reasonable basis for disqualifying each submission. Petitioners suggest that the commissioner's rejection of all of the studies stems from his prejudicial bias that OPEs cannot possibly work. We find no evidence of such a bias. Moreover, the rejection of all of the studies is just as consistent with the possibility that, in fact, OPEs do not work.

Our task is not to resolve the scientific question of the mythological correctness of the submitted studies, but the legal question whether the commissioner's rejection of the studies is supported by substantial evidence [see *Smithkline Corporation v. FDA*, 190 U.S. App. D.C. 210, 587 F.2d 1107, 1119 (D.C. Cir. 1978)]. Were we to reverse the commissioner's order merely because of an asserted improbability in his reasoning, we would be discarding the commissioner's expertise in favor of our own inexpert judgment. Such a course would contravene a clear congressional judgment to leave to the agency's expertise the primary decision as to drug effectiveness.

*List the options open to you. That is, answer the question, "What could you do?"*

- 
- 
- 
-

*Choose the best solution from an ethical point of view, justify it, and respond to possible criticisms. That is, answer the question, "What should you do, and why?"*

- 
- 
- 
- 

*Select one member of your PBL group to role-play as a Warner or ARW representative and have another member of your PBL group role-play as an FDA representative. How might the two converse about different ways of thinking and techniques for conflict management?*

- 
- 
- 
- 

*Again, please select one member of your PBL group to role-play as a Warner or ARW representative and have another member of your PBL group role-play as an FDA representative. How might a Warner or ARW representative use what is known about stages of change and about motivational interviewing to solve what you consider the major problem presented in the case?*

- 
- 
- 
- 

## Part three

In summary, we conclude that the policies behind delegation to administrative agencies, particularly the policy underlying the 1962 amendments to the Food, Drug, and Cosmetic Act requiring that drug manufacturers produce substantial evidence of the effectiveness of their drugs, support the commissioner's position that he had authority to make the requisite determinations. We also conclude that the commissioner did not err as a legal matter in ruling that each study could be evaluated to determine if the results were therapeutically significant rather than merely statistically significant. The commissioner's conclusion that petitioners had not made the requisite showing [**51] that their drugs will have the purported or representative effect is supported by substantial evidence in the record. Finally, we conclude that the commissioner was not precluded by the stipulation with Warner from considering the use of concomitant medicine in rejecting the studies proffered by Warner in support of its drug, and the commissioner did not abuse his discretion in upholding the ALJ's ruling excluding the expert testimony of the Warner witnesses who failed to appear for oral cross-examination.

For the reasons set forth herein, we affirm the order of the commissioner withdrawing approval for the new drugs at issue and deny the drug manufacturers' petition for review.

## Conclusion

Both the Nuremberg Code, which focuses on the human rights of research subjects, and the Declaration of Helsinki, which focuses on the review of research protocols prior to the start of the experiment, have served as models for current U.S. federal research regulations to prevent any more torturous human experiments from occurring in the future.

As a member of the society, one must recognize the important role of the Declaration of Helsinki. It is one document that is still valid in providing guidance to biomedical researchers. There are suggestions that the declaration should be revised in such a way to "encompass and provide guidance for changing realities in global health issues." Others still hold firm and state that the declaration should be strengthened and followed regardless of how advanced society has become. As future health care professionals, we must be aware of all issues that have evolved and use the best judgment to act in protecting the welfare of patients.

The Belmont Report made it clear that certain individuals cannot be discriminated against based on their ethnicity, economic standing, health, or social standing. Their rights as humans must be protected first and foremost. Research should only be conducted when the benefits clearly outweigh the risks for the human subject.

Government and institutional regulations state that, to receive approval in conducting human research, the rights and welfare of human research subjects should be protected. Informed consent requirements must be documented if the FDA inspects their records.

# case thirteen

# Scientific integrity

This problem-based learning session is based on the following: *United States ex rel. Berge v. Bd. of Trustees*, No. 95-2811, U.S. Court of Appeals for the Fourth Circuit, 104 F.3d 1453; 1997 U.S. App. Lexis 935; 41 U.S.P.Q.2D (BNA) 1481. December 4, 1996, Argued. January 22, 1997, Decided. Counsel Amended February 11, 1997. Certiorari Denied October 14, 1997. Reported at: 1997 U.S. Lexis 6071. It is reprinted here with permission of LexisNexis.

## Objectives

The objectives of this problem-based learning case are:

- To examine how record keeping affects the profession of pharmacy
- To examine preceptors' responsibility for the development of technicians and interns as professionals
- To understand what scientific misconduct is and how it affects the medical profession
-
- To understand the impact that conflicts of interest can have on the health care system

## Introduction

Throughout the case, you will need to keep four things in mind:

1. The true character of a pharmacist can be shown through personal record-keeping styles.
2. Preceptors can mold future professionals if proper techniques are implemented.
3. Scientific misconduct can lead to the loss of public trust in medical professionals.
4. Conflicts of interest can lead to biases in medical studies.

## Part one

Defendants–appellants appeal from a denial of their motion for judgment as a matter of law following a jury verdict awarding the United States, after trebling and the imposition of a civil penalty, $1.66 million, 30% of which ($498,000) is to be awarded to relator–appellee Pamela A. Berge (Berge) on a False Claims Act claim, and Berge is to be awarded $265,000 in compensatory and punitive damages on a pendent state law claim for conversion of intellectual property. We reverse.

At the time the events at issue occurred, Pamela Berge was a doctoral candidate in nutritional sciences at Cornell University. The individual defendants–appellants Sergio Stagno, Charles Alford, and Robert Pass were medical researchers and professors at defendant–appellant the University of Alabama at Birmingham (UAB). Defendant–appellant Karen Fowler was a doctoral candidate at UAB supervised by Pass.

Scientists at UAB have been studying cytomegalovirus (CMV), the most common infectious cause of birth defects, since 1971 and over the years have accumulated the leading database on maternal and congenital CMV in the world. A significant part of the funding for this research has been provided by grants from the National Institutes of Health (NIH), in particular grant HD-10699, "Perinatal Infections, Immunity and Maldevelopment Research Program Project," administered by NIH's National Institute of Child Health and Human Development (NICHD). This grant is renewable every 5 years, with Years 11 to 15 relevant to this case. Alford was the principal investigator for this project, although Stagno and Pass were closely associated with it. All three are internationally recognized as leading authorities on CMV.

Berge decided to do her dissertation on CMV as a possible cause of low birth weight. She arranged access to and extensive assistance with UAB's database through Stagno, and she worked closely with Stagno and his colleagues while she was in residence as a visiting graduate student at UAB from February to August 1987. After Berge returned to Cornell, she resisted the attempts of others to use the collected data and began to complain about Cornell faculty members, including her thesis chair. She made three further trips to Birmingham, during which she made presentations of her work. She completed her thesis in May 1989 and received her Ph.D. Berge thereafter attempted to publish papers based on her thesis, but she was rejected repeatedly by the *Journal of the American Medical Association, Epidemiology,* and *Journal of Infectious Diseases.*

In the meantime, defendant–appellant Fowler decided in June 1988 to do her dissertation on the relationship between CMV and sexually transmitted diseases and began working with Pass. After Fowler had begun her data analysis, based in part on UAB's existing database and in part on original medical records, she consulted completed theses, including Berge's, to choose a format. She defended her dissertation in May 1990. The following month, Fowler presented her research at a meeting of the Society of Epidemiological Research. Berge was in the audience and became shocked at what she considered to be plagiarism of her work by Fowler.

Berge brought her allegations to Stagno's attention, but did so in such a way that ultimately Stagno and his colleagues determined they could no longer collaborate with her. Two investigations of the allegations were conducted at UAB, but the allegations were found to be baseless. Unsatisfied with these results, as well as those produced from the other avenues she pursued, Berge next obtained copies of UAB's grant applications through a Freedom of Information Act (FOIA) request and then brought this litigation.

As the basis for her qui tam action under the False Claims Act (31 U.S.C. §§ 3729–3733), Berge alleged that UAB had made false statements to NIH in its annual progress reports under its grant. In particular, these false statements were that (1) UAB misled NIH in Year 11 about the amount of data that had been computerized; (2) UAB had included an abstract of Berge's work in Year 12 without mentioning her name, thereby overstating UAB's competence and progress in epidemiology; (3) UAB, although including Berge's name on the abstracts in Years 13 and 14, had "submerged" her research so that serious questions about one of UAB's central theses would not be noticed; and (4) UAB misled NIH in Year 15 by including abstracts of Fowler's work that plagiarized Berge's. Although Berge also alleged a number of pendent state law claims, only the conversion of intellectual property is at issue on this appeal.

After this action was filed, the government naturally investigated to determine whether it would choose to prosecute the matter on its own behalf. The Office of the Inspector General (OIG) of the Department of Health and Human Services (HHS) conducted such an investigation and recommended that no action be taken. Its report stated:

> *This investigation, which has involved the interview of NICHD grant officials, interview of University officials, and the examination of documents of relator, NICHD and the University of Alabama, has found no evidence that the subjects committed a criminal violation in connection with grant applications or progress reports submitted to the Government. Information has been obtained however, which shows many of the assumptions behind the relator's allegations to be in error or exaggerations of the truth. The government accordingly declined to become involved in the litigation. This OIG report was never submitted into evidence at trial. The parties make various contentions as to why this is so and whether the district court abused its discretion in failing to allow it. Given our disposition of this case, we do not reach this issue.*

After a ten-day jury trial, the jury returned a verdict in favor of Berge, finding False Claims Act liability against all defendants except Fowler, but assessing damages only against UAB in the amount of $550,000. Pursuant to 31 U.S.C. § 3729(a), this amount was trebled to $1.65 million, and the district court imposed a civil fine of $10,000 against all the defendants, jointly and severally, except Fowler. Pursuant to § 3730(d)(2), the district court awarded Berge, as relator, 30% of the total recovery of the United States, or $498,000. The jury also found the four individual defendants liable for conversion of intellectual property in differing amounts, imposing a total of $50,000 in compensatory damages and $215,000 in punitive damages. The district court, without opinion, denied defendants' motions for judgment as a matter of law and a new trial. This appeal followed.

## Make a list of the major problems presented in this case

- 
- 
- 
- 

## Hypothesis and mechanism

For the problems in your list above, give a cause or a reason for them to happen:

- 
- 
- 
- 

## Learning issues

Make a list of learning issues in the form of questions. Remember, your goal is to gather the medical, social, and all other relevant facts that may apply to the case.

What records should we, as health care practitioners, be careful to protect?
    General patient information
    Physician information
    Drug history
    Past medical history
    Disease state/history
    Current medical problems and management of disease (recording lab
        results, blood pressure, etc.)
    Comments pertaining to patients' specific needs
    Controlled substances and inventory

How should we maintain and safeguard patient data?

Keep current records.

Keep prescriptions in an organized manner, such that they can be obtained at any time — accountability is the key.

Do not break confidentiality.

Keep organized records in a location such that only pharmacists and interns can view them.

What type of supervision occurs in health care settings (e.g., pharmacies)?

Licensed pharmacists are responsible in all aspects for the supervision of technicians and interns.

A *pharmacy intern* is a person who is currently registered in and attending a duly accredited school or college of pharmacy and who is duly and properly registered with the board provided by these rules.

A *technician* is a person to whom a licensed pharmacist may delegate duties, tasks, and functions that do not fall within those of a pharmacist or pharmacist intern.

Who should a pharmacist be held acountable for supervising?

One pharmacist cannot supervise more than two technicians.

Pharmacists are held accountable for everything an intern and technician do.

Increasing the interaction between the preceptor and the intern/technician tends to increase the atmosphere of professionalism.

What supervisory skills should a health care practitioner cultivate?

Developmental goals for interns:

Professional competency

Problem-solving skills

Values, attitudes, beliefs

Judgment

Sense of purpose

Self-esteem

Leadership development

Responsibility and accountability

Dealing with conflict and the risk of failure

Communication skills

Literature review

Ethics

Trust

What are examples of scientific misconduct?

Padding resumé

Suppressing data

Altering data

Duplicating data to skew opinion

How can scientists deter this kind of misconduct?
    Supervise trainees.
    Set up laboratory procedures on data recording.
    Personally handle data analysis and interpretation.
    Allow peer reviewers to see data.

What is conflict of interest?
    Conflict of interest occurs when a principal investigator is or may be in
        a position to influence business, research, or other decisions in ways
        that could lead to any form of personal gain for the principal inves-
        tigator or give improper advantage to others.
    Examples of results from a conflict of interest:
        Biased results
        Altered data to retain funding
        Suppression of data that reflects badly on affiliated parties
    The National Science Foundation (NSF), the NIH, the Public Health
        Service (PHS), and HHS were formed to protect the integrity of
        publicly funded research. They have set up policies and procedures
        to prevent the conflict of interest that may arise in certain financial
        situations.

What actions can the PHS and the HHS take if misconduct occurs?
    Debarment from federal funds
    Prohibition from PHS advisory committees
    Loss of certification of data by affiliated institutions
    Required submission of corrected data
    Retraction of published article

## Literature review

To help you get ready to answer certain questions you anticipate being asked
during the second part of the case, look in the local medical library and on
the World Wide Web for helpful information. Please indicate in the spaces
below (1) several helpful articles or books you found and (2) several helpful
Web sites you found.

- **Helpful articles:**
    Appelbaum, P.S., Threats to the confidentiality of medical records —
        no place to hide, *JAMA*, 15, 795–797, 2000.
    Krimsky, S. and Rothenberg, L.S., Financial interest and its disclosure
        in scientific publication, *JAMA*, 280, 225–226, 1998.
    Mastroianni, A.C. and Kahn, J.P., The importance of expanding cur-
        rent training in the responsible conduct of research, *Acad. Med.*,
        73, 1249–1254, 1998.
    Wilson, A.L., Hiring pharmacists and technical personnel: Part 2,
        Interviewing, *Top. Hosp. Pharm. Manage.*, 13(3): 37–45, 1993.

- **Helpful Web sites:**
  Eastern Michigan University Graduate Studies and Research: www.gradord.emich.edu.
  Harvard Medical School guidelines for investigations in clinical research: www.hms.harvard.edu/integrity/clinical.html
  American Association for the Advancement of Science – Scientific Freedom Responsibility Law: www.aaas.org/spp/dspp/sfrl
  Duke University policy and procedures governing misconduct in research: www.ors.duke.edu/policies/miscond.htm

## Identify all relevant values that play a role in the case and determine which values, if any, conflict

Nonmaleficence:

Beneficence:

Respect for persons:

Loyalty:

Distributive justice:

## Learning issues for next student-centered problem-based learning session

- List the options open to you. That is, answer the question, "What could you do?"

- Choose the best solution from an ethical point of view, justify it, and respond to possible criticisms. That is, answer the question, "What should you do, and why?"
- What are the different ways of thinking about the problem? Which conflict management techniques can be used in the situation?

## Part two

Berge instituted the action below under the False Claims Act, 31 U.S.C. §§ 3729–3733. Subject matter jurisdiction of the district court was thus based on the federal question statute, 28 U.S.C. § 1331. Supplemental jurisdiction over the pendent state law claims was pursuant to 28 U.S.C. § 1367. This appeal arises from a final judgment below, and thus we possess appellate jurisdiction under 28 U.S.C. § 1291.

Normally, that would end our jurisdictional inquiry, but the defendants and various amici raise issues concerning the constitutionality of the False Claims Act, whether qui tam relators possess standing, and whether state instrumentalities can be held liable pursuant to the act under the Eleventh Amendment. None of these issues was raised below, but to the extent they partake of jurisdictional matters, we may properly consider them. Because we reverse on the facts of this case, we naturally see no need to reach the issue of the constitutionality of the act itself. We do, however, briefly address why we consider the general issue of standing to be unproblematic and why the government, as the real party in interest, possesses standing under the facts of this case.

We have previously held that the "United States is the real party in interest in any False Claims Act suit, even where it permits a qui tam relator to pursue the action on its behalf." Although *Milam* arose in the pre-*Seminole* context of a claim of Eleventh Amendment immunity, which was denied since states may be sued in federal court by the United States, we see *Milam* as resolving the general issue of standing in this circuit. The Seventh Circuit has concluded that "once we accept the premise that the United States is the real plaintiff in a qui tam action, it stands to reason that challenges to the standing of the government's representative are beside the point" [*United States ex rel. Hall v. Tribal Development Corporation*, 49 F.3d 1208, 1213 (7th Cir. 1995)].

Similarly, the Ninth Circuit has analyzed extensively whether the qui tam provisions of the False Claims Act conflict with Article III or violate the principle of separation of powers, the Appointments Clause, or the Due Process Clause, points which various amici raise again here, and our sister circuit concluded they do not [*United States ex rel. Kelly v. Boeing Co.*, 9 F.3d 743, 747–60 (9th Cir. 1993), cert. denied, 510 U.S. 1140, 127 L. Ed. 2d 433, 114 S. Ct. 1125 (1994)]. That court has recently affirmed its rejection of these same arguments in *United States ex rel. Schumer v. Hughes Aircraft Company* [63 F.3d 1512, 1520–1521 (9th Cir. 1995), cert. granted in part, 117 S. Ct. 293, 136 L. Ed. 2d 212 (U.S. Oct. 15, 1996)], and we note that the Supreme Court has granted certiorari to consider, *inter alia*, whether the lower courts erred "in asserting jurisdiction over this action under qui tam provisions of FCA" [117 S. Ct. 293, 136 L. Ed. 2d 212 (U.S. 1996)]. Although we would not hazard to predict what the Supreme Court may do in *Schumer* or whether it will even reach the question on which certiorari was granted, given that our disposition reverses the liability of the defendants *in toto*, we decline to enter into a long disquisition on the standing issue.

However, it must be admitted that, notwithstanding a qui tam relator's general standing as the government's representative, the government, as the real party in interest, must still have suffered an injury in fact [see *Lujan v. Defenders of Wildlife*, 504 U.S. 555, 119 L. Ed. 2d 351, 112 S. Ct. 2130 (1992)]. Amicus Association of American Medical Colleges contends that Berge lacks standing because the United States suffered no injury in fact, as evidenced by the OIG report. We find this argument meritless. In the first place, the OIG report was more concerned with possible criminal violations, which would put the government to a higher burden of proof than in a civil action as here.

Second, and most important, the plain language of the act clearly anticipates that, even after the attorney general has "diligently" investigated a violation under 31 U.S.C. § 3729, the government will not necessarily pursue all meritorious claims; otherwise, there is little purpose to the qui tam provision permitting private attorneys general. Compare id. at § 3730(a), "If the Attorney General finds that a person has violated or is violating section 3729, the Attorney General may bring a civil action under this section against the person" with id. at § 3730(c)(3), "If the Government elects not to proceed with the action, the person who initiated the action shall have the right to conduct the action;" see also *United States ex rel. McGough v. Covington Techs. Co.*, 967 F.2d 1391, 1397 (9th Cir. 1992), stating that "to hold that the government's initial decision not to take over the qui tam action is the equivalent of its consent to a voluntary dismissal of a defendant with prejudice would require us to ignore the plain language of § 3730(b)(1)." The OIG report is not an admission by the United States that it has suffered no injury in fact, but rather it amounts to a cost–benefit analysis. Here, the government surmised — and, as we decide this case, it turns out rightly — that the costs of proceeding on Berge's claims outweighed the anticipated benefits.

Finally, we note that injury in fact is not to be judged *post hoc*. The logical outcome of amicus's position is that any losing plaintiff–relator would not have possessed standing in the first place. In this context, it is worth noting that the district court determined in a lengthy memorandum that Berge's allegations of false statements were sufficient to overcome a motion for summary judgment [see *United States ex rel. Berge v. Board of Trustees of the University of Alabama*, Civil No. N-93-158 (D. Md. filed Mar. 14, 1995), at 9–14].

As a final jurisdictional matter, we recognize that no court has yet considered the interposition of the Eleventh Amendment to the False Claims Act in the wake of *Seminole*. Amici Regents of the University of Minnesota et al. make an interesting case that the False Claims Act was not intended to apply to the states, which they think takes on added significance post-*Seminole*. Amici American Council on Education et al. also suggest we need to take another look at Eleventh Amendment immunity in the qui tam context. We disagree. *Seminole's* relevant holding here is its reconfirmation that Congress must use unequivocal statutory language if it intends to abrogate the sovereign immunity of states in suits brought by and for private parties (*Seminole*, 134 L. Ed. 2d at 266).

But, as we already said in *Milam*, this is a nonissue in the False Claims Act context (*Milam*, 961 F.2d at 50). There is simply no question of abrogation of immunity here. *Seminole* certainly left intact what is beyond purview: the federal government may sue states in federal court [*Seminole*, 134 L. Ed. 2d at 276, citing *United States v. Texas*, 143 U.S. 621, 644–645, 36 L. Ed. 285, 12 S. Ct. 488 (1892), for the proposition that such power is necessary to the "permanence of the Union"; see also *West Virginia v. United States*, 479 U.S. 305, 311, 93 L. Ed. 2d 639, 107 S. Ct. 702 (1987)]. The United States is the real party in interest. The act itself states that the "action shall be brought in the name of the Government" [31 U.S.C. § 3730(b)(1)]. We affirm our reasoning in *Milam*: "The states have no Eleventh Amendment immunity against the United States *ab initio*. Therefore, there is no reason Congress would have displaced it in the False Claims Act" (*Milam*, 961 F.2d at 50).

Turning to the merits, appellants assign at least seven points of error to the district court below. We reach only three of them in reversing the entire judgment below: the lack of materiality to the government's funding decisions of the alleged false statements; the insufficiency of the evidence that appellants even made false statements to the government, as merged into the first issue on the False Claims Act claim; and the preemption, by federal copyright law, of the state law conversion of intellectual property claim. We address the materiality and insufficiency of evidence issues in this section and the preemption issue in the next section.

The civil False Claims Act provides in relevant part:

> *Any person who —*
>
> 1. *knowingly makes, uses, or causes to be made or used, a false record or statement to get a false or fraudulent claim paid or approved by the Government; . . .*
>
> 2. *is liable to the United States Government for a civil penalty of not less than $5000 and not more than $10,000, plus 3 times the amount of damages which the Government sustains because of the act of that person.*

[31 U.S.C. § 3729(a)]. We have previously suggested that the civil False Claims Act requires a materiality element [see *United States v. Snider*, 502 F.2d 645, 652 n.12 (4th Cir. 1974) (construing the FCA's predecessor statute, 31 U.S.C. § 231)]. If previously unclear, we now make explicit that the current civil False Claims Act imposes a materiality requirement [see also *Tyger Construction Co. v. United States*, 28 Fed. Cl. 35, 55 (1993), "The FCA covers only those false statements that are material"].

On this materiality issue, however, we must initially determine whether the issue is to be properly decided by the court. In the context of the criminal false statements statute (18 U.S.C. § 1001), we had previously held that materiality is a question of law for which the test is "whether the false statement has a natural tendency to influence agency action or is capable of influencing agency action" [*United States v. Norris*, 749 F.2d 1116, 1122 (4th Cir. 1984) (citations omitted), cert. denied, 471 U.S. 1065, 85 L. Ed. 2d 496, 105 S. Ct. 2139 (1985)]. In the criminal context, that holding can no longer stand as a result of *United States v. Gaudin* [132 L. Ed. 2d 444, 115 S. Ct. 2310 (1995)]. In *Gaudin*, a unanimous Court held that the materiality of false statements was an element of the crime under 18 U.S.C. § 1001 to which a defendant has a constitutional right under the Fifth and Sixth Amendments for a jury to determine guilt beyond a reasonable doubt (id. at 458). Berge's expansive interpretation that *Gaudin*'s rationale must apply even in civil cases for which there is a right to jury trial under the Seventh Amendment is unwarranted. The Court expressly declined to reach that issue, stating that "the courts' power to resolve mixed-law-and-fact questions in civil cases is not at issue here; civil and criminal juries' required roles are obviously not identical, or else there could be no directed verdicts for civil plaintiffs" [id. at 454; see also id. at 460, stating that the "Court properly acknowledges that other mixed questions of law and fact remain the proper domain of the trial court" (Rehnquist, C.J., concurring)]. Moreover, the Court refused to overrule its unanimous opinion in *Kungys v. United States* [485 U.S. 759, 99 L. Ed. 2d 839, 108 S. Ct. 1537 (1988)], a civil denaturalization case, that the "materiality requirement under . . . statutes dealing with misrepresentations to public officers" is one for the court (id. at 772 [citations omitted]), since the constitutional ramifications were different (*Gaudin*, 132 L. Ed. 2d at 458).

In addition, we have already indicated our reluctance to construe *Gaudin* broadly. See, for instance, *United States v. Daughtry* [91 F.3d 675, 675 (4th Cir. 1996)], stating that "Gaudin held only that in prosecutions for violations of [18 U.S.C.] § 1001, the element of materiality must be submitted to the jury;" see also *United States v. Klausner* [80 F.3d 55, 61 (2d Cir. 1996)], holding that even in some criminal contexts, materiality remains a purely legal question after *Gaudin*. Thus, in light of our earlier determination that the materiality of false statements is a legal question and of our inclination not to give an expansive interpretation to *Gaudin*, we hold that, in the context of the civil False Claims Act, the determination of materiality, although partaking of the character of a mixed question of fact and law, is one for the court. See also *United States ex rel. Butler v. Hughes Helicopter Company* [No. CV 89-5760 SVW, 1993 U.S. Dist. Lexis 17844, (C.D. Cal. Aug. 25, 1993)], holding that the materiality of false statements under the False Claims Act is a legal question for the court [aff'd on other grounds, 71 F.3d 321 (9th Cir. 1995)].

Moreover, we see no reason to depart from the test we enunciated in *Norris*, even though the remainder of its holding cannot stand post-*Gaudin*; that is, the materiality of the false statement turns on "whether the false statement has a natural tendency to influence agency action or is capable of influencing agency action" (Norris, 749 F.2d at 1122; see also *Kungys*, 485 U.S. at 770, recognizing that a "misrepresentation is material if it has a natural tendency to influence, or was capable of influencing, the decision of the decision-making body to which it was addressed" [internal quotation marks omitted]).

In any event, even the *Gaudin* Court acknowledged that there always remains as a threshold question of law whether the case for materiality is "so weak that no reasonable juror could credit it" (*Gaudin*, 132 L. Ed. 2d at 454). In the instant case, our *de novo* review [see, e.g., *Benedi v. McNeil-P.P.C., Inc.*, 66 F.3d 1378, 1383 (4th Cir. 1995), "We review a denial of a motion for judgment as a matter of law *de novo*" (citation omitted)], of the alleged false statements plainly shows they were not material to NICHD's funding decisions, and furthermore, are so lacking in materiality, indeed, are not even false, that no reasonable jury could have so found.

As a general matter, NICHD's program officer with responsibility for UAB's grant testified that Berge's contributions were not central to UAB's project, and that the progress reported by UAB was satisfactory for a recommendation of continued funding without Berge's contribution. As even the government notes in its brief as intervenor on appeal, "NICHD determined that the information Berge alleged was false or misrepresented was not material to its funding decisions" (Br. of United States as intervenor at 34).

More particularly, Berge's assertion of UAB's alleged misstatement concerning the extent of computerization in Year 11 is belied by the fact that information on upward of 20,000 patients had been computerized by that time. Even accepting Berge's assertion that only 124 cases of congenitally infected babies were computerized, that fact is irrelevant to the greater computerization effort and, moreover, is one fully consistent with Berge's own dissertation claim that congenital infection affects only 0.2–2.4% of all live births. Furthermore, the program officer testified that the principal purpose of the project was the collection of data, not its computerization. Thus, not only did UAB not mislead NIH about the extent of computerization, but also UAB fully reported the number of subjects of the project every year and thereby complied with NIH's expectation on the collection of data. In fact, the program officer stated that UAB's data collection "is considered to be the largest single source of information on maternal and congenital CMV in the world."

Second, the Year 12 omission of Berge's name from an abstract submitted as part of the progress report cannot possibly be material. In the first place, NIH did not even require the inclusion of her name or anyone's name. There can only be liability under the False Claims Act when the defendant has an obligation to disclose omitted information. More important, the abstract itself was included, and was required to be included, because Stagno appeared on the abstract as a coauthor. Berge expended considerable effort in attempting to convince us, both in her briefs and at oral argument, that the jury properly found this failure to attribute the abstract to her and obtain her permission to use it was a material false statement. The report, in fact, did not attribute the abstract to any of its authors; it simply "abstracted" the study for the purpose of reporting on project activity. Co-owners are treated as tenants in common, with each co-owner having an undivided, independent right to use the work, subject only to a duty of accounting for profits to other co-owners. Thus, it was perfectly proper for Stagno to use the abstract as he did, and that use therefore is not a false statement, let alone a material one capable of affecting NIH's funding decision.

Third, Berge's claim of the "submergence" of her work in the progress reports for Years 13 and 14 is inexplicable. In each year's progress report, fully half of the discussion of activity under Specific Aim # 1 of Project 1 is given over to quoting in full from Berge's abstracts, with attribution. If Berge's work supported the hypothesis that there was a downside risk to · a live vaccine, the development of which she claims was a central goal of UAB's project, then it was incumbent on her to note that implication in her work, which she did not. The omission is her own fault, not UAB's. An *ex post facto* realization of the possible importance of this implication cannot support a charge of falsity at the time the report was submitted. Moreover, NIH's expectation that only the abstract would be included in the progress report cannot form the basis for liability for an omission in any event. While it is true that the reports mistakenly referred to Berge as a "postdoctoral graduate student from the Department of Biostatistics" at Cornell, when, in fact, she was in Year 13 as a doctoral candidate in nutritional sciences and by Year 14 had obtained her Ph.D., no reasonable jury could conclude that such trivial errors were materially capable of influencing NIH's funding decision.

As to Berge's final asserted false statement by UAB, that NIH was misled by including an abstract of Fowler's work in Year 15, which allegedly plagiarized Berge's own work and about which plagiarism UAB knew, the evidence is patently clear that there was no plagiarism by Fowler and thus no false statement by UAB. The government itself points out that "none of the scientific or administrative bodies to which complained found that Fowler had plagiarized Berge's work." As Berge herself concedes, "Ms. Fowler's ultimate hypothesis and conclusions were different from [mine]."

But, if the hypothesis and conclusions were different, what was plagiarized? Certainly not independently obtained data sets extracted from UAB's own collection; the case control method, one of the most frequently used research designs in epidemiology; the textbook statistical methodologies employed; the risk factors, derived from the scientific literature, commonly used in perinatal studies; or even the organization of Fowler's and Berge's tables, which do nothing more than reflect UAB's own clinic forms. None of these "ideas" was original to Berge, and thus none of these could have been taken by Fowler from Berge and passed off as her own.

The ideas that were original to Berge were her hypotheses and conclusions concerning the relationship between CMV infection and low birth weight, but these ideas are concededly different from Fowler's hypotheses and conclusions concerning the relationship between sexually transmitted diseases and maternal CMV infection. As the Public Health Service's Office of Research Integrity has determined, plagiarism does not include credit disputes. But, once the surface is scratched, there is nothing to Berge's claim except her complaint that Fowler did not give Berge's work the notice she felt she deserved. If that is scientific misconduct, it is far too attenuated to any federal right for us, or any federal court, to decide.

Berge also makes much of the fact that the Year 15 review had to be performed three times before UAB could allegedly get its grant renewed. Indeed, she claims it is "difficult to imagine a more concrete demonstration of the materiality of the false statements." However, the record clearly shows that the first review had to be rejected because of a conflict of interest by one of the reviewing scientists, and the second had to be rejected because it impermissibly had access to the first review. The third review was thus the only clean review, and it recommended funding the project. Thus, Berge's most concrete demonstration of materiality rests on no foundation whatsoever.

In addition to this allegation-by-allegation analysis that demonstrates the lack of materiality (as well as the lack of falsity) of the statements, we also decide that no reasonable jury could possibly conclude that a multimillion-dollar grant, continually renewed over a period of more than a decade, undertaken by three internationally respected scientists engaged, in part, in the collection of the world's leading database on CMV, would be reduced or eliminated due to UAB's lack of expertise in an area. It seems difficult to believe that the grant process could be bolstered by the work of an unknown graduate student in nutritional sciences — work that, when reviewed by independent scientists at peer-reviewed journals, was determined to be "scarcely comprehensible, extremely difficult to read and even more difficult to evaluate, and so cavalier in its design and conduct as to induce great skepticism in "any findings reported from it." The hubris of any graduate student to think that such grants depend on the results of her work is beyond belief. That is not the way Big Science works. Assuming arguendo that all of Berge's allegations were true, and UAB had made these false statements, it is hard to imagine that NIH's decision making would have been influenced by them.

Reviewing all this evidence in the light most favorable to Berge, it is abundantly clear that substantial evidence on which the jury could have found for Berge is lacking. Her evidence amounts at most to a scintilla, which is insufficient to sustain the verdict. At best, Berge fails on her burden of showing materiality; at worst, she cannot even show the statements were false. In either case, judgment as a matter of law is appropriate for appellants on the False Claims Act claim since Berge has "failed to make a showing on an essential element of [her] case with respect to which she had the burden of proof." We reverse the judgment below on the False Claims Act claim in its entirety.

We turn now to the claim of conversion of intellectual property under Alabama law. The Alabama conversion statute provides:

> *The owner of personality is entitled to possession thereof. Any unlawful deprivation of or interference with such possession is a tort for which an action lies. Whether federal copyright law preempts a state law claim is a question of law that we review de novo.* Rosciszewski v. Arete Assocs., Inc., 1 F.3d 225, 229 (4th Cir. 1993).

Berge's conversion claim in this instance is clearly preempted by federal copyright law. Section 301(a) of the Copyright Act provides in pertinent part:

> *All legal or equitable rights that are equivalent to any of the exclusive rights within the general scope of copyright as specified in section 106 in works of authorship that are fixed in a tangible medium of expression and come within the subject matter of copyright as specified by sections 102 and 103 . . . are governed exclusively by this title. [After January 1, 1978], no person is entitled to any such right or equivalent right in any such work under the common law or statutes of any State.*

[17 U.S.C. § 301(a)]. We have recently held that the statute thus sets up a two-prong inquiry to determine when a state law claim is preempted: first, the work must be "within the scope of the 'subject-matter of copyright' as specified in 17 U.S.C. §§ 102, 103," and second, "the rights granted under state law" must be "equivalent to any exclusive rights within the scope of federal copyright as set out in 17 U.S.C. § 106" (*Rosciszewski*, 1 F.3d at 229 [quotation marks and citation omitted]).

There can be no doubt that Berge's work — her dissertation, to which she affixed a copyright mark; her abstracts; her drafts, and so on — falls within the scope of the subject matter of copyright. All of these written works are clearly "original works of authorship fixed in a tangible medium of expression" [17 U.S.C. § 102(a)]. Berge's argument that her conversion claim is not preempted because it is her "ideas and methods," which are specifically excluded from copyright protection [see id. at § 102(b)], that have been converted rests on a fallacious interpretation of the Copyright Act. In other words, Berge wants to argue that ideas embodied in a work covered by the Copyright Act do not fall within the scope of the act because the act specifically excludes them from protection. But, scope and protection are not synonyms. Moreover, the shadow actually cast by the act's preemption is notably broader than the wing of its protection.

The second prong of the preemption test is satisfied unless there is an "extra element" that changes the nature of the state law action so that it is "qualitatively different from a copyright infringement claim" [*Rosciszewski*, 1 F.3d at 229–230 (emphasis in original) (internal quotation marks and citation omitted); see also *Trandes Corp. v. Guy F. Atkinson Co.*, 996 F.2d 655, 659–660 (4th Cir.), cert. denied, 510 U.S. 965, 126 L. Ed. 2d 377, 114 S. Ct. 443 (1993)]. It is hornbook law that a "state law action for conversion will not be preempted if the plaintiff can prove the extra element that the defendant unlawfully retained the physical object embodying plaintiff's work" [Goldstein, P., *Copyright, Patent, Trademark and Related State Doctrines 777*, 3rd ed., 1993, (quoting Paul Goldstein, Copyright 1989)]. See also Melville B. Nimmer & David Nimmer, Nimmer on Copyright § 1.01[B](1)(i) (1995), "The torts of conversion and trespass relate to interference with tangible rather than intangible property."

However, § 301(a) will preempt a conversion claim "where the plaintiff alleges only the unlawful retention of its intellectual property rights and not the unlawful retention of the tangible object embodying its work" [Goldstein, supra, at 777; see *Dielsi v. Falk*, 916 F. Supp. 985, 992 (C.D. Cal. 1996), holding that a claim for conversion of a television script was preempted since there was no extra element to the essential claim that the ideas were misappropriated; compare *Patrick v. Francis*, 887 F. Supp. 481, 482, 484 (W.D.N.Y. 1995), holding a conversion claim preempted when the action actually sought to recover for unauthorized copying of the work, concepts, and ideas of a research paper, with *Oddo v. Ries*, 743 F.2d 630, 635 (9th Cir. 1984), conversion of tangible property not preempted]. It could hardly be clearer that Berge's conversion claim is preempted. We have already dismissed Berge's argument that her "ideas and methods" are not within the scope of copyright's protection or preemption as to the first prong (see supra). As to the second prong, what is crucial is that Berge makes no claim that appellants converted any tangible objects embodying her intellectual property.

Berge attempts to salvage her conversion claim first by claiming that *Alabama* recognizes the conversion of intangible property and, second, by claiming that the extra element is unauthorized use. She must founder on both attempts. Although the Alabama Supreme Court has held that "in appropriate circumstances, intangible personal property can be converted" [*National Surety Co. v. Applied Systems, Inc.*, 418 So. 2d 847, 850 (Ala. 1982)], it was a specific computer program that was converted, at a time when the manner of the applicability of copyright law to computer programs was unclear. If *National Surety* holds only that intellectual property may be converted in particular circumstances, then it is unexceptional. However, if it holds that such intellectual property can be converted without an extra element beyond copyright infringement, then it must be repudiated as contrary to the Copyright Act under the Supremacy Clause.

Perhaps recognizing the weakness of that reed, Berge also grasps onto *G.S. Rasmussen & Associates v. Kalitta Flying Service* [958 F.2d 896 (9th Cir. 1992), cert. denied, 508 U.S. 959, 124 L. Ed. 2d 678, 113 S. Ct. 2927 (1993)].

But *Kalitta* only held that a conversion claim did not run afoul of copyright preemption when an unauthorized copy of a supplemental type certificate from the Federal Aviation Administration (FAA) had been used improperly to obtain an airworthiness certificate from the FAA (958 F.2d 896 at 904). In distinguishing *Kalitta*, the Fifth Circuit properly recognized in *Daboub v. Gibbons* [42 F.3d 285 (5th Cir. 1995)], that when the core of the state law theory of recovery, as in conversion, goes to wrongful copying, in its case, the plagiarism of an entire song, it is preempted.

Recognizing the broad and absolute preemption of § 301, "stated in the clearest and most unequivocal language possible, so as to foreclose any conceivable misinterpretation of its unqualified intention that Congress shall act preemptively, and to avoid the development of any vague borderline areas between State and Federal protection" [H.R. Rep. No. 1476, 94th Cong., 2d Sess. (1976) reprinted in 1976 U.S.C.C.A.N. 5659, 5746], the *Daboub* court concluded that "if the language of the act could be so easily circumvented, the preemption provision would be useless, and the policies behind a uniform Copyright statute would be silenced." Berge's charge of plagiarism and lack of attribution can only amount to, indeed, are tantamount to, a claim of copyright infringement, for Berge has certainly not been prevented from using her own ideas and methods [see *Garrido v. Burger King Corp.*, 558 So. 2d 79, 82 (Fla. Dist. Ct. App. 1990), holding that when the gravamen of a conversion claim was the unauthorized taking or use of ideas, the elements of the claim were not qualitatively different from copyright infringement].

Berge complains that, if the Copyright Act's idea–expression dichotomy [see 17 U.S.C. § 102(b)] and § 301's preemption provision be read this way, then there is "no legal remedy for the theft of [my] intellectual property. Intellectual property which can be stolen without fear of legal punishment ceases to be property" (Br. of appellee at 41). But, what Berge fails to realize is that, as a general proposition, ideas are simply part of the public domain [see, e.g., *Hoehling v. Universal City Studios, Inc.*, 618 F.2d 972, 979–980 (2d Cir.), holding that, in nonfiction works, since facts, themes, and research "have been deliberately exempted from the scope of copyright protection to vindicate the overriding goal of encouraging contributions to recorded knowledge, the states are pre-empted from removing such material from the public domain," cert. denied, 449 U.S. 841, 66 L. Ed. 2d 49, 101 S. Ct. 121 (1980); see also *Nimmer and Nimmer*, supra, at § 16.01, stating that "the concept that ideas are 'free as air' is of ancient origin, and is well rooted in our jurisprudence" (footnotes omitted)]. It is not that this form of intellectual property ceases to be property, rather it is just not intangible personality [see, e.g., *Richter v. Westab, Inc.*, 529 F.2d 896, 902 (6th Cir. 1976), "The law does not favor the protection of abstract ideas as the property of the originator"]. Berge wants to fence off the commons, but the only part she may rightly claim is the original expression of her ideas fixed in a tangible medium. The law recognizes her stake there and accords it copyright protection.

Berge's conversion claim is preempted by federal copyright law. We therefore reverse the judgment below on this claim in its entirety.

*List the options open to you. That is, answer the question, "What could you do?"*

- 
- 
- 
- 

*Choose the best solution from an ethical point of view, justify it, and respond to possible criticisms. That is, answer the question, "What should you do, and why?"*

- 
- 
- 
- 

*Select one member of your PBL group to role-play as Pamela Berge and have another member of your PBL group role-play as a representative of VAB. How might the two converse about different ways of thinking and techniques for conflict management?*

- 
- 
- 
- 

*Again, please select one member of your PBL group to role-play as Pamela Berge and have another member of your PBL group role-play as a representative of VAB. How might Pamela Berge use what is known about stages of change and about motivational interviewing to solve what you consider the major problem presented in the case?*

- •
- •
- •
- •

## Part three

For the foregoing reasons, we hold that the district court erred when it improperly denied appellants' motion for judgment as a matter of law, both as to Berge's False Claims Act claim and to her conversion claim. The judgment of the district court is therefore reversed.

## Conclusion

Medical professionals must have good and honest record-keeping skills to protect the integrity of their profession. Altering records or storing data irresponsibly damages the character of the individual, as well as the profession as a whole. By teaching leadership, responsibility, ethics, communication, and problem-solving skills, a preceptor can develop trust with the trainee that is crucial for an effective learning environment. This will give interns/technicians the ability to contribute to the profession. This allows them to contribute to their professional community and show the individual integrity that is developed.

Integrity in scientific research relies on the scientific method. Scientific misconduct appears when it is not used properly. Research should not be persuaded by conflicts of interest. The foundation of trust and honesty between the academic world and the public crumbles when scientific misconduct occurs. This is why government foundations have been set up to regulate and protect the credibility of publicly funded research.

# Research on human subjects

This problem-based learning session is based on the following: *McNeil v. United States*, No. 92 C 0339, U.S. District Court for the Northern District of Illinois, Eastern Division, 1992 U.S. Dist. Lexis 7665. May 29, 1992, Decided. June 2, 1992, Docketed. It is reprinted here with permission of LexisNexis.

## Objectives

The objectives of this problem-based learning case are to:

- Make the subjects of a research project aware of their rights
- Understand the role of the institutional review boards (IRBs)
- Understand the ethical issues involved in selecting subjects and research in special populations — specifically, less-developed countries
- Understand the components of an informed consent form

## Introduction

Human subjects are commonly unaware of their rights when involved in a study. Many times, an informed consent form is used that is confusing to the subject. It is important that the researcher fully disclose the purpose, duration, risks, and benefits of the study in the informed consent. Institutional review boards make sure that the investigator conducts the study in an ethical and lawful manner.

## Part one

Willie E. McNeil brings this self-styled *pro se* class action pursuant to the Federal Torts Claims Act (FTCA) [28 U.S.C. §§ 1346(b), 2671–2680] on behalf of himself and 42 other inmates of the Stateville Correctional Center. The complaint charges the federal government (Department of Health and Human Services [HHS]) with conducting medical experiments on the prisoners at Stateville without first obtaining permission from them. The experiments allegedly were designed to "study . . . the prevalence of HTLV-III/LAV and HBV infections among adult males entering [the Illinois] prison system and the likelihood of transmission (incidence) of HTLV-III/LAV and HBV infections among these inmates." Plaintiffs claim they were exposed to these viruses as a result of the study. Only McNeil has filed a motion to proceed *in forma pauperis*. McNeil has submitted the instant claim "as attorney for the class."

This is not the first time McNeil has attempted to peddle this claim in this district. In fact, the Seventh Circuit recently affirmed Judge Alesia's dismissal of an identical claim by McNeil on timeliness grounds [*McNeil v. United States of America*, Case No. 91-1303 (7th Cir. May 20, 1992)]. Moreover, the same claim, different plaintiff, was resolved on the merits by Judge Shadur in 1989 [*Wilson v. United States Public Health Service*, 731 F.Supp. 844 (N.D.Ill. 1989)].

As in the Wilson case, the plaintiffs in this case claim to have been exposed to infectious diseases as a result of a study performed pursuant to a contract between the U.S. government and the Illinois Department of Corrections (DOC). According to the instant complaint:

> *prison authorities were forcing the plaintiffs herein to par-*
> *ticipate in human research and experimentation conducted*
> *by the "government" . . . [sic] To investigate the spread of*
> *infectious diseases among these plaintiffs, (where per order*
> *of the government all incidences were not traceable to the*
> *cause). Once prison authorities determined who was active*
> *carriers [sic] and how meny prison [sic] was being release*
> *[sic] into the general prison population, this information*
> *was forwarded to the government . . . [sic] And prison*
> *authorities destroyed the list of the carriers, so only the*
> *government knew by identification number issued by Abt*
> *Associates, who was active as carriers and who suffered a*
> *transmission. So at this time all the herein plaintiffs must*
> *be considered as prisoners who suffered a incidence, [sic]*
> *without their informed consent to participate.*

Further in the complaint, plaintiffs allege they were "purposefully exposed to these infectious diseases. By forcing known active carriers of said diseases into the population for the purpose of infecting known healthy prisoners ... and then guess at how many [sic] will suffer a incedences [sic]."

Plaintiffs have attached to their complaint a portion of what purports to be the contract between the federal government and the DOC; it outlines the procedures for conducting the study. The contract, *inter alia*, provides as follows:

*The prevalence [of HTLV-III/LAV and HBV infections] should be estimated by determining the percentage of males who are seropositive on entry into the prison. The incidence should be estimated by determining the percentage of inmates who test negative for antibody to these viruses on specimens collected at the beginning of the study and test positive on specimens collected 6 to 24 months later.*

*For the initial prevalence study test a sample of 500 sera from inmates who have been incarcerated in a correctional facility (not necessarily the study prison) for at least 3 consecutive months before entering the study. . . . All personal identifiers should be removed before specimens are tested for this part of the study.*

*For the incidence study, collect paired sera from all study participants, and brief demographic information, including age group, race, and duration of incarceration. Serum from inmates who have been continuously incarcerated for at least 3 months will be collected and frozen. . . . Repeat specimens will be collected 6 to 24 months later and matched with the previously collected specimen. The specimen pairs may be given unique identifiers which link them to each other, but not to a specific prisoner. The second specimen from each pair would then be tested for HTLV-III/LAV and HBV. If the second specimen is positive, the first will be tested to determine if seroconversion occurred during the study period.*

## Make a list of the major problems presented in this case

- 
- 
- 
- 

## Hypothesis and mechanism

For the problems in your list above, give a cause or a reason for them to happen:

- 
- 
- 
-

## Learning issues

Make a list of learning issues in the form of questions. Remember, your goal is to gather the medical, social, and all other relevant facts that may apply to the case.

What is the Belmont Report?

> The Belmont Report, published in 1979, outlined three basic ethical principles of informed consent:
>
> > Beneficence: identifies the need to maximize benefits and minimize risks associated with research participation
> >
> > Respect for persons: addresses the importance of treating individuals as autonomous agents and protecting those who have diminished autonomy (for example, prisoners, children, or persons with physical or mental disabilities) .
> >
> > Justice: focuses on the need to ensure fairness and equity in the selection of research participants and in the distribution of the costs and benefits of research

What are the elements of an informed consent?

> On June 18, 1991, the *Federal Policy for the Protection of Human Subjects* put forth the following elements of an informed consent:
>
> - Statement that the study involves research, along with an explanation of the purpose, procedures, and expected duration of participation
> - Explanation of the procedures to be followed in the medical experiment and any drug or device to be used
> - Description of alternative treatments or procedures that may be advantageous
> - Description of foreseeable risks as well as benefits
> - Explanation of extent to which confidentiality will be maintained
> - If research involves more than minimal risk, an explanation of treatment and compensation availability
> - Who to contact in the event of research-related injury or questions
> - A copy of a signed and dated written consent form given to subject
> - Statement that participation is voluntary and that the subject may discontinue participation at anytime without prejudice
> - Statement that the study may be discontinued at any time

What is an institutional review board (IRB)?

> An IRB is a diverse group of scientific and nonscientific individuals who conduct the initial and ongoing review of clinical research studies to ensure the protection of the rights, safety, and well-being of human subjects participating in those trials.

IRB's have the authority to: approve, require modifications, and disapprove of the proposed study protocols and consent forms for research that involves human subjects.

What are the responsibilities of IRBs?

The investigator for the research is reviewed and approved or disapproved.

Progress of ongoing research is monitored.

Food and Drug Administration and HHS regulations require an IRB to consist of at least five members, with varied backgrounds, representing both scientific and nonscientific fields.

IRBs ensure that technical and scientific terms of an informed consent are adequately explained, or that common terms are substituted so that a typical subject can read and comprehend them.

What are the responsibilities of investigators?

Submit a submission letter for initial IRB review

Submit a study status report to the IRB for continuing review

Submit a final study status report to the IRB when study is closed or canceled

Obtain IRB approval of advertisement/recruitment material before use

Report serious adverse events that occur during study to IRB

Get IRB approval before all changes to informed consent forms

What are some of the ethical issues of conducting clinical studies in third world countries?

Regarding ethical issues that face investigators in conducting clinical studies in less-developed countries, we chose to analyze the relevance of the three aforementioned principles outlined in the Belmont Report. We attempt to explore both sides of the ethical issues as they apply to the following two HIV studies conducted in sub-Saharan Africa, as discussed below:

1. Reduction of material transmission of human immunodeficiency virus type 1 (HIV-1) with zidovudine treatment

2. Viral load and heterosexual transmission of HIV-1

In the United States and other developed countries, the placebo-controlled trial design of this study would not be permitted and would be viewed as unethical. In developed countries, it would be viewed as a blatant disregard of the well-being of participants not to allow them access to readily available antiviral drugs. There is no justification for the potential loss of infant life due to maternal transmission that may have been prevented by antiviral therapy.

Therefore, how can a clinical study conducted in a less-developed country be viewed as ethically viable, yet at the same time be considered unethical in developed countries? Is it morally right to argue that different standards are justified by social and economic conditions within the region in which the studies are conducted?

Reduction of maternal transmission of HIV-1 with zidovudine treatment:

Zidovudine was shown to decrease maternal–infant transmission by two thirds, although this is of no direct beneficence to population groups in sub-Saharan Africa. Local health care systems cannot absorb the high costs of antiviral therapy; therefore, the zidovudine regimen is not a viable option to reduce maternal–infant transmission in this population group.

HIV research in sub-Saharan Africa is justified due to the devastating epidemic nature of this disease. Proper research should be conducted that is relevant to the population from which subjects are utilized. There was no mutual beneficence or justice to local populations because the outcome of this study could not be incorporated into local health care systems. The acquired data from this study bear no significant use to indigenous populations of sub-Saharan Africa.

What this study meant to participants is that, for up to 30 months, several hundred people with HIV were observed and untreated. One half of the study population was not given inexpensive antibiotics to treat sexually transmitted diseases such as syphilis or gonorrhea. In addition, many participants were found to have other sexually transmitted diseases, and they were left to seek their own treatment.

In the United States, such a study would not be permitted because it would be expected that patients with HIV and sexually transmitted diseases would be treated. Thus, this clinical study was unethical because it lacked beneficence to its participants. This study is an example of an ongoing ethical dilemma because of the issue whether researchers should adhere to ethical standards in the country (less-developed country) in which the study is conducted or the ethical standards of the host country (developed country).

This brings up another important question: Are investigators obligated to provide better care for human subjects than is generally available in the region from which they are drawn? Therefore, is it ethical to justify not treating subjects with HIV since antiviral drugs are not available in rural Uganda?

This prospective study did not obligate the investigator to inform seronegative subjects that their partners tested seropositive to HIV-1. This responsibility to inform was left to seropositive partners in couples discordant for HIV-1. The Ugandan government mandated this policy. This policy places voluntary subjects at unnecessary risk without regard to their well-being and leaves questionable justification for participating in the study.

This ethical issue brings up the following questions: How much responsibility do investigators assume for the well-being of their subjects? Also, do human subjects have certain irreducible fundamental rights that are not relative to the political, social, and economic conditions in which the studies are conducted?

## Literature review

To help you get ready to answer certain questions you anticipate being asked during the second part of the case, look in the local medical library and on the World Wide Web for helpful information. Please indicate in the spaces below (1) several helpful articles or books you found and (2) several helpful Web sites you found.

- **Helpful articles:**
  Angell, M., The ethics of clinical research in the third world, *N. Engl. J. Med.*, 337, 847–849, 1997.
  Angell, M., Investigators' responsibilities for human subjects in developing countries, *N. Engl. J. Med.*, 342, 967–968, 2000.
  Bunch, W.H., Informed consent, *Clin. Orthop. Relat. Res.*, 378, 71–77, 2000.
  Cassell, E.J., The principles of the Belmont Report revisited, *Hastings Cent. Rep.*, 30, 12–21, 2000.
  Connor, E.M. et al., Reduction of maternal–infant transmission of human immunodeficiency virus type I with zidovudine treatment, *N. Engl. J. Med.*, 331, 1173–1179, 1994.
  Harrison, L., Issues related to the protection of human research participants, *J. Neurosci. Nurs.*, 25, 187–193, 1993.
  Lurie, P., Unethical trials of interventions to reduce perinatal transmission of the human immunodeficiency virus in developing countries, *N. Engl. J. Med.*, 337, 853–855, 1997.
  Macklin, R., Understanding informed consent, *Acta Oncol.*, 38, 83–87, 1999.
  Moreno, J. et al., Updating protections for human subjects involved in research, *JAMA*, 280, 1951–1958, 1998.
  Quinn, T.C. et al., Viral load and heterosexual transmission of human immunodeficiency virus type I, *N. Engl. J. Med.*, 342, 921–929, 2000.
  Silverman, W.A., The myth of informed consent: in daily practice and in clinical trials, *J. Med. Ethics*, 15, 6–11, 1981.
  Varmus, H., Ethical complexities of conducting research in developing countries, *N. Engl. J. Med.*, 337, 1003–1005, 1997.

- **Helpful Web sites:**
  Copernicus Group: www.copernicusgroup.com

Western Institutional Review Board: www.wirb.com
Deem Corporation: www.humansubjects.com
National Institutes of Health — Office of Human Subjects Research:
www.ohsr.od.nih.gov/guidelines.php3

## *Identify all relevant values that play a role in the case and determine which values, if any, conflict*

Nonmaleficence:

Beneficence:

Respect for persons:

Loyalty:

Distributive justice:

## *Learning issues for next student-centered problem-based learning session*

- List the options open to you. That is, answer the question, "What could you do?"
- Choose the best solution from an ethical point of view, justify it, and respond to possible criticisms. That is, answer the question, "What should you do, and why?"
- What are the different ways of thinking about the problem? Which conflict management techniques can be used in the situation?

## Part two

As can be seen from an examination of the documents attached to plaintiffs' complaint, the government gave detailed instructions concerning the collection of specimens and the computation of data derived from those specimens. Nowhere, however, is it suggested that prison officials purposely expose healthy inmates to infected inmates to somehow inflate the incidence of infection. The study appears to be designed with the purpose of determining the rate of transmission of certain infectious diseases in the course of normal prison life. How inmates are housed and how they interact with each other (which is really what plaintiffs are complaining about) is controlled by the DOC in the normal course of managing the prison, not by the federal government. Simply collecting blood specimens from a random sampling of inmates does not contribute to the spread of infectious diseases.

The FTCA waives sovereign immunity for certain conduct committed by "any employee of the Government while acting within the scope of his office or employment." Plaintiffs claim that the agreement between the federal government and the DOC creates an employment relationship between the federal government and the DOC, and thus the conduct of the DOC is attributable to the United States. Even if this court were to give plaintiffs the benefit of the doubt and find that, for purposes of conducting the study of prison inmates, the DOC was acting as an agent of the federal government, as discussed above, the study itself did not subject the inmates to any higher risk of infection. Thus, any DOC conduct attributable to the federal government cannot be said to have caused the plaintiffs' alleged injuries.

*List the options open to you. That is, answer the question, "What could you do?"*

- 
- 
- 
- 

*Choose the best solution from an ethical point of view, justify it, and respond to possible criticisms. That is, answer the question, "What should you do, and why?"*

- 
- 
- 
-

Select one member of your PBL group to role-play as an inmate of the
    Stateville Correction Center and have another member of your
    PBL group role-play as Willie E. McNeil. How might the two
    converse about different ways of thinking and techniques for
    conflict management?

- 
- 
- 
- 


Again, please select one member of your PBL group to role-play as
    Willie E. McNeil and have another member of your PBL group
    role-play as a representative of HHS. How might Willie E.
    McNeil use what is known about stages of change and about
    motivational interviewing to solve what you consider the major
    problem presented in the case?

- 
- 
- 
- 


## Part three

As the Supreme Court recently stated in *Denton v. Hernandez* [60 U.S.L.W.
4346, 4347 (May 4, 1992)], a district court, when deciding whether to allow
a plaintiff to proceed *in forma pauperis*, "is not bound, as it usually is when
making a determination based solely on the pleadings, to accept without
question the truth of the plaintiff's allegations." In the instant case, the
plaintiffs' bald assertion that the federal study caused them to be exposed
to infectious diseases simply does not withstand logical scrutiny. Similarly,
the plaintiffs' contention that the contract between the federal government
and the DOC somehow gave the federal government the authority to direct
the housing and movement of inmates in the Stateville Correctional Center
lacks an arguable basis in fact. Absent such control, the United States cannot
be held liable for any of the conduct that may have caused plaintiffs' alleged
injuries.

Accordingly, finding no arguable legal basis for the complaint, the court
denies plaintiffs' motion for leave to file and dismisses this action.

## Conclusion

It is important, when conducting a research study, that the researcher properly address all the components of an informed consent: beneficence, justice, and respect. Institutional review boards are developed to help protect the subject from any type of harm during a study. IRBs also make sure the study is carried out in a valid and ethical manner. Finally, political and social-economic factors should not preclude the conductance of ethical studies as they pertain to the relevance of the study population for which they are conducted.

# Research/testing on animals

This problem-based learning session is based on the following: *MSM Investments Company, LLC v. Carolwood Corporation*, 00-1092, U.S. Court of Appeals for the Federal Circuit, 259 F.3d 1335; 2001 U.S. App. Lexis 17881; 59 U.S.P.Q.2D (BNA) 1856. August 9, 2001, Decided. It is reprinted here with permission of LexisNexis.

## Objectives

The objectives of this problem-based learning case are:

- To become familiar with professional and institutional regulations and guidelines concerning responsible research on animals
- To understand and apply assessment criteria for conducting responsible research on animals, including:
  - The nature and measurement of pain and suffering in animals
  - The purpose of the experiment
  - Policies on pain and death
  - Alternatives to the use of animals

## Introduction

The humane use of laboratory animals in research testing and education is an integral part of the work of most companies, such as Allergram, Del Laboratories, Johnson & Johnson, Proctor & Gamble, and others. By testing products on animals, companies are able to determine possible dangers to human health and avoid product liability suits. The industry of animal testing promises to cure human diseases through animal experimentation. Medical science's great advances could not have been made without animal testing. Society would be plagued if animal testing were stopped.

## Part one

MSM Investments is the assignee of the '878 patent, which relates to a method of using methylsulfonylmethane to enhance the diet of an animal ('878 patent, col. 1, ll. 26–28). Claims 1 and 5, the only independent claims at issue, read in relevant part as follows:

> A method of feeding . . . an animal which comprises provid-
> ing to the animal for ingestion a beneficial amount of meth-
> ylsulfonylmethane which is in addition to any amount
> present as a naturally occurring constituent in the foodstuff
> ingested by the animal.

> A method of increasing the amount of metabolizable sulfur
> ingested by an animal which comprises providing to the
> animal for ingestion thereby a beneficial amount of methyl-
> sulfonylmethane which is exogenous to and which is in
> addition to any amount thereof which is present as a natu-
> rally occurring ingredient of the foodstuff sources thereof
> ingested by the animal.

During prosecution, the applicant amended Claim 1 by replacing the phrase "enhancing the diet of" with the term "feeding" to overcome an indefiniteness rejection under 35 U.S.C. § 112, P 2. *MSM Investments*, 70 F. Supp. 2d at 1046–1047; Paper No. 4 at 1.

According to the written description, MSM has "multiple functions in the body" ('878 patent, col. 3, ll. 67–68). Specifically, "at low levels of inges-tion, it functions as a normal dietary ingredient, viz., as a food or food ingredient; at higher levels it functions as a pharmaceutically active agent" (id. at col. 3, l. 68 to col. 4, l. 3). In addition to disclosing the use of MSM as a dietary supplement for nutritional purposes, the written description also discloses multiple examples of pharmacological benefits derived from the ingestion of MSM (see, e.g., id. at col. 13, l. 53 to col. 14, l. 62).

The '878 patent claims priority from a chain of nine earlier-filed appli-cations and has an effective filing date of September 14, 1982 (*MSM Invest-ments*, 70 F. Supp. 2d at 1047). More than 1 year prior to that date, Dr. Stanley Jacob publicly administered MSM, via oral ingestion, to human patients at the Oregon Health Sciences University (OHSU) clinic (id. at 1048). As early as February 1981, Dr. Jacob administered MSM as a pain reliever by mixing up to one-half teaspoon (roughly 2 g) of MSM in powdered form with water or orange juice.

Prior to assigning his rights to MSM Investments, Robert J. Herschler, the sole named inventor of the '878 patent, filed suit against Foodscience Corporation, alleging, *inter alia*, infringement of U.S. Patent 4,616,039, a related patent in the chain of priority of the '878 patent [(*Herschler v. Food-science Corp.*, No. 90-84 (D. Vt. Nov. 5, 1992) ("Foodscience I")]. In Foodscience I, the district court held that the asserted claims were valid and infringed. Claims 1 and 5 of that patent read:

> *A method of providing a source of metabolizable sulfur to an animal whose diet comprises sufficient processed food to render the animal's diet deficient in metabolizable sulfur, which comprises physically admixing with one or more food-stuffs ingested daily by the animal, prior to the ingestion thereof by the animal, an amount of methylsulfonylmethane to at least 0.01 mg/kg of body weight per day.*

> *A method of improving the overall state of health and resistance to disease of an animal maintained on a diet which supplies naturally occurring methylsulfonylmethane in amounts insufficient to maintain body levels thereof in the animal of at least 1 ppm, which comprises administering orally thereto and thereby adding to the diet of the animal an amount of methylsulfonylmethane effective to maintain these body levels at least 1 ppm.*

('039 patent, col. 28, ll. 44–51, 58–66). With respect to validity, the court concluded that Foodscience had failed to prove that the claims of the '039 patent were invalid based on prior public use at the OHSU clinic. On appeal, this court affirmed the district court's judgment on infringement, but reversed part of the judgment on validity [*Herschler v. Foodscience Corp.*, 1995 U.S. App. Lexis 24348, No. 93-1138, 1995 WL 490283 (Fed. Cir. Aug. 16, 1995) (table) ("Foodscience II")]. We concluded that the claims of the '039 patent that were limited to nonhuman use (i.e., use by a herbivore) were not invalid, whereas the claims that included human use were invalid "based on prior public use at the [OHSU clinic]" (id. at *1). The claims that included human use in that patent were quite similar to those at issue here, reciting methods of "providing a source of metabolizable sulfur" and "improving the overall state of health and resistance to disease of an animal" ('039 patent, col. 28, ll. 44–45, 58–59). Such language was held to encompass the prior public pharmaceutical use.

MSM Investments brought the present suit against Nurgetics and several other defendants (collectively, "Defendants"), alleging infringement of claims 1–8 of the '878 patent (*MSM Investments*, 70 F. Supp. 2d at 1045). In response, Defendants moved for summary judgment of invalidity under 35 U.S.C. § 102(b) based on Dr. Jacob's public use more than 1 year prior to the effective filing date of the '878 patent (id.). The district court granted Defendants' motion, concluding that Dr. Jacob's activities at the OHSU clinic constituted a prior "public use" under 35 U.S.C. §

102(b) that rendered the claims invalid (id. at 1057). MSM Investments now appeals from that decision. We have jurisdiction pursuant to 28 U.S.C. § 1295(a)(1) (1994).

## Make a list of the major problems presented in this case

- 
- 
- 
- 

## Hypothesis and mechanism

For the problems in your list above, give a cause or a reason for them to happen:

- 
- 
- 
- 

## Learning issues

Make a list of learning issues in the form of questions. Remember, your goal is to gather the medical, social, and all other relevant facts that may apply to the case.

What are the alternatives to animal testing?
   Alternatives to the use of animals in consumer product testing are available. In 1959, *The Principles of Humane Experiment Technique* was published in London; it defined the concept of animal testing alternatives as the "three R's."
   The three R's consist of:
      Refinement
      Reduction
      Replacement

What are the specific alternatives to animal testing?
   Alternatives to animal testing can be narrowed down to the following:
      Physical–chemical testing
      Computer mathematical analysis
      Microbiological systems
      Tissue/organ culture preparation
      Epidemiological surveys
      Plant analysis

What are the general ethical principles for animal testing/research?
Formulated by Marshall Hall in 1831:

1. *We should never have recourse to experiment in cases in which observation can afford us the information required.*
2. *It must be assumed that no experiment should be performed without a distinct and definite objective.*
3. *We should not needlessly repeat experiments that we have already been performed by physiologists of reputation.*
4. *A given experiment should be instituted with the least possible infliction of suffering.*
5. *Every experiment should be performed under such circumstances as will secure due observation and attestation of its results.*

What are the policies on pain and death regarding animal research?

The care, use, and transportation of animals should be in accordance with the Animal Welfare Act (7USC2131 et seq.) and other applicable federal laws, guidelines, and policies. Procedures with animals that may cause more than slight pain or distress should be performed with appropriate analgesia, sedation, or anesthesia.

Animals that would otherwise suffer severe pain or distress that cannot be relieved should be painlessly killed at the end of the procedure or, if appropriate, during the procedure. Proper use of animals involves: avoidance or minimization of discomfort, stress, and pain.

Discuss the purpose of animal experiments.

The experiments should have relevance to human or animal health, the advancement of knowledge, or the good of society.

The animals selected for a procedure should be an appropriate species and quality and the minimum number required to obtain valid results.

The classification of animal research techniques as to pain and distress are:

Animals subjected to procedures that will not involve pain or distress greater than that associated with standard injections, routine blood sampling, or induction of anesthesia.

Animals under anesthesia to be subjected to procedures involving minor pain or distress of short duration such as: surgical/diagnostic procedures; exposure of blood vessels; and procedures involving short-term restraint.

Animals receiving appropriate anesthetics, analgesics, or tranquilizing drugs will be subject to procedures involving significant but unavoidable pain or distress.

Animals without appropriate anesthetic, analgesic, or tranquilizing drugs will be used in procedures involving significant pain or distress. (All procedures in this item must be accompanied with written justification for producing unalleviated pain or distress.)

*In vivo* studies of tumor growth and metastatic phenomena require careful experimental planning. The tumor transplant site is also important since significant suffering can be avoided by careful selection of an appropriate site.

End-point death studies require special consideration and scientific justification. However, in the face of distinct signs that such studies are causing irreversible pain and distress, alternate end points should be sought to satisfy both the requirements of the study and the needs of the animal.

## Literature review

To help you get ready to answer certain questions you anticipate being asked during the second part of the case, look in the local medical library and on the World Wide Web for helpful information. Please indicate in the spaces below (1) several helpful articles or books you found and (2) several helpful Web sites you found.

- **Helpful articles:**
  Cotton, P., Animals and science benefit from "replace, reduce, refine" effort, *JAMA*, 270, 2905–2907, 1993.
  Crimm, N.J., From lawsuits to laboratories: new funding source for pharmacologic research, *J. Clin. Psychopharmacol.*, 15, 241–242, 1995.
  Dickety, S., Animal testing is a slippery slope, *Nurs. Stand.*, 13, 12, 1998.
  Fano, A., Animal testing, *J. R. Soc. Med.*, 90, 710, 1997.
  Grotenl, J.P. et al., TNO Network alternatives to animal experiment (TNA): aims and activities, *Pharmacol. Toxicol.*, Suppl. 80, 182–183, 1997.
  Lamberg, L., Researchers urged to tell public how animal studies benefit human health, *JAMA*, 282, 619–621, 1999.
  Nurses vote to end medical animal testing, *Nurs. Stand.*, 13, 5, 1998.
  Puppy love can be therapeutic too, *JAMA*, 274, 1897, 1995.
  Roe, F., Lethal laws: animal testing, human health and environmental policy, *J. R. Soc. Med.*, 90, 521–522, 1997.
  Russell, S.M. and Nicoll, C.S., A dissection of the chapter "Tools for research" in Peter Singer's *Animal Liberation*, *Proc. Soc. Exp. Biol. Med.*, 211, 109–138, 1996.
  Should we ban all animal testing? *Nurs. Stand.*, 13, 5, 1998.

- **Helpful Web sites:**
  RDS Online — understanding animal research in medicine: www.rds-online.org.uk

Guidelines for ethical conduct in the care and use of animals: www.apa.org/science/anguide.html

Association for the Assessment and Accreditation of Laboratory Animal Care: www.aaalac.org

## *Identify all relevant values that play a role in the case and determine which values, if any, conflict*

Nonmaleficence:

Beneficence:

Respect for persons:

Loyalty:

Distributive justice:

## *Learning issues for next student-centered problem-based learning session*

- List the options open to you. That is, answer the question, "What could you do?"
- Choose the best solution from an ethical point of view, justify it, and respond to possible criticisms. That is, answer the question, "What should you do, and why?"
- What are the different ways of thinking about the problem? Which conflict management techniques can be used in the situation?

## Part two

Summary judgment is appropriate "if the pleadings, depositions, answers to interrogatories, and admissions on file, together with the affidavits, if any, show that there is no genuine issue as to any material fact and that the moving party is entitled to a judgment as a matter of law" (Fed. R. Civ. P. 56(c)). For purposes of the motion, "the evidence of the nonmovant is to be believed, and all justifiable inferences are to be drawn in his favor" [*Anderson v. Liberty Lobby, Inc.*, 477 U.S. 242, 255, 91 L. Ed. 2d 202, 106 S. Ct. 2505 (1986)]. We review a district court's grant of a motion for summary judgment *de novo* [*Ethicon Endo-Surgery, Inc., v. U.S. Surgical Corp.*, 149 F.3d 1309, 1315, 47 U.S.P.Q.2D (BNA) 1272, 1275 (Fed. Cir. 1998)].

On appeal, MSM Investments argues that the district court erred in granting Defendants' motion for summary judgment of invalidity because the claims of the '878 patent are limited to the nutritional use of MSM, whereas Dr. Jacob's activities at the OHSU clinic were limited to pharmaceutical or pharmacological uses of MSM. MSM Investments contends that the district court misconstrued Claims 1 and 5 by concluding that they were not limited to nutritional uses of MSM. MSM Investments asserts that, given its ordinary meaning, the term "feeding" in Claim 1 means "to give food to; to supply with nourishment." MSM Investments also contends that the phrase "a beneficial amount of methylsulfonylmethane" in Claims 1 and 5 should be construed as meaning "the amount of MSM that produces a nutritional benefit."

Nurgetics responds that the district court did not err in determining that the term feeding does not limit Claim 1 to the use of MSM for nutritional purposes. Nurgetics also asserts that the district court properly interpreted the phrase "beneficial amount of methylsulfonylmethane" in Claims 1 and 5 to mean "any nonzero amount of methylsulfonylmethane that does not occur naturally in food actually eaten by an animal." Nurgetics further responds that, because the claims do not include a nutritional use limitation, they are rendered invalid under 35 U.S.C. § 102(b) by the prior public use of MSM by Dr. Jacob at the OHSU clinic.

Because the parties do not dispute that Dr. Jacob publicly used MSM to treat pain more than 1 year prior to the effective filing date of the '878 patent, the sole issue on appeal is one of claim construction: whether the terms "feeding" and "beneficial amount" limit the claims to the use of MSM for nutritional purposes. Claim construction is an issue of law [*Markman v. Westview Instruments, Inc.*, 52 F.3d 967, 970–971, 34 U.S.P.Q.2D (BNA) 1321, 1322 (Fed. Cir. 1995) (*en banc*), aff'd, 517 U.S. 370, 134 L. Ed. 2d 577, 116 S. Ct. 1384 (1996)] that we review *de novo* [*Cybor Corp. v. FAS Techs., Inc.*, 138 F.3d 1448, 1456, 46 U.S.P.Q.2D (BNA) 1169, 1172 (Fed. Cir. 1998) (en banc)]. In interpreting claims, a court "should look first to the intrinsic evidence of record, i.e., the patent itself, including the claims, the specification and, if in evidence, the prosecution history" [*Vitronics Corp. v. Conceptronic, Inc.*, 90 F.3d 1576, 1582, 39 U.S.P.Q.2D (BNA) 1573, 1577 (Fed. Cir. 1996)]. Claim terms are to be given their ordinary and accustomed meaning "unless it appears from the specification or the file history that they were used differently by the inventor" [*Carroll Touch, Inc., v. Electro Mech. Sys., Inc.*, 15 F.3d 1573, 1577, 27 U.S.P.Q.2D (BNA) 1836, 1840 (Fed. Cir. 1993)].

As always, our claim construction analysis begins with the actual words of the claim, such as *Optical Disc Corporation v. Del Mar Avionics*, 208 F.3d 1324, 1334, 54 U.S.P.Q.2D (BNA) 1289, 1295 (Fed. Cir. 2000), "We begin the claim construction process by considering the words of the claim itself" [citing *Bell Communications Research, Inc., v. Vitalink Communications Corp.*, 55 F.3d 615, 619–620, 34 U.S.P.Q.2D (BNA) 1816, 1819 (Fed. Cir. 1995)]; *Vitronics*, 90 F.3d at 1582, 39 U.S.P.Q.2D (BNA) at 1577, "First, we look to the words of the claims themselves, both asserted and nonasserted, to define the scope of the patented invention." We agree with MSM Investments that the ordinary meaning of the term "feeding" would indicate that the method in Claim 1 entails supplying or providing food or nourishment. See, for instance, *Webster's Second New Riverside University Dictionary* (p. 469, 1988), which defines feed as "1. a. To supply with nourishment . . . b. To provide as food or nourishment"). Thus, the ordinary meaning of the term "feeding" provides some support for the argument of MSM Investments that the method in Claim 1 is limited to the use of MSM for nutritional purposes.

However, claim language must always be construed in light of the specification [*Vitronics*, 90 F.3d at 1582, 39 U.S.P.Q.2D (BNA), "It is always necessary to review the specification to determine whether the inventor has used any terms in a manner inconsistent with their ordinary meaning"; *Markman*, 52 F.3d at 979, 34 U.S.P.Q.2D (BNA) at 1330, "Claims must be read in view of the specification, of which they are a part"]. Contrary to the ordinary meaning arguably suggested by its dictionary definition, when viewed in light of the specification, we conclude that the term "feeding" does not limit Claim 1 to nutritional uses and does not exclude the use of MSM for pharmaceutical or pharmacological purposes [see *Vitronics*, 90 F.3d at 1584 n.6, 39 U.S.P.Q.2D (BNA) at 1578 n.6, "Judges may . . . rely on dictionary definitions when construing claim terms, so long as the dictionary definition does not contradict any definition found in or ascertained by a reading of the patent documents"].

While the written description does not specifically define the term "feeding," it does disclose that MSM may be used "as a food and as a normalizer of biological function ('878 patent, col. 7, ll. 53–56), and although its use as a "food" suggests that MSM may be used for nutritional purposes, the written description broadly defines the word food as meaning "a nutritive material taken into an organism for growth, work, protection, repair, restoration and maintenance of vital processes" (id. at col. 8, ll. 20–23). This expansive definition of the word food, coupled with the disclosed use of MSM as a "normalizer of biological function," clearly suggests that the claimed method of feeding includes both nutritional and pharmacological uses. Indeed, in addition to stating that MSM may be used as a "normal dietary ingredient," the specification also explicitly states that MSM has "multiple functions in the body" and that "at higher levels [of ingestion] it functions as a pharmaceutically active agent" (id. at col. 3, l. 67 to col. 4, l. 3). The written description explains that "the major differences between the use of [MSM] as a food and as a normalizer of biological function is the concentration and amount employed, dosage forms, and routes of systemic entry" (id. at col. 7, ll. 53–56).

Furthermore, the written description provides numerous examples of specific pharmacological benefits derived from the ingestion of MSM (e.g., id. at col. 13, l. 53 to col. 14, l. 62, "The following are pharmacological benefits from the ingestion of exogenous methylsulfonylmethane"). These examples range from relieving various types of pain and treating parasitic infections to improving the overall health of animals (id.). The specification states that these pharmacological benefits may be effectuated by adding MSM to the "daily diet" of the patient (id. at col. 20, ll. 3–11) or by administering MSM "in admixture with one or more foodstuffs ingested daily by the patient, e.g., milk, coffee, tea, cold desserts, etc." (id. at col. 22, ll. 60–68). It is also clear that animals may be administered pharmaceuticals by including them in their animal feed (e.g., id. at col. 10, l. 58 to col. 13, l. 52). Such examples erase the distinction that MSM Investments attempts to create between the use of MSM as a nutritional food or dietary supplement and the use of MSM for pharmacological purposes.

MSM Investments argues that the examples of pharmacological uses of MSM in the specification "were actually examples of different inventions claimed in different, but related, patents," and that the district court's "improper reliance" on these examples led to an erroneous claim construction. However, that argument is unpersuasive. According to its own written description, the '878 patent discloses additional examples of pharmacological benefits that were not disclosed in patent applications (id. at col. 2, l. 67 to col. 3, l. 5, "In addition to the pharmacologically beneficial effects [of] methylsulfonylmethane . . . which are specifically disclosed in my patent applications, it is useful in the treatment of a surprising variety of other diseases and adverse physiological conditions, as disclosed in detail hereinafter").

Moreover, the fact that other related patents have claims that are limited to certain pharmacological uses (e.g., treatment of gastrointestinal upset, nocturnal muscle cramps, etc.) does not compel the conclusion that the claims of the '878 patent must be limited to nutritional uses. While a patent specification may contain a description of separately patentable inventions that end up claimed in multiple patents, the specification of this patent indicates that the generic term "feeding" encompasses the administering of pharmaceuticals. The specification commingles pharmaceutical uses with nutritional uses and does not describe nutritional benefits and pharmacological benefits as mutually exclusive. Thus, when reading the claim language in light of the specification, the term "feeding" in Claim 1 of the '878 patent covers both nutritional and pharmacological uses of MSM.

With respect to the beneficial amount limitation, MSM Investments contends that this limitation should be interpreted as "the amount of MSM that produces a nutritional benefit." We disagree. While the district court's construction of "a beneficial amount of methylsulfonylmethane" as meaning "any nonzero amount of methylsulfonylmethane that does not occur naturally in food actually eaten by an animal," [*MSM Investments Co. v. Carolwood Corp.*, No. C 98-20238 EAI, slip op. at 8 (N.D. Cal. Jul. 23, 1999), order regarding claim construction], misses the implication of the word beneficial that the amount must "promote a favorable result" for the animal, the claim language plainly encompasses both pharmacological and nutritional benefits. Furthermore, the written description explains that, while it is desirable to ingest "from about 0.5–1.0 milligram/kg body weight/day" to maintain optimum good health, "any lower level will serve some benefit" (id. at col. 4, ll. 60–66). The specification discloses many of such benefits, which include pharmacological benefits. We therefore conclude that the district court's construction of the phrase "a beneficial amount of methylsulfonylmethane," while incomplete, at most constituted harmless error.

*List the options open to you. That is, answer the question, "What could you do?"*

- 
- 
- 
- 

*Choose the best solution from an ethical point of view, justify it, and respond to possible criticisms. that is, answer the question, "What should you do, and why?"*

- 
- 
- 
-

*Select one member of your PBL group to role-play as a representative of MSM Investments and have another member of your PBL group role-play as a representative of Norgetics. How might the two converse about different ways of thinking and techniques for conflict management?*

- 
- 
- 
- 

*Again, please select one member of your PBL group to role-play as a representative of MSM Investments and have another member of your PBL group role-play as a representative of Norgetics. How might the representative of MSM Investments use what is known about stages of change and about motivational interviewing to solve what you consider the major problem presented in the case?*

- 
- 
- 
- 

## Part three

MSM Investments Company LLC appeals from the decision of the U.S. District Court for the Northern District of California granting the motion of Nurgetics, Inc., for summary judgment that the claims of U.S. Patent 5,071,878 are invalid under 35 U.S.C. § 102(b) [*MSM Investments Co. v. Carolwood Corp.*, 70 F. Supp. 2d 1044 (N.D. Cal. 1999), order granting defendants' motion for summary judgment of invalidity]. Because the district court did not err in concluding that the claims of the '878 patent are invalid under 35 U.S.C. § 102(b), we affirm.

Accordingly, we agree with Nurgetics that the district court correctly concluded that Claims 1 and 5 are not limited to nutritional uses of MSM. Moreover, because the parties do not dispute that Dr. Jacob publicly administered MSM as a pain reliever more than 1 year prior to the effective filing date of the '878 patent, the district court did not err in granting summary judgment that the claims of the '878 patent are invalid under 35 U.S.C. § 102(b). We therefore affirm.

## Conclusion

Animal testing has been a controversial issue for years, and there are many laws and regulations surrounding this specific topic. There have been many policies implanted in regard to pain and suffering of animals, as well as the ethical issues behind the use of animals.

In conclusion, there are many national, state, and institutional rules and regulations concerning the controversial issue of animal testing. These regulations and guidelines must be followed to prevent unnecessary pain and suffering to animals. People will continue to fight to stop animal testing; however, by following strict and practical guidelines, scientists can assure the public that animal testing is being used accurately, appropriately, and ethically.

*case sixteen*

# Intellectual property

This problem-based learning session is based on the following: *Eli Lilly and Company v. American Cyanamid Company*, 95-1489, U.S. Court of Appeals for the Federal Circuit, 82 F.3d 1568; 1996 U.S. App. Lexis 10935; 38 U.S.P.Q.2D (BNA 1705). May 10, 1996, Decided. Rehearing Denied and In Banc Suggestion Declined July 2, 1996. Reported at: 1996 U.S. App. Lexis 18004. It is reprinted here with permission of LexisNexis.

## Objectives

The objectives of this problem-based learning case are:

- To define a patent
- To define whom patents affect
- To explore the process of obtaining a patent

## Introduction

The methods by which patents are obtained are unique to every country. The idea of patenting in the United States is over 200 years old. Patents were first implemented while Thomas Jefferson was Secretary of State. In 1793, the U.S. Congress passed a patent act that provided for the registration of products without examination.

Depending on an individual's perspective, patents could or could not be a benefit in the medical field. Patents involve almost everyone, if not everyone, in society. In this presentation, we show both the positive and the negative aspects related to patents and how they affect society as a whole.

## Part one

The pharmaceutical product at issue in this case is a broad-spectrum antibiotic known as cefaclor. Cefaclor is a member of the class of cephalosporin antibiotics, all of which are based on the cephem nucleus. Although there are many different cephem compounds, only a few have utility as antibiotic drugs. Each of the known commercial methods for producing cefaclor requires the production of an intermediate cephem compound known as an enol. Once the desired enol cephem intermediate is obtained, it is then subjected to several processing steps to produce cefaclor.

Lilly developed cefaclor and patented it in 1975. Until recently, Lilly has been the exclusive manufacturer and distributor of cefaclor in this country. In addition to its product patent on cefaclor, Lilly obtained several patents covering different aspects of the manufacture of cefaclor, including processes for producing enol cephem intermediates. Many of those patents have now expired.

In 1995, Lilly purchased the patent at issue in this case, U.S. Patent No. 4,160,085 (the '085 patent). Claim 5 of that patent defines a method of producing enol cephem compounds, including what is called Compound 6, an enol cephem similar to the one Lilly uses in its process for manufacturing cefaclor. The '085 patent expired on July 3, 1996.

Compound 6 differs from cefaclor in three respects. Although both Compound 6 and cefaclor are based on the cephem nucleus, Compound 6 has a hydroxy group at the 3-position on the cephem nucleus, a para-nitrobenzyl carboxylate ester at the 4-position, and a phenylacetyl group at the 7-position. Cefaclor has different groups at each of those positions: it has a chlorine atom at the 3-position, a free carboxyl group at the 4-position, and a phenylglycyl group at the 7-position. Each of those differences between Compound 6 and cefaclor contributes to the effectiveness of cefaclor as an orally administered antibiotic drug. The free carboxyl group at the 4-position is believed important for antibacterial activity; the chlorine increases cefaclor's antibiotic potency; and the phenylglycyl group enables cefaclor to be effective when taken orally.

To produce cefaclor from Compound 6 requires four distinct steps. First, the hydroxy group is removed from the 3-position and is replaced by a chlorine atom, which results in the creation of Compound 7. Second, Compound 7 is subjected to a reaction that removes the phenylacetyl group at the 7-position, which results in the creation of Compound 8. Third, a phenylglycyl group is added at the 7-position, which results in the creation of Compound 9. Fourth, the para-nitrobenzyl carboxylate ester is removed from the 4-position, which results in the creation of cefaclor.

On April 27, 1995, defendants Zenith Laboratories, Inc. (Zenith), and American Cyanamid Company (Cyanamid) obtained permission from the Food and Drug Administration (FDA) to distribute cefaclor in this country. Defendant Biocraft Laboratories, Inc. (Biocraft), had applied for FDA approval to manufacture and sell cefaclor in the United States, but had not yet obtained that approval. All three have obtained large quantities of cefaclor that were manufactured in Italy by defendant Biochimica Opos, S.p.A. (Opos).

On the same day that Zenith and Cyanamid obtained FDA approval to sell cefaclor in this country, Lilly obtained the rights to the '085 patent and filed suit against Zenith, Cyanamid, Biocraft, and Opos. In its complaint, Lilly sought a declaration that the domestic defendants' importation of cefaclor manufactured by Opos infringed Lilly's rights under several patents, including the '085 patent. Lilly also requested a preliminary injunction, based on the alleged infringement of Claim 5 of the '085 patent, to bar the defendants from importing or inducing the importation of cefaclor manufactured by Opos.

The district court held a 3-day hearing on the motion for a preliminary injunction. Following the hearing, the court denied the motion in a comprehensive opinion. The court devoted most of its attention to the question whether Lilly had met its burden of showing that it was likely to prevail on the merits of its claim that the defendants were liable for infringing Claim 5 of the '085 patent.

Based on the evidence presented at the hearing, the district court concluded that Lilly had shown that it was likely to prevail on the issue of the validity of the '085 patent. With respect to the infringement issue, however, the court held that Lilly had not met its burden of showing that it was likely to prevail.

The district court correctly framed the issue as whether, under the Process Patent Amendments Act of 1988 (Pub. L. No. 100-418, §§ 9001–9007), the importers of cefaclor infringed Claim 5 of the '085 patent, which granted U.S. patent protection to the process that Opos used to make Compound 6. The Process Patent Amendments Act makes it an act of infringement to import, sell, offer to sell, or use in this country a product that was made abroad by a process protected by a U.S. patent [35 U.S.C. § 271(g)]. The act, however, does not apply if the product made by the patented process is "materially changed by subsequent processes" before it is imported [35 U.S.C. § 271(g)(1)].

The district court found that Compound 6 and cefaclor differ significantly in their structure and properties, including their biological activity. Citing the Senate Report on the Process Patent Amendments Act, the district court found that, because the processing steps necessary to convert Compound 6 to cefaclor "'change the physical or chemical properties of the product in a manner which changes the basic utility of the product'" [896 F. Supp. at 857, 36 U.S.P.Q.2D (BNA) at 1016, citing S. Rep. No. 83, 100th Cong., 1st Sess. 50 (1987)], Lilly was not likely to succeed on its claim that the defendants infringed Lilly's rights under Claim 5 of the '085 patent by importing and selling cefaclor.

The district court also found that Lilly had failed to prove that it would suffer irreparable harm in the absence of a preliminary injunction. The presumption of irreparable harm that is available when a patentee makes a strong showing of likelihood of success on the merits was not available here, the court held, because of Lilly's failure to make such a showing on the issue of infringement. In addition, the court was not persuaded by Lilly's arguments that it faced irreparable economic injury if it were not granted immediate equitable relief. Under the circumstances of this case, the district court found that an award of money damages would be an adequate remedy in the event that Lilly ultimately proves that the importation of cefaclor made by the Opos process infringes the '085 patent. In light of Lilly's failure to establish either a likelihood of success on the merits or irreparable harm, the court found it unnecessary to articulate findings regarding the other factors bearing on the propriety of preliminary injunctive relief — the balance of the hardships and the effect of the court's action on the public interest.

The Process Patent Amendments Act of 1988 was enacted to close a perceived loophole in the statutory scheme for protecting owners of U.S. patents. Prior to the enactment of the 1988 statute, a patentee holding a process patent could sue for infringement if others used the process in this country, but had no cause of action if such persons used the patented process abroad to manufacture products and then imported, used, or sold the products in this country. In that setting, the process patent owner's only legal recourse for such products was to seek an exclusion order from the International Trade Commission under Section 337a of the Tariff Act of 1930 [19 U.S.C. § 1337a (1982)]. By enacting the Process Patent Amendments Act, the principal portion of which is codified as 35 U.S.C. § 271(g), Congress changed the law by making it an act of infringement to import into the United States, or to sell or use within the United States, "a product which is made by a process patented in the United States . . . if the importation, sale, or use of the product occurs during the term of such process patent."

A concern raised during Congress's consideration of the process patent legislation was whether and to what extent the new legislation would affect products other than the direct and unaltered products of patented processes — that is, whether the new statute would apply when a product was produced abroad by a patented process, but then modified or incorporated into other products before being imported into this country. Congress addressed that issue by providing that a product that is "made by" a patented process within the meaning of the statute "will . . . not be considered to be so made after — (1) it is materially changed by subsequent processes; or (2) it becomes a trivial and nonessential component of another product" [35 U.S.C. § 271(g)].

That language, unfortunately, is not very precise. Whether the product of a patented process is a trivial and nonessential component of another product is necessarily a question of degree. Even less well defined is the question whether the product of a patented process has been materially changed before its importation into this country. While applying that statutory language may be relatively easy in extreme cases, it is not at all easy in a closer case such as this one.

Lilly argues that the materially changed clause of Section 271(g) must be construed in light of its underlying purpose, which is to protect the economic value of U.S. process patents for their owners. Prior to the enactment of the Process Patent Amendments Act, the value of a U.S. process patent could be undermined by a manufacturer who used the process abroad and then imported the product into this country. Because the purpose of the process patent legislation was to protect against such subversion of protected economic rights, Lilly argues that the statute should be read to apply to any such scheme that undercuts the commercial value of a U.S. process patent. In Lilly's view, the product of a patented process therefore should not be considered materially changed if the principal commercial use of that product lies in its conversion into the product that is the subject of the infringement charge. Because cefaclor is the only product of Compound 6 that is sold in the United States market, Lilly argues, the change in Compound 6 that results in cefaclor — no matter how significant as a matter of chemical properties or molecular structure — is not a material change for purposes of Section 271(g).

Although we are not prepared to embrace Lilly's argument, we acknowledge that it has considerable appeal. Congress was concerned with the problem of the overseas use of patented processes followed by the importation of the products of those processes, and a grudging construction of the statute could significantly limit the statute's effectiveness in addressing the problem Congress targeted. That is especially true with respect to chemical products, for which simple, routine reactions can often produce dramatic changes in the products' structure and properties.

Nonetheless, while the general purpose of the statute informs the construction of the language Congress chose, purpose cannot displace language, and we cannot stretch the term materially changed as far as Lilly's argument would require. The problem is that the language of the statute refers to changes in the product; the statute permits the importation of an item that is derived from a product made by a patented process as long as that product is materially changed in the course of its conversion into the imported item. The reference to a changed product is very hard to square with Lilly's proposed test, which turns on the quite different question of whether the use or sale of the imported item impairs the economic value of the process patent.

The facts of this case demonstrate how far Lilly's test strays from the statutory text. While Lilly notes that there are only four steps between Compound 6 and cefaclor, and that all four steps involve relatively routine chemical reactions, Lilly does not suggest any limiting principle based on the structure of the intermediate product or the nature of the steps necessary to produce the imported product. Thus, even if there were ten complex chemical reactions that separated Compound 6 from cefaclor, Lilly's test would characterize the two compounds as not materially different as long as the primary commercial use of Compound 6 in this country was to produce cefaclor.

Besides not responding to the natural meaning of the term changed, Lilly's construction of the materially changed clause would create a curious anomaly. Lilly's value-based construction of the clause turns in large measure on Lilly's contention that the only commercial use for Compound 6 in this country is to produce cefaclor; that is, Lilly views Compound 6 and cefaclor as essentially the same product because Compound 6 has no commercial use in the U.S. market except to produce cefaclor. Under that approach, however, the question whether Compound 6 was materially changed in the course of its conversion to cefaclor would depend on whether and to what extent other derivative products of Compound 6 are marketed in this country. Thus, under Lilly's theory, Compound 6 would become materially different from cefaclor if and when Compound 6 came to have other commercial uses in the United States, even though the respective structures and properties of the two compounds remained unchanged.

That is asking the statutory language to do too much work. We cannot accept the argument that the question whether one compound is materially changed in the course of its conversion into another depends on whether there are other products of the first compound that have economic value. We therefore do not adopt Lilly's proposed construction of Section 271(g). We look instead to the substantiality of the change between the product of the patented process and the product that is being imported.

In the chemical context, a material change in a compound is most naturally viewed as a significant change in the compound's structure and properties. Without attempting to define with precision which classes of changes would be material and which would not, we share the district court's view that a change in chemical structure and properties as significant as the change between Compound 6 and cefaclor cannot lightly be dismissed as immaterial. Although Compound 6 and cefaclor share the basic cephem nucleus, which is the ultimate source of the antibiotic potential of all cephalosporins, the cephem nucleus is common to thousands of compounds, many of which have antibiotic activity, and many of which are dramatically different from others within the cephem family. Beyond the cephem nucleus that they have in common, Compound 6 and cefaclor are different in four important structural respects, corresponding to the four discrete chemical steps between the two compounds. While the addition or removal of a protective group, standing alone, might not be sufficient to constitute a material change between two compounds (even though it could dramatically affect certain of their properties), the conversion process between Compound 6 and cefaclor involves considerably more than the removal of a protective group. We therefore conclude that the statutory text of Section 271(g) does not support Lilly's contention that it is likely to prevail on the merits of its infringement claim.

In aid of their differing approaches to the issue of statutory construction, both sides in this dispute seek support for their positions in the legislative history of the 1988 statute. As is often the case, there is something in the legislative history for each side. On Lilly's side, for example, are characterizations of the legislation as creating process patent protection that is "meaningful and not easily evaded" [H.R. Rep. No. 60, 100th Cong., 1st Sess. 13 (1987)] and as excluding products only if they "cease to have a reasonable nexus with the patented process" [S. Rep. No. 83, 100th Cong., 1st Sess. 36 (1987)]. On the other side are directions for applying the statute to chemical intermediates — directions that suggest a narrower construction of the statute than Lilly proposes. On balance, while we do not find the legislative history dispositive, we conclude that it does not unequivocally favor Lilly's position and thus does not raise doubts about the district court's statutory analysis as applied to the facts of this case.

Congress considered proposals for process patent reform for many years before the Process Patent Amendments Act was finally enacted in 1988. The 1966 report of the President's Commission on the Patent System recommended extending patent protection to the imported products of patented processes, and bills proposing such a measure were introduced in several sessions of Congress thereafter [see "To Promote the Progress of . . . Useful Arts," Report of the President's Commission on the Patent System 35–36 (1966); S. Rep. No. 642, 94th Cong., 1st Sess. 5–7 (1976), surveying patent law reform proposals in the 90th through the 94th Congresses].

In 1983, efforts to enact process patent legislation resumed with the introduction of a number of bills in both houses of Congress. The bills varied in many respects, but with respect to the issue presented in this case, they were largely alike. The language contained in one of the bills was typical: it gave the patentee an action for infringement against anyone who, without authority, used or sold in the United States "a product produced by [a patented] process," even if the product in question was manufactured abroad [S. 1841, 98th Cong. 1st Sess. (1983)]. None of those bills became law, in part because of disputes concerning procedural issues over which various advocacy groups differed sharply.

The question of how to define the required relationship between the product of the patented process and the imported product came to the fore during the 99th Congress's consideration of process patent legislation. In 1985, the Commissioner of Patents and Trademarks told a Senate subcommittee that the proposed legislation should specifically provide that the product must be the "direct" product of the patented process "to lay to rest arguments that, for example, a product resulting from a series of processes would be covered by a process patent for an intermediate step." [Process Patents: Hearing on S. 1543 before the Subcomm. on Patents, Copyrights and Trademarks of the S. Comm. on the Judiciary, 99th Cong., 1st Sess. 9 (1985).] The commissioner pointed out that inserting the word "directly" in the proposed statute would make U.S. law consistent with the laws of many foreign countries, which protect only the "direct" products of patented processes (id. at 15). The Pharmaceutical Manufacturers Association agreed that the proposed limiting language would be appropriate as long as it was understood that "immaterial and minor later steps such as salt formation or removal of protective [groups] should not be construed in such a way that importation of the final product of that added step would not be an infringement" (id. at 71). Other interest groups likewise offered support for the proposed limiting language, subject to similar qualifications (see id. at 63, statement of the Intellectual Property Owners, Inc.; id. at 186, statement of the American Intellectual Property Law Association).

The following year, the administration again suggested, this time in a hearing before a House committee, adding the term "directly" to the proposed statute [see Intellectual Property and Trade: Hearings before the

Subcomm. on Courts, Civil Liberties, and the Admin. of Justice of the H. Comm. on the Judiciary, 99th Cong., 2d Sess. 58–59 (1986)]. The National Association of Manufacturers (NAM) agreed that the scope of process patent protection should be limited, but regarded the word "directly" as too restrictive; instead, NAM suggested that the statute "not apply to products materially changed chemically by subsequent steps or processes from the product resulting from the patented process" (id. at 275–276). That language, according to the NAM representative, would cover the case of "a chemical intermediate made abroad by a patented process," but then "subjected to a common chemical reaction" [*1575] and converted into "a salt or amino-derivative" (id. at 275; see also id. at 280).

The drafters of subsequent process patent bills embraced the administration's suggestion to restrict the scope of the statute, but they did so by using the language suggested by NAM. Thus, the term materially changed was adopted to exclude from the reach of the proposed statute those products that were significantly altered before their importation.

The House report on the 1986 version of the process patent legislation was the first committee report to discuss the meaning of the materially changed clause. It explained that, if the patented process is for chemical X, and "subsequent modifications change the basic structure of chemical X so that a clearly different chemical Y results, the connection between the patented process and the product, chemical Y, is broken" [H.R. Rep. No. 807, 99th Cong., 2d Sess. 21 (1986)]. The report noted, however, that chemical X would not be materially changed within the meaning of the statute if the subsequent modifications of chemical X were only "trivial or conventional in nature," such as "modifications which result in the formation of simple derivatives, including salts or esters, or the removal of impurities," or if the subsequent processing steps "only change [the] shape, size or form" of the product, such as by being diluted or put in tablet form (id. at 21–22).

Efforts to enact process patent legislation continued the following year; those efforts ultimately bore fruit in 1988 with the enactment of the Process Patent Amendments Act. Although several persons during the 1987 Senate hearings called attention to the need to clarify the materially changed clause in light of the difficulty of applying it to chemical intermediates [see Process Patent Legislation: Hearing on S. 568, S. 573, and S. 635 before the Subcomm. on Patents, Copyrights and Trademarks of the S. Comm. on the Judiciary, 100th Cong., 1st Sess. 114 (1987), statement on behalf of the Intellectual Property Owners, Inc.; id. at 146], the bills considered during 1987 and 1988 continued to employ the prior language without modification.

The pertinent portion of the 1987 House report on the process patent bill was identical to the portion of the 1986 House report summarized above, except for some new material that was inserted into one paragraph of the 1987 report. The new material appears to have been intended to express the notion that, under certain circumstances, significant changes in the properties or structure of a chemical product do not render the product materially changed within the meaning of the statutory language. The principal portion of the added matter explained that a hypothetical chemical product, chemical X, is not materially changed if chemical X is an important intermediate product, such as a polymer, that can materially be changed into an end product, albeit by trivial or conventional processes. In this respect, a product will be considered made by the patented process, regardless of any subsequent changes, if it would not be possible or commercially viable to make that product but for the use of the patented process. In judging the commercial viability, the courts shall use a flexible standard that is appropriate to the competitive circumstances [H.R. Rep. No. 60, 100th Cong., 1st Sess. 13–14 (1987)].

The inserted language is not easy to interpret, in part because it purports to identify some products that can "materially be changed" without being "materially changed." In any event, however, the inserted language appears not to apply to the present case as it seems to contemplate that when an intermediate that is the product of a patented process undergoes significant changes in the course of conversion into an end product, the end product will be deemed to be made by the patented process if (and only if) it would not be commercially feasible to make the end product other than using the patented process. In this case, Lilly concedes that it is both possible and commercially viable to make cefaclor by methods that do not include the process defined by Claim 5 of the '085 patent. Therefore, even if the explanatory language from the 1987 House report were accorded equal status with the language of the statute itself, the explanatory language would not require that Section 271(g) be read to reach the defendants' conduct in this case.

Lilly seizes on the statement in the House report that suggests that a change in "the basic structure" of the intermediate is necessary to break "the connection between the patented process and the [final, imported] product" (H.R. Rep. No. 60, supra, at 13). Because both Compound 6 and cefaclor share the core cephem nucleus, Lilly contends that the process of converting Compound 6 to cefaclor does not alter the basic structure of Compound 6, and that Compound 6 is therefore not materially changed by the process of converting it into cefaclor.

While Lilly's argument on this point cannot be lightly dismissed, we do not think the use of the term "basic structure" in the House report limits the materially changed clause, as applied to a cephem compound, to a change that alters the core cephem nucleus. If adopted, Lilly's argument would mean that there would never be a material change resulting from the conversion of one cephem compound to another. Lilly's argument would also leave open the question whether even a change in the cephem nucleus would be sufficiently "basic" if, for example, the initial and end products both contained the beta lactam ring, which is one of the components of the cephalosporin nucleus, and thus were members of the beta lactam "superfamily" of compounds. The effect of Lilly's construction of Section 271(g)(1), both within the family of cephem compounds and within other families of compounds that are based on a common nucleus, would be sweeping. Absent clearer congressional direction, we decline to adopt so broad a principle. We therefore decline Lilly's invitation to find the answer to this case in the House report's reference to changes in the basic structure of chemical intermediates.

Like the House report, the 1987 Senate report contains a detailed elaboration on the statutory term "material change." In fact, the Senate report contains what may best be described as a detailed set of instructions to courts called on to construe that term as it applies to particular fields of technology. The report noted that many foreign patent statutes extending process patent protection to a product require that the product in question be made directly from the patented process and suggested that the term "materially changed" in Section 271(g) was intended to embody a similar, but somewhat broader, scope of protection; as the Senate Committee explained, the term "directly" was not used because it might have been read to "exempt too many products that have been altered in insignificant ways after manufacture by the patented process" [S. Rep. No. 83, 100th Cong., 1st Sess. 49 (1987)].

Acknowledging that the task of determining whether a product was materially changed prior to its importation would ultimately be left to the courts, the committee then set out a "two-phased test" to "give the courts Congressional guidance in what may be a difficult determination" (S. Rep. No. 83, supra, at 50). The first part of the test restated the test set forth in the House report, that is, that a product "will be considered made by the patented process . . . if it would not be possible or commercially viable to make that product but for the use of the patented process."

The Senate report provided an analysis of how the first part of the test should be applied in the case of chemical intermediates. The report explained (S. Rep. No. 83, supra, at 51):

> *If the only way to have arrived at Y is to have used the patented process at some step, e.g., producing X as an intermediate, Y is infringing.*
>
> *If there is more than one way to have arrived [at] Y, but the patented process is the only commercially viable way to have done so, Y is infringing.*
>
> *If there are commercially viable non-infringing processes to have arrived at X, the connection between the patented process for producing chemical X and the ultimate product, chemical Y, is broken, and Y would be a non-infringing product having satisfied both phases of the test.*

As we noted above, the record makes clear that there is at least one commercially viable process for making cefaclor that does not involve the patented method of synthesizing enol cephems (including Compound 6). Opos does not use that noninfringing process, but under the test set forth in the Senate report, it is enough to defeat the claim of infringement that there is another way of producing the intermediate, even if the alleged infringer does not use that alternative process.

The Senate committee described the second portion of the two-part test for identifying a material change as follows (S. Rep. No. 83, supra, at 50):

> *A product will be considered to have been made by a patented process if the additional processing steps which are not covered by the patent do not change the physical or chemical properties of the product in a manner which [\*\*28] changes the basic utility of the product [produced] by the patented process. However, a change in the physical or chemical properties of a product, even though minor, may be "material" if the change relates to a physical or chemical property which is an important feature of the product produced by the patented process. Usually a change in the physical form of a product (e.g., the granules to powder, solid to liquid) or minor chemical conversion, (e.g., conversion to a salt, base, acid, hydrate, ester, or addition or removal of a protection group) would not be a "material" change.*

It seems fairly clear that, under this second part of the test, the change from Compound 6 to cefaclor would be regarded as a material change. The chemical properties of the two compounds are completely different, the basic utility of the products is different, and the chemical structure of the two products is significantly different. The changes between Compound 6 and cefaclor go far beyond the minor changes that the report described as not material, such as the conversion to a salt, base, acid, hydrate, or ester or the removal of a protective group.

Lilly interprets the references in the Senate report to the basic utility and properties of the product of the patented process in a quite different manner. The basic utility and principal property of Compound 6 in the U.S. market, according to Lilly, is to serve as an intermediate for the production of cefaclor. Because the defendants have "exploited" that utility or property, Lilly argues, Compound 6 cannot be regarded as undergoing a material change in the course of its conversion to cefaclor.

Lilly's argument distorts the terms "utility" and "properties" beyond recognition. The chemical and biological properties of Compound 6 are plainly different from those of cefaclor, and the utility of the two compounds, as that term is conventionally used, is quite different. Cefaclor is a powerful oral antibiotic, with a set of chemical and biological properties that give it great utility in that regard; Compound 6 has no such properties, and it has no significant utility as an antibiotic. Moreover, the premise of Lilly's argument — that Compound 6 has utility only as an intermediate in the preparation of cefaclor — is flawed. As the district court noted, Compound 6 can be used to produce a variety of cephalosporin antibiotics, of which cefaclor is only one. While Lilly claims that cefaclor was the only derivative of

Compound 6 that was on the commercial market in the United States at the time of the district court's decision in this case, other cephalosporin antibiotics that are producible from Compound 6 were on sale in other countries, and proceedings were pending to obtain authorization to market at least one of those antibiotics in this country. Thus, despite Lilly's creative effort to draw support from the references to utility and properties in the Senate report, the two-part test in the Senate report appears to offer no aid to Lilly's statutory argument.

The conference report on the process patent bill contained only a short discussion of the material change issue, but that report reiterated the test found in both the House and Senate reports: infringement can be found, even in the case of a significant change in the imported product, if "it would not have been possible or commercially viable to make the different [product] but for the patented process" [H.R. Conf. Rep. No. 576, 100th Cong., 2d Sess. 1087 (1988); see also *Bio-Technology General Corp. v. Genentech, Inc.*, 80 F.3d 1553 (Fed. Cir. 1996), slip op. 14–15, citing the same test, in the biotechnology context, from the Senate report]. Again, because there is at least one known commercial method for making cefaclor that does not use the patented process, the language in the conference report on the Process Patent Amendments Act does not help Lilly.

At the end of this Long March through the legislative history, we cannot claim that the legislative background of the 1988 act provides a conclusive answer to the question of how the "materially changed" clause should be construed in general and how it should be applied to the facts of this case in particular. What we are able to say, however, is that the legislative history does not compel adoption of Lilly's proposed analysis of the statute. In fact, to the extent that Congress intended the courts to look to the committee reports for guidance in construing the "materially changed" clause, the reports support the conclusion that the district court reached and that we uphold: Compound 6 is likely to be found to have been materially changed in the process of its conversion into cefaclor, and that the importation and sale of cefaclor is therefore not likely to be held to infringe Lilly's rights under Claim 5 of the '085 patent.

*Make a list of the major problems presented in this case*

- 
- 
- 
- 

## Hypothesis and mechanism

For the problems in your list above, give a cause or a reason for them to happen:

- 
- 
- 
- 

## Learning issues

Make a list of learning issues in the form of questions. Remember, your goal is to gather the medical, social, and all other relevant facts that may apply to the case.

What is a patent?
 A patent is a legal right granted by a government for a time period.
 The length of patents is 17 years from the issue or 20 years from the filing date if filed before June 1995.
 Patents prevent others from making or selling an invention.

What types of patents are available?
 *Invention* — protects how technology works. Patent can protect such diverse things as articles of manufacture, new chemical compounds, and methods of making them.
 *Design* — protects how things look.
 *Utility* — protects the functional aspects of products.

Whom do patents affect?
 Professionals in the medical field are affected. They are given the option to choose from many drug products. They must choose the most effective medical treatment, while keeping the cost and affordability for the patient in mind.
 Almost everybody is affected by patents. Patients are affected in a positive manner because patents could improve the quality of life due to expert treatment and maintenance of their diseases. For example, in the past, a patient would have to undergo surgery and have to recover in the hospital. Today, a course of tablets can treat certain disease states at far less cost to the patient and the medical system.
 Innovators of products are limited by many factors, for example, the extensive time and effort put into applying for a patent and the limited time they have regarding their rights.
 Generic manufacturers are affected because there is a specified time that dictates when they can and cannot make available medications that are affordable to the public.
 Patents also dictate how manufacturers are able to make drugs that are therapeutically equivalent to the patented drug, so that it can be substituted with the innovators' drug.

How is a patent obtained?

Requirements: the product must be new, novel, or useful.

Inventorship: legal determinants of single or joint inventors.

Costs: fees, filing, attorney, research, development, and time.

Steps toward obtaining a patent: Initial, Phase I, Phase II, Phase III, and Phase IV.

Where does the money go?

Pharmaceutical companies argue that the high prices for new drugs that enter the market are the result of costs for research and development.

In 1996, the ten companies thought to have the strongest pipelines for new pharmaceuticals spent approximately $14 billion on research and development.

There are at least 350 pharmaceutical agents in a late stage (Phase II or later) of clinical development, and they are estimated to be worth more than $61 billion at their peak.

The average major global pharmaceutical company spent 11% of its revenue base, or $16 billion, on new drug discovery in 1997. Spending for 1998 increased by 10%.

What questions should be asked to determine which drugs will be marketed?

Will the drug be in high demand?

Will there be a significant number of people who would benefit from the drug?

Will the drug treat a common or rare disease?

Will the drug be affordable?

## Literature review

To help you get ready to answer certain questions you anticipate being asked during the second part of the case, look in the local medical library and on the World Wide Web for helpful information. Please indicate in the spaces below (1) several helpful articles or books you found and (2) several helpful Web sites you found.

- **Helpful articles:**
  Angell, M., The pharmaceutical industry — to whom is it accountable? *N. Engl. J. Med.*, 342, 1902–1904, 2000.
  Barton, J.H., Reforming the patent system, *Sci. Drug Discovery*, 287, 1933–1934, 2000.
  The bigger companies for better drugs? *Lancet*, 346, 585, 1995
  Chirac, P. et al., AIDS: patent rights versus patient's right, *Lancet*, 356, 502, 2000.
  Mattes, J.A., Patent laws: could changes enhance drug development? *Arch. Gen. Psychiatry*, 54, 970, 1997.

Mehl, B. and Santell, J.P., Projecting future drug expenditures—1998, *Am. J. Health-Syst. Pharm.*, 55, 127–136, 1998.

Rees, J., Patents and intellectual property: a salvation for patient-oriented research? *Lancet*, 356, 849–850, 2000.

Savage, L.M., IBC's Fifth Annual World Congress puts drug discovery into perspective: record number of attendees get a taste of the past and future of biomedical research, *Drug Market Dev.*, 11, 370–372, 2000.

Schull, M., Medecins Sans Frontieres/Doctors Without Borders (Canada). Effect of drug patents in developing countries, *BMJ*, 321, 833–834, 2000.

- **Helpful Web sites:**
  Body and soul: the price of biotech: www.purefood.org/patlaw.html
  Ladas and Parry: intellectual property — patent perspectives: www.ladas.com/patpers.html
  Pharmaceutical Research and Manufacturers (PhRMA) policy papers: intellectual property: www.phrma.org/issues

## *Identify all relevant values that play a role in the case and determine which values, if any, conflict*

Nonmaleficence:

Beneficence:

Respect for persons:

Loyalty:

Distributive justice:

*Learning issues for next student-centered problem-based learning
     session*

- List the options open to you. That is, answer the question, "What
  could you do?"
- Choose the best solution from an ethical point of view, justify it, and
  respond to possible criticisms. That is, answer the question, "What
  should you do, and why?"
- What are the different ways of thinking about the problem? Which
  conflict management techniques can be used in the situation?

## Part two

Lilly also challenges the district court's conclusion that it failed to show
that it would suffer irreparable harm if the district court did not grant a
preliminary injunction in this case. We conclude that the court did not
commit clear error in finding that Lilly failed to prove irreparable harm;
the court therefore acted within its discretion in denying Lilly's request for
preliminary relief [see *New England Braiding Co. v. A.W. Chesterton Co.*, 970
F.2d 878, 882, 23 U.S.P.Q.2D (BNA) 1622, 1625 (Fed. Cir. 1992); *H.H. Rob-
ertson Co. v. United Steel Deck, Inc.*, 820 F.2d 384, 391, 2 U.S.P.Q.2D (BNA)
1926, 1930 (Fed. Cir. 1987)].

Because Lilly has not made a strong showing on the issue of infringement, it is not entitled to a presumption of irreparable harm [see *High Tech
Medical Instrumentation v. New Image Indus., Inc.*, 49 F.3d 1551, 1556, 33
U.S.P.Q.2D (BNA) 2005, 2009 (Fed. Cir. 1995)]. The district court also did not
commit clear error in rejecting Lilly's arguments that, apart from the presumption, it would suffer irreparable harm in the absence of a preliminary
injunction. In particular, the district court found that, under the specific
circumstances of this case, "an award of money damages would be an adequate remedy in the event that Lilly ultimately establishes" infringement
[896 F. Supp. at 860, 36 U.S.P.Q.2D (BNA) at 1019]. In light of the structure
of the cefaclor market, the court found that calculating lost profits would be
a relatively simple task. The court also found that the two distributors who
have been authorized by the FDA to sell cefaclor in this country have adequate assets to satisfy any judgment likely to be awarded if Lilly were to
prevail on the merits of its infringement claim.

Lilly contends that the loss of profits on sales of cefaclor because of competition from the appellees will result in irreparable injury to Lilly's overall
pharmaceutical research efforts. As the district court pointed out, however,
that claim of injury is not materially different from any claim of injury by a
business that is deprived of funds that it could usefully reinvest. If a claim of
lost opportunity to conduct research were sufficient to compel a finding of
irreparable harm, it is hard to imagine any manufacturer with a research and
development program that could not make the same claim and thus be equally

entitled to preliminary injunctive relief. Such a rule would convert the "extraordinary" relief of a preliminary injunction into a standard remedy, available whenever the plaintiff has shown a likelihood of success on the merits. For that reason, adopting the principle that Lilly proposes would "disserve the patent system" [*Illinois Tool Works, Inc., v. Grip-Pak, Inc.*, 906 F.2d 679, 683, 15 U.S.P.Q.2D (BNA) 1307, 1310 (Fed. Cir. 1990)].

We have examined Lilly's other claims of irreparable injury based on the effects of generic competition in the cefaclor market during the remaining life of the '085 patent, and we do not find them sufficiently compelling to justify overturning the district court's conclusion on the issue of irreparable harm. We also are not persuaded by Lilly's argument that the district court erred in finding that both Zenith and Cyanamid would be able to satisfy a monetary judgment against them if Lilly were to prevail on the merits. While there is some ambiguity in the record about whether Zenith would have to call on its parent corporation in the event of a judgment against it and whether the parent would be obligated to respond to such a judgment, the president of Zenith testified that the parent corporation would stand behind Zenith with respect to a judgment entered against it for patent infringement. The district court's finding on the "sufficient assets" issue therefore cannot be held to be clearly erroneous.

*List the options open to you. That is, answer the question, "What could you do?"*

- 
- 
- 
- 

*Choose the best solution from an ethical point of view, justify it, and respond to possible criticisms. That is, answer the question, "What should you do, and why?"*

- 
- 
- 
- 

*Select one member of your PBL group to role-play as a representative of Lilly and have another member of your PBL group role-play as a representative of Zenith Labs or Cyanamid. How might the two converse about different ways of thinking and techniques for conflict management?*

- •
- •
- •
- •

*Again, please select one member of your PBL group to role-play as a
representative of Lilly and have another member of your PBL
group role-play as a representative of Zenith Labs or
Cyanamid. How might a representative of Lilly use what is
known about stages of change and about motivational
interviewing to solve what you consider the major problem
presented in the case?*

- •
- •
- •
- •

## Part three

The ongoing struggle between "pioneer" drug manufacturers and generic
drug distributors has once more come before our court. Eli Lilly and Company (Lilly), the pioneer drug manufacturer in this case, has filed suit for
patent infringement against the appellees, who are involved in various ways
in the distribution of a particular generic drug. Lilly sought a preliminary
injunction, arguing that the importation and sale of the generic drug in this
country infringed Lilly's patent on a process for making a related compound.
After a hearing, the U.S. District Court for the Southern District of Indiana
denied Lilly's request for a preliminary injunction. The court found that Lilly
had failed to show that it was likely to prevail on the merits of its infringement claim and had failed to show that it would suffer irreparable harm in
the absence of preliminary injunctive relief [*Eli Lilly and Co. v. American
Cyanamid Co.*, 896 F. Supp. 851, 36 U.S.P.Q.2D (BNA) 1011 (S.D. Ind. 1995)].
Because Lilly has failed to overcome the substantial hurdle faced by a party
seeking to overturn the denial of a preliminary injunction, we affirm.

In sum, we do not agree with Lilly that the district court erred in finding
an absence of irreparable harm in this case. For that reason, and because we
agree with the district court that Lilly has failed to establish that it is likely
to succeed on the merits of its infringement claim, we hold that the district
court did not abuse its discretion in declining to enter a preliminary injunction pending the resolution of this case on the merits.

I concur in the result reached by the majority because Lilly did not show
irreparable harm. On that basis, the district court did not abuse its discretion.
I depart from the court's reasoning and conclusion about the material change
standard under 35 U.S.C. § 271(g).

The court's majority places great emphasis on the legislative history to resolve the meaning of "material change" — a curious approach given its recognition that the legislative history contains "something . . . for each side." The enactment history is far from dispositive in this case. The record of the enactment of this provision evinces a bitter battle between the pharmaceutical industry and its generic industry competitors.

In the first place, neither combatant could convince either house of Congress to enact a statutory standard clearly favorable to their segment of the industry. The hearings before the various subcommittees considering intellectual property components of the bill highlight some of the positions taken by industry and trade groups. [See A Bill to Protect Patent Owners from Importation into the United States of Goods Made Overseas by Use of a United States Patented Process: Hearings on S. 1543 Before the Subcomm. on Patents, Copyrights and Trademarks of the Senate Comm. on the Judiciary, 99th Cong., 1st Sess. 9, 15, 71, 186–187 (1985), advocating various degrees of limitation on initial broad statute: — PMA (Pharmaceutical Manufacturers Association) favoring "direct products" with legislative history allowing for trivial changes; AIPLA [American Intellectual Property Law Association] — opposing "direct" alone as creating loophole without detailed explanation; Intellectual Property Rights: Hearings on S. 1860 and S. 1869 Before the Subcomm. on International Trade of the Senate Comm. on Finance, 99th Cong., 2d Sess. 175, 182 (1986), arguing on behalf of the International Anti-Counterfeiting Coalition against "direct" limitation as too narrow and for liability for "obvious use of the innovator's patent"; Intellectual Property and Trade: Hearings Before the Subcomm. on Courts, Civil Liberties, and the Admin. of Justice of the House Comm. on the Judiciary, 99th Cong., 2d Sess. 275–276 (1986), arguing on behalf of NAM against direct limitation and for "materially changed chemically by subsequent steps."]

Without a clear resolution in the statutory language, the battleground shifted to the committee reports. On this front, each combatant could find lobbyists to lace the reports with tutorials to the courts about applying the ambiguous provisions of Section 271(g) in future litigation.

With a focus on future litigation, these committee reports became particularly unenlightening as an aid to interpret statutory language. These reports surrendered any pretext of informing members of Congress about the meaning of pending bills before a vote on the floor. Instead, these tutorials, by their own admission, addressed judicial officers, not legislative officers. And, the legislative officers ignored them. In fact, the floor debates during passage of the Process Patents Act do not refer to any of the relevant portions of the committee reports.

In the House debates preceding passage of H.R. 4848, only two committee reports were even cited. Both were cited in a discussion unrelated to the process patent portion of the omnibus bill. [See 134 Cong. Rec. 17880–18063 (1988), citing H.R. Rep. No. 40, Pt. 1, 100th Cong., 1st Sess. 124 (1987) and S.R. Rep. No. 71, 100th Cong., 1st Sess. 123 (1987).] Moreover, in all of the debate on the floor of the House, no member discussed (or appears to have even mentioned) material change. The debate in the Senate preceding passage of H.R. 4848 contains even less. No senator cites any committee report or mentions material change [see 134 Cong. Rec. 20104 (1988)].

Moreover, the reports show all the signs of unresolved conflict evident in the statutory language. Early versions of the bill were silent on the scope of protection. Senate Bill 1535 refers only to the importation of "a product produced [**39] by such process" [S. Rep. No. 663, 98th Cong., 2d Sess. 30 (1984)]. In the analysis, the report indicates that the goal of the bill is to prevent importation of "products produced by a process covered by the patent" (id. at 5). The Senate committee notes: "The principle effect of these changes is to prevent competitors of a patent owner from avoiding the patent by practicing the patented process outside the United States and marketing the resulting product in this country" (id.).

By 1986, "material change" had crept into the statute (see H.R. 4899). The committee explains the addition: "Without such limitations, liability could attach, for example, to the seller of a car in which the steel was made from iron ore that was mined by a patented process, or in which the reflective surface used on the rear view mirror was made by a patented process" [H.R. Rep. 807, 99th Cong., 2d Sess. 20 (1986)]. Clearly, the House was concerned with notions akin to proximate cause — that is, how far down the line should we cut off potential liability.

The 1987 report accompanying H.R. 1931 sets forth significantly greater and more confusing detail concerning material change [H.R. Rep. 60, 100th Cong., 1st Sess. 13–14 (1987)]. The committee states that it "intends to provide protection to process patent owners which is meaningful and not easily evaded" (id.). The report then suggests no liability would attach when the "basic structure" of the product is changed by a subsequent process (id. at 13). However, the next paragraph notes: "the subsequent processing modifications of chemical X may only be trivial or of a conventional nature even though a material change occurred in chemical X" (id.). Such a nonmaterial change would occur, for example, where "chemical X is an important intermediate product . . . which can materially be changed into an end product" (id.). By this test, the House sets forth a commercial viability test that looks to the efficiency of making the end product absent use of the infringing process (id. at 13–14). This same report goes on to identify at least two more tests for material change, an active ingredient test and an integral or important component test (id. at 14).

Likewise, the related Senate report accompanying Senate Bill S. 1200 provides immense detail on the definition of material change [S. Rep. No. 83, 100th Cong., 1st Sess. (1987)]. In this report, the committee explains that S. 1200 "introduces" a "new phrase, materially changed" to restrict the scope of the bill "to exclude ultimate products that, because of intervening manufacturing steps, cease to have a reasonable nexus with the patented process" (id. at 36). The committee also recognized that "the courts will have to assess the permutations of this issue of proximity to or distance from the process on a case-by-case basis" [id. at 46; see *Bio-Technology General Corp. v.*

*Genentech, Inc.*, 80 F.3d 1553, 1996 WL 163035, at *6 (Fed. Cir. 1996), recognizing Congress intended the courts to resolve the question of "proximity to the product of the patented process on a case-by-case basis"]. Interestingly, this statement follows the debate over the scope of the act, suggesting Congress chose an intentionally vague limitation such as "material change" as a compromise between the pharmaceuticals and generics.

The report then sets forth a two-phase test that looks to the commercial viability of making the end product absent use of the infringing process coupled with a basic utility test (id. at 50). This test, like others in the enactment history, provides little practical utility in assessing material change. As with its House counterpart, the directly conflicting and confusing tests set forth in the section analysis leave little doubt that they were inserted by lobbyists for use in future litigation by their clients. In sum, the enactment history maps all the graves on this inconclusive legislative battleground, but shows no route away from the combat zone. If anything, the enactment history "is more conflicting than the text [of the statute] is ambiguous" [*Wong Yang Sung v. McGrath*, 339 U.S. 33, 49, 94 L. Ed. 616, 70 S. Ct. 445 (1950)].

With no real enlightenment about the meaning of "material change" in the enactment history, this court should interpret this language in light of the overriding purpose of the statute. As recognized by this court's majority, the Process Patents Act sought to afford meaningful protection to owners of U.S. process patents. Before the act, foreign entities could import goods made from patented processes used abroad without liability for patent infringement. The act sought to plug this loophole.

Sadly, this decision will create another massive loophole in the protection of patented processes. This decision will, in effect, deny protection to holders of process patents on intermediates as opposed to "final" products. This decision denies protection to a patented process any time it is not the only way to make an intermediate, even if it is the most economically efficient way to produce the intermediate.

In view of the purpose of the statute, Compound 6 and cefaclor are essentially the same product. Compound 6 has no commercial use in the U.S. market except to make cefaclor. The patented process is thus in use to make Compound 6 — a product only four simple, well-known steps from cefaclor. The record shows no other current commercial use of Compound 6.

Rather than attempting to distill an elixir from this intoxicating witches brew of enactment history, this court should interpret "material change" consistent with the overriding purpose of the act — to provide protection to process patent holders. With its eye firmly fixed on the purpose of the act, this court would avoid eliminating processes for intermediates from the protections of the 1988 act.

## Conclusion

Basically, you can be pro-patent or antipatent. Below are arguments concerning these two viewpoints.

*Pro-Patent*

Patents encourage research of innovative medical products because new
   areas of research are explored.
Patents encourage competition. Successful inventors are rewarded and
   are encouraged to develop innovative products.
Patents decrease medical costs and enhance health.
Patents enable generic manufacturing of drugs.

*Antipatent*

Patents inhibit research by keeping a particular invention "off limits"
   for a certain period of time.
Patents create monopolistic situations because they prevent others from
   selling the patented product.
Patents inflate the price of pharmaceuticals.

The pros and cons of patents are going to continue to grow in the
future. We cannot avoid the controversy. Currently, patents seem to serve
as a protection that is fundamental for ensuring financial rewards after
time-consuming and costly research and development. But, patents also
contribute to the prices that are sometimes unaffordable for citizens in need
of the lifesaving/improving benefits a new drug can offer. Without patents,
companies would not have the financial incentive to create innovative
drugs. In addition, citizens may not have drugs available to improve their
particular disease state. Ultimately, patent controversy is inevitable.

*case seventeen*

# Germline therapy

This problem-based learning session is based on the following: *United States v. Loran Medical Systems,* No. CV 96-4283 SVW (CWx), U.S. District Court for the Central District of California, 25 F. Supp. 2d 1082; 1997 U.S. Dist. Lexis 22701. December 17, 1997, Opinion Filed. It is reprinted here with permission of LexisNexis.

## Objectives

The objectives of this problem-based learning case are:

- To present a background of germline therapy
- To examine the broad range of relevant issues germline therapy raises
- To explore the national and international standards in current use

## Introduction

In germline therapy, the parents' egg and sperm cells are changed with the goal of passing on changes to their offspring. This therapy offers a multitude of potential opportunities for the elimination of inherited diseases, such as cancers. Currently, human germline therapy is decades away from any realistic application. This is the time to discuss the potential ethical issues that this and other potential therapies can raise.

## Part one

On June 20, 1996, this court granted a temporary restraining order enjoining defendants Loran Medical Systems, Inc., Bent Formby, and Ernest Thomas, M.D. ("Defendants") from importing neonatal rabbit and human fetal cells (the "Cell Product") from Russia for use in the treatment of human diabetes. Defendants claim that injection of the Cell Product into diabetic patients can stimulate the body's production of insulin.

On July 1, 1996, the court entered a preliminary injunction against Defendants' importation and use of the Cell Product on the grounds that the government had demonstrated a reasonable probability of success on the merits of its claim — that the Cell Product fell within the Food and Drug Administration's (FDA's) regulatory authority pursuant to the federal Public Health Service (PHS) Act (42 U.S.C. § 201 et seq. and the Food, Drug and Cosmetic Act, 21 U.S.C. § 301 et seq.).

Now before the court are the parties' cross motions for summary judgment. Plaintiff seeks a permanent injunction against the unregulated use of the Cell Product, while Defendants argue that the Cell Product is outside the FDA's regulatory authority. For the reasons stated below, the court finds that the FDA has authority over the Cell Product and grants Plaintiff's request for a permanent injunction.

### Summary judgment standard

Summary judgment is appropriate when there is "no genuine issue as to any material fact and ... the moving party is entitled to judgment as a matter of law" [Fed. R. Civ. P. 56(c)]. In this case, the parties agree that there are no questions of fact. The case thus hinges on a purely legal question, an appropriate use of the summary judgment procedure.

## Analysis

The gravamen of this case is whether the Cell Product falls within the regulatory ambit of the FDA. The government argues that it does, pointing to regulations defining "biological product," which the FDA regulates pursuant to its authority under the Public Health and Service Act; and regulations involving "drugs" and "new drugs," which the FDA regulates under its Food and Drug Act authority.

We review the decisions of administrative agencies according to the two-part test established in *Chevron v. Natural Resources Defense Council* [467 U.S. 837, 81 L. Ed. 2d 694, 104 S. Ct. 2778 (1984)]. Under *Chevron*, the first inquiry is whether Congress has directly spoken on the issue before the court (467 U.S. at 842–843). The parties agree that there is no statutory authority that directly speaks to the FDA's authority over the Cell Product. Under the second prong of the *Chevron* test, the court must determine whether the agency's position is a permissible construction of the relevant statute (id.). The court may only overturn the agency's interpretation if it finds that the interpretation "is not one that Congress would have sanctioned" [id. at 845, quoting *United States v. Shimer*, 367 U.S. 374, 383, 6 L. Ed. 2d 908, 81 S. Ct. 1554 (1961)].

## The Cell Product is a biological product

A biological product is any "virus, therapeutic serum, toxin, antitoxin or analogous product applicable to the prevention, treatment or cure of human diseases or injuries" [21 C.F.R. § 600.3(h); see also 42 U.S.C. § 262(a)]. A product is analogous to a toxin or antitoxin if, irrespective of its source or origin, it can be used in the treatment of disease through a "specific immune process" [21 C.F.R. § 600.3(h)(5)(iii)].

The human immune system will naturally react to the injection of any cellular material, whether obtained from a human or nonhuman source. Defendants inject the Cell Product into an area of the abdomen selected specifically to evade this response and thus reduce the chance that the cells will be rejected. This procedure purportedly allows the rabbit cells to begin producing insulin immediately while the human fetal cells mature.

The government argues that this attempt at evading the body's natural immune system is a specific immune process as required by the FDA's regulations. Defendants read the regulation more narrowly. Defendants rely on the Court of Custom and Patent Appeals opinion in *Certified Blood Donor Services, Inc., v. United States* [62 C.C.P.A. 66, 511 F.2d 572 (1975)] in support of their argument that a substance analogous to a toxin or antitoxin must be used to treat diseases through specific immunization. Defendants' reliance, however, is misplaced. The issue before the court in *Certified* was whether a serum used for diagnosis rather than treatment fell within the regulatory definition of biological product (511 F.2d at 575). Moreover, the regulatory language cited, but not relied on, by the court in *Certified* is an outdated version of the regulation. The current language was adopted by the FDA in 1973. Accordingly, *Certified* does not bear on this case.

Defendants also argue that the PHS Act only authorizes the FDA to regulate products that immunize against a specific disease, such as polio or smallpox. The court disagrees. As described in greater detail below, Congress conferred on the FDA the broad statutory authority to regulate products analogous to toxins, antitoxins, vaccines, blood, and the like [see 42 U.S.C. § 262(a)]. The FDA's assertion of authority over immunological agents such as the Cell Product is a reasonable construction of the PHS Act.

## The Cell Product is analogous to a toxin or antitoxin

Defendants next argue that, even if the Cell Product does use a specific immune process, the FDA does not have regulatory authority under the PHS Act because the Cell Product is not analogous to a toxin or antitoxin. Defendants rely on the Fifth Circuit's decision in *Blank v. United States* [400 F.2d 302 (1968)], which held that blood and plasma were not analogous to therapeutic serums because they were not employed for immunological purposes; they merely replaced blood lost through disease or injury (400 F.2d at 304). Accordingly, the *Blank* court held that the FDA did not have regulatory authority over blood and plasma (id. at 305). Defendants argue that, like blood, the Cell Product merely replaces cells that have been lost to disease, in this case diabetes.

*Blank* rested heavily on the fact that the FDA had not promulgated regulations that could be read to include blood within the definition of a product analogous to a therapeutic serum (400 F.2d at 303–304). In this case, however, the regulations defining products analogous to toxins and antitoxins appear to encompass the Cell Product [see 21 C.F.R. § 0600.3(h)(5)(iii), a product is analogous to a toxin or antitoxin if, irrespective of source or origin, it is applicable to the treatment of human disease through a specific immune process]. Thus, to the extent the *Blank* analysis relied on the paucity of regulatory authority, it does not apply in this case.

The *Blank* court also noted that blood transfusions were unknown to Congress when it enacted the PHS Act in 1902; therefore, it could not have intended blood to be analogous to a therapeutic serum (400 F.2d at 303). Defendants argue that the Cell Product was similarly unknown to Congress when it last amended the PHS Act. *Blank*, however, was contrary to the Supreme Court's holding in *In re Permian Basin Area Rate Cases* [390 U.S. 747, 20 L. Ed. 2d 312, 88 S. Ct. 1344 (1968)] that administrative agencies must be able to adapt to changing circumstances (390 U.S. at 784; see also *Chevron*, 467 U.S. at 862, an agency should have broad discretion to implement the policies of the organic acts]. The FDA has construed its mandate under the PHS Act to include a broad spectrum of biological products used in the treatment of disease. The court cannot say that the FDA's construction was unreasonable.

## Whether the Cell Product is biologically or chemically altered is irrelevant to whether it is a biological product

Defendants argue that the Cell Product cannot be a biological product under 42 U.S.C. § 262(a) because it is not biologically or genetically altered in any way. Somatic cell therapy — medical treatment using biologically altered cells — is regulated under the FDA's authority to regulate biological products (see 58 Fed. Reg., 53250; FDA, *Points to Consider in Human Cell Therapy and Gene Therapy,* 4, Aug. 27, 1991, which lists examples of somatic cell therapy). But nothing in the regulation requires alteration before a product is to fall under the FDA's purview.

Accordingly, the court finds that the FDA's conclusion that the Cell Product is a biological product that uses a specific immune process is reasonable, and thus the Cell Product is properly under the FDA's authority.

## The Cell Product is properly classified as a new drug under the FD&C Act: the Cell Product is a drug

The FD&C (Food, Drug, and Cosmetic) Act defines drugs as, *inter alia,* "articles intended for use in the diagnosis, cure, mitigation, treatment or prevention of disease in [humans]" (21 U.S.C. § 321). The Cell Product was developed for use in the treatment of diabetes. Thus, it meets the statutory definition of a drug.

Defendants argue that the statutory definition is overbroad — that it encompasses a wide variety of items that fall outside the plain meaning of the word drug. Defendants' argument relies on two cases, both inapposite to the present case. First, Defendants argue that under *Juneau v. Interstate Blood Bank of Louisiana* [333 So. 2d 354 (La. App. 1976)], tissue samples are not drugs under the Louisiana State Food and Drug Act (333 So. 2d at 357). It may very well be true that the Louisiana definition of drug excludes the Cell Product; however, that definition has no relevance to this case. The question before the court is whether the federal FD&C Act's definition properly encompasses the Cell Product.

Second, Defendants argue that there is a conflict between the plain language of the statute and the intent of Congress when it was enacted. Accordingly, although the Cell Product clearly falls within the plain language of the FD&C Act's definition of drug, the plain wording does not control. Defendants argue that the 1951 case of *62 Cases of Jam v. United States* [340 U.S. 593, 95 L. Ed. 566, 71 S. Ct. 515 (1951)] somehow supports their argument. In *62 Cases of Jam*, however, the court addresses the problem of conflicting statutory definitions (340 U.S. at 594). Here, there is no conflict — only a broad statutory definition of "drug." Defendants have provided no authority for why the statutory definition should not apply.

In contrast, Plaintiffs correctly argue that Congress intended an expansive definition of "drug." "Congress fully intended that the [FD&C] Act's coverage be as broad as its literal language indicates" [*United States v. An Article of Drug . . . Bacto-Unidisk*, 394 U.S. 784, 798–799, 22 L. Ed. 2d 726, 89 S. Ct. 1410 (1969), which holds that an "antibiotic sensitivity disk," a device used in laboratories to help choose particular antibiotics for treatment, was a drug according to the statutory definition]. "Remedial legislation such as the Food, Drug and Cosmetic Act is to be given a liberal construction consistent with the Act's overriding purpose to protect the public health" [*Grand Laboratories, Inc. v. Harris*, 660 F.2d 1288, 1291 (8th Cir. 1981) (en banc), which holds that animal biologics — products prepared from animal tissue for the treatment of disease in animals — were drugs under the statutory definition]. "In interpreting the FD&C Act, the court's duty is to avoid any construction which would result in the free marketing of drugs which might well be unsafe" [*United States v. Western Serum*, 666 F.2d 335, 341 (9th Cir. 1982)]. Classifying the Cell Product as a drug is consistent with the intent of Congress to give the FDA broad authority in this important area.

*Make a list of the major problems presented in this case*

- 
- 
- 
-

## Hypothesis and mechanism

For the problems in your list above, give a cause or a reason for them to happen:

- 
- 
- 
- 

## Learning issues

Make a list of learning issues in the form of questions. Remember, your goal is to gather the medical, social, and all other relevant facts that may apply to the case.

What is the goal of germline therapy?

It is to alleviate human suffering and disease by curing disorders for which available therapies are unsatisfactory. To pursue this goal within the ethical tradition of medicine, guidelines have been adopted nationally and internationally. The current position of the Recombinant DNA Advisory Committee is that "it will not at present entertain proposals for germline alteration." Similar guidelines have been adopted in the United Kingdom and in India.

What are the policies of other countries involving germline therapy?

All institutions in the United States receiving federal funds are prohibited from engaging in research that will make germline modifications.

Any private sector germline study falling under the scope of the FDA would similarly not be approved.

The National Health and Medical Council of Australia stated that germ-cell therapy was ethically unacceptable.

In Australia and Germany, germline intervention is a criminal act.

The European Council has passed a recommendation that every individual has a right to a genetic constitution that has not been interfered with.

What are the recommendations of the American Medical Association concerning any future germline therapy?

Informed consent

Genetic manipulations only for therapeutic purposes

Only when other therapies are insufficient

Complete elimination of viral agents from vector

What might be the effect on future generations of germline therapy?

One concern about somatic gene therapy is that the genetic material from
a vector might insert into the genome of the recipient's reproductive
cells, inadvertently affecting the germline.

The American Association for the Advancement of Sciences (AAAS) feels
that germline therapy remains problematic because unintended genetic changes could be passed to a new child along with the intended
benefits.

Discuss the differences between using germlines for therapy and enhancement.

There is a sharp line to be drawn between germline therapy for enhancement and germline therapy to fight disease.

The possible harmful effects of manipulating the germline are unknown,
and researchers have a duty to use this powerful technology only for
the treatment of disease and not for any other purpose.

What religious issues are concerned with germline therapy?

Many religious traditions take a "developmental" view of personhood,
believing that the early embryo or fetus only gradually becomes a
full human being and thus may not be entitled to the same moral
protections as it will later.

Others hold that, while the embryo represents human life, that life may
be taken for the sake of saving and preserving other lives in the
future.

Others believe that the use of human embryos other than for achieving
pregnancy is unethical.

What economic issues are concerned with germline therapy?

Federal funding would automatically trigger a set of oversight mechanisms now in place to ensure that the conduct of biomedical research
is consistent with broad social values and legal requirements.

Federal funding for stem cell research is necessary to promote invest-
ment in this promising line of research, to encourage sound public
policy, and to foster public confidence in the conduct of such research.

Federal funds also offer a basis for public review, approval, and monitoring through well-established oversight mechanisms that will promote the public's interest in ensuring that stem cell research is
conducted in a way that is both scientific and ethical.

Discuss the issues involving informed consent and germline therapy.

Federal common rule governing human subjects research provides for
local and federal agency review of research proposals in such circumstances, weighing the risks against benefits and requiring involved and voluntary consent.

The most ethical source of human primordial stem cells is embryos
produced for the process of *in vitro* fertilization whose progenitors

have decided not to implant them and have given full and informed consent for the use of these embryos for research purposes.

Two potential sources of donation:

Embryos with poor quality that makes them inappropriate for transfer

Embryos remaining when couples have definitely completed their family

Procurement of germline cells:

The extraction of embryonic stem cells from the inner mass of blastocytes raises ethical questions for those who consider the loss of embryonic life by intentional means morally wrong.

The derivation of embryonic germ cells from the gonadal tissue of aborted fetuses is problematic for those who oppose abortion.

## *Literature review*

To help you get ready to answer certain questions you anticipate being asked during the second part of the case, look in the local medical library and on the World Wide Web for helpful information. Please indicate in the spaces below (1) several helpful articles or books you found and (2) several helpful Web sites you found.

- **Helpful articles:**
  Gulcher, J. and Stefansson, K., Population genomics. Laying the groundwork for genetic disease modelling and targeting, *Clin. Chem. Lab. Med.*, 36, 523–527, 1998.
  Peters, T., 'Playing God' and germline intervention, *J. Med. Philos.*, 20(4): 365–387, 1995.
  Willgoos, C., FDA regulation: an answer to the questions of human cloning and germline gene therapy, *Am. J. Law Med.*, 27, 101–125, 2001.

- **Helpful Web sites:**
  U.S. Department of Energy — Humane Genome Project information: www.ornl.gov/hgmis/medicine/genetherapy.html
  American Association for the Advancement of Science and Institute for Civil Society stem cell research and applications: www.aaas.org/spp/dspp/sfrl/projects/stem/findings.html
  Engineering the Human Germline Symposium: www.ess.ucla.edu/huge/report.html

*Identify all relevant values that play a role in the case and determine which values, if any, conflict*

Nonmaleficence:

Beneficence:

Respect for persons:

Loyalty:

Distributive justice:

## Learning issues for next student-centered problem-based learning session

- List the options open to you. That is, answer the question, "What could you do?"
- Choose the best solution from an ethical point of view, justify it, and respond to possible criticisms. That is, answer the question, "What should you do, and why?"
- What are the different ways of thinking about the problem? Which conflict management techniques can be used in the situation?

## Part two

### The Cell Product is a new drug

All new drugs must undergo premarket review by the FDA [21 U.S.C. § 355(a)]. A new drug is any drug that is not already generally recognized among medical experts as safe and effective for its intended use [21 U.S.C. § 321(p)]. The exception for "generally recognized" drugs is very narrow [*United States v. Undetermined Quantities . . . Equidantin*, 675 F.2d 994, 1000

(9th Cir. 1982)]. The court's task is to determine whether the drug has a general reputation in the scientific community for safety and effectiveness, not to make an independent determination of these characteristics (id.).

The inquiry into whether a drug is generally recognized has three parts:

> *(1) There must be a consensus of expert opinion that drug product is safe and effective for its labeled indications.* Weinberger v. Hynson, Westcott, and Dunning, *412 U.S. 609, 632, 37 L. Ed. 2d 207, 93 S. Ct. 2469 (1973);*

> *(2) That expert consensus must be based upon adequate and well-controlled clinical investigations conducted on the drug product in issue. Id. at 630;*

> *(3) The studies conducted on the drug must be published in the medical literature and available to experts generally.* Equidantin, *675 F.2d at 1000.*

A proponent's failure to provide substantial evidence on any of these conditions means that the substance is a new drug as a matter of law [*United States v. Articles of Drug (Promise Toothpaste), 826 F.2d 564, 569 (7th Cir. 1987)*]. The Cell Product fails all three. While Defendants make sweeping arguments about the worldwide acceptance of the product, they fail to provide specific examples of successful clinical trials or published studies. Moreover, while Defendants provide anecdotal evidence of clinical success, the declarations of Plaintiffs' experts demonstrate that there is a marked lack of consensus in the medical community as to the effectiveness of the Cell Product [see *Simeon Management Co. v. FTC, 579 F.2d 1137, 1142 (9th Cir. 1978)*, anecdotal evidence or a doctor's belief that a drug is effective is not substantial evidence of general acceptance].

Accordingly, the court finds that the FDA has acted reasonably in classifying the Cell Product as a new drug.

## The experimental use of the Cell Product is not the "practice of medicine"

The court disposes quickly of Defendants' argument that the FDA's exercise of authority over the Cell Product is an attempt to regulate the practice of medicine — an area traditionally left to the states. While the FD&C Act "was not intended to regulate the *practice of medicine*, it was obviously intended to control the availability of drugs for prescribing by physicians" [*United States v. Evers, 643 F.2d 1043, 1048 (1981)*]. The court has already determined that the Cell Product is a drug. Accordingly, the FDA has the authority to regulate its use.

*List the options open to you. That is, answer the question, "What could you do?"*

- 
- 
- 
- 

*Choose the best solution from an ethical point of view, justify it, and respond to possible criticisms. That is, answer the question, "What should you do, and why?"*

- 
- 
- 
- 

*Select one member of your PBL group to role-play as Dr. Formby and have another member of your PBL group role-play as a representative of the FDA. How might two converse about different ways of thinking and techniques for conflict management?*

- 
- 
- 
- 

*Again, please select one member of your PBL group to role-play as Dr Formby and have another member of your PBL group role-play as a representative of the FDA. How might Dr. Formby use what is known about stages of change and about motivational interviewing to solve what you consider the major problem presented in the case?*

- 
- 
- 
-

## Part three

The Cell Product is both a biologic product and a new drug; thus, the FDA has regulatory authority over the Cell Product under the PHS Act and the FD&C Act. The Court grants the government's motion for summary judgment and enters a permanent injunction against Defendants' importation, use, and sale of the Cell Product.

## Conclusion

Human germline therapy and therapies like it are exciting efforts to increase our knowledge of the human family and its evolution, history, diversity, and essential unity; however, it has much potential for use and misuse. Several principles have guided our consideration of the ethical issues raised by this project: the effect on future generations, religious issues, economic issues, informed consent, and procurement of germline cells.

It is crucial that these therapies be conducted according to the highest ethical standards. There may be no other scientific project that has the capacity to touch so many lives and minds. The United States currently has no law that would prohibit this kind of manipulation for any purpose. These types of therapy are in their infancy. However, open discussion should be started early and include the public as well as the scientific community.

# case eighteen

# Medical surveillance

This problem-based learning session is based on the following: *Griel v. Franklin Medical Center,* Civil Action No. 97-30285-MAP, U.S. District Court for the District of Massachusetts, 71 F. Supp. 2d 1; 1999 U.S. Dist. Lexis 18140; 11 Am. Disabilities Cas. (BNA) 459. November 23, 1999, Decided. It is reprinted here with permission of LexisNexis.

## Objectives

The objectives of this problem-based learning case are:

- To inform the pharmacy profession of employee/employer rights toward drug testing before and after joining a private company
- To determine the control of medical surveillance data and if it may be used against the participant

## Introduction

The Drug Free Workplace Act of 1988, supported by insurance companies that discount workman's compensation rates, has compelled many employers to develop "no-drug policies." The American Civil Liberties Union (ACLU) states that workplace drug testing is up 277% from 1987. In many states, no laws exist to define employee/employer rights for "on-the-job" drug testing. On testifying to Congress on drug testing in the workplace, the ACLU claimed that performing drug tests without grounds of suspicion as "unfair and unnecessary."

Employers cite the benefit of drug testing as a medical screening device for monitoring employee performance. If drug screening results are maintained in a database and reviewed periodically, as in noting trends and effectiveness of current workplace strategies, then these results are termed *medical surveillance.* The Occupational Safety and Health Administration (OSHA) defines medical surveillance as the analysis of health information to look for problems that may be occurring in the workplace that require targeted prevention and thus serve as a feedback loop to the employer.

## *Part one*

The relevant material facts, taken in the light most favorable to plaintiff, are as follows. Defendant Franklin Medical Center ("Franklin") is a corporation with its place of business in Greenfield, Massachusetts. Defendant William Garrand resides in Hadley, Massachusetts, and began working at Franklin on January 6, 1996, as the intensive care unit (ICU) nurse manager. Plaintiff, Dolores Griel, is a registered nurse who lives in Charlemont, Massachusetts.

In July 1992, Franklin hired Griel to work 32 hours per week as a critical care nurse in Franklin's ICU. During her interview with Mary Brown, the then-manager of the ICU nurses, Griel revealed that she was a recovering drug addict who previously worked at Mercy Hospital, but was terminated for diverting narcotics. Moreover, she revealed that she was presently enrolled in the Massachusetts Nursing Association's (MNA's) Substance Abuse Rehabilitation Program (SARP) — a 5-year program designed to assist nurses who have diverted narcotics.

During her first 3 years at Franklin, Griel received favorable personnel evaluations and a commendation for her role in preventing the suicide of a patient. On November 2, 1995, however, Griel injured her back when she was lifting a patient. As a result, she had to stop working for approximately 1 year. During that time, she remained active in SARP and graduated in March 1996.

Because of her back injury, Griel, under the care of Dr. Michael Sanders, began taking the narcotic Percocet for pain control. She continued taking Percocet even as the time approached for her to return to work. Concerned, she considered the idea, suggested to her by other medical professionals in recovery, of setting up a "safety net" by which her coworkers would administer narcotics to her patients for her if she felt she needed the help on a particular occasion. Although she decided against the safety net, the idea itself appeared to have raised enough concern that Deborah Palmeri, the then-acting manager of the ICU, asked the ICU staff "to keep an eye" on Griel.

Nevertheless, 1 year after her back injury, on November 2, 1996, Griel returned to work at Franklin. On her return she took part in an orientation aimed at refreshing her procedural skills, and after 2 weeks, she resumed all of her previous duties as a critical care nurse.

Soon after her return, however, a coworker raised concerns about Griel's nursing practices. During the week of December 29, 1996, Gail Shattuck, an ICU nurse, approached Palmeri with concerns regarding three specific patients. After reviewing the patients' charts, Palmeri had concerns about Griel's assessment of the patients' needs and administration of narcotics. For example, patients under plaintiff's care seemed to receive an excessive amount of narcotics, and narcotics seemed to be the first line of intervention when alternatives were available. Palmeri reviewed six more of Griel's patient charts, "but found nothing dramatic in these" (defendants' statement of material facts at 13, Docket No. 39). After consulting with Karen Moore (vice president of patient care), Mike Saracino (clinical director of pharmacy), and Robert Oldenburg (employee assistance program director), on January 3, 1996, Griel was suspended for 3 days with pay pending an investigation.

On January 6, 1996, Franklin hired defendant William Garrand as the nurse manager for Franklin's ICU nurses. On his second day of employment, Palmeri informed him that she had already suspended Griel for alleged poor nursing practices. Palmeri was scheduled to meet with Griel, and Palmeri asked Garrand if he wished to get involved. Since he was going to be taking over the unit, he agreed to review the patient charts. He reviewed the nine patient charts concerning the patients that Griel had medicated with morphine. He agreed with Palmeri that three charts raised concerns about Griel's ability to assess properly patients' needs and to administer narcotics. Thus, they recommended, as a condition for returning to work, that Griel refrain from dispensing narcotics for 3 months and submit to random urine testing.

On January 8, 1997, plaintiff agreed to sign a confidential memorandum setting forth these conditions. After signing the memorandum, plaintiff returned to work and informed her coworkers on her shift about the restrictions. In addition, Garrand called a staff meeting and informed Griel's colleagues about the restrictions. By this time, Garrand had "very strong suspicions that [Griel] was diverting [drugs]" (plaintiff's exhibits, Docket No. 45, Exhibit 8, Garrand deposition at 74).

On January 10, 1997, soon after returning from her 3-day suspension, another incident occurred. Margaret Kelly-House, a nurse's aide working in the ICU, reported seeing plaintiff on her hands and knees in the utility room doorway rummaging through discarded medication bottles. The nurse's aide reported the incident to Garrand on January 15. Garrand contacted Human Resource Director Mike Derose for guidance, and after Derose spoke with Oldenburg, they instructed Garrand to contact Griel and ask her to go for a drug test pursuant to the conditions of her return.

On January 15, Garrand attempted to contact Griel at home because she had called in sick. After about eight attempts within a 2-hour period, Garrand became concerned for her physical well-being, having also learned that she had not been to work since the utility closet incident. He contacted the police and asked them if they would check on her and ask her to call the hospital. After the two state troopers found her at home, Griel contacted Garrand and informed him that she was all right. When asked about the utility closet incident, she explained that she was cleaning up broken bottles. He responded by asking her to take a urine test. She complied, and the result was negative.

On March 4, 1997, Franklin lifted Griel's restrictions, and soon after, Garrand confronted her with protocol violations arising during her care of two patients. On or about March 12, 1997, while caring for patient C.W., Lucy Leete, an ICU nurse, reported to Garrand that Griel drew up a narcotic (Demerol) for C.W., but then asked Leete to administer the drug. Leete reported the incident because Griel's handling of the matter violated a nursing rule against allowing one nurse to administer medications another has drawn up. Garrand disciplined Leete for this violation, although the level of discipline was reduced based on Leete's inexperience and forthrightness. Griel, however, initially denied the story, telling Garrand that Leete had asked her to administer the narcotic. But, when further questioned, Griel conceded that she drew up the medication and asked Leete to administer it because the patient was lying on her side and the task was physically more convenient for Leete. Moreover, in subsequently reviewing C.W.'s chart, Garrand questioned Griel's decision to administer the Demerol in the first place. Although the dosage was technically permitted by the doctor's orders, other shifts were only medicating C.W. with Tylenol. Garrand believed that Griel's assessment of C.W. was similar to the January assessment problems for which she was placed on restrictions.

On or about March 18, 1997, Griel allegedly violated two other nursing protocols while administering four doses of morphine to a second ICU patient (E.W.). First, she failed to obtain the required cosignature for surplus narcotics that she "wasted." Second, she did not record one of the morphine doses in the medication administration record (MAR) or in her nurse's notes, which allows subsequent shifts to know which medications have been given at what time. At a disciplinary meeting, plaintiff claimed that she asked another nurse to cosign, but the nurse failed to do so. In addition, Griel explained that she did not document the dosage in the MAR because she was busy taking care of a patient, and she had verbally informed the incoming nurse that she had given the dose.

After the disciplinary meeting, Garrand consulted with Derose and Moore. While they remained convinced about the possibility that Griel's failure to comply with nursing protocols resulted from a possible diversion of narcotics, they did not rest their decision regarding Griel on this basis. They did, however, conclude that, because of patient safety concerns, termination was the appropriate course of action. Griel was suspended on March 24, 1997, and a disciplinary hearing was held on March 27. On April 3, 1997, citing unacceptable risks to patient safety, Franklin terminated Griel. Griel then brought suit on the ground that the defendants' decision reflected discrimination against her based on her disability, that is, her status as a recovering drug-dependent person.

*Make a list of the major problems presented in this case*

- 
- 
- 
-

## *Hypothesis and mechanism*

For the problems in your list above, give a cause or a reason for them to happen:

- 
- 
- 
- 

## *Learning issues*

Make a list of learning issues in the form of questions. Remember your goal is to gather the medical, social, and all other relevant facts that may apply to the case.

What does it mean for the employer to be responsible for the health and safety of all employees?
> Creates a safe and drug-free environment for all employees, patients, customers, and visitors within their facility
> Uses drug testing procedures to maintain pharmacists in a mentally alert state to serve the public properly
> Vicariously held liable for negligent acts of an employee based on the negligence of the employer in selecting or dealing with their employees
> Uses ten-panel drug screening test

What are the effects of employee impairment (focus on a pharmacist)?
> An impaired pharmacist may:
>> Dispense the wrong medication
>> Dispense the wrong strength of a medication
>> Make a labeling error
>> Fail to detect a serious drug–drug interaction

What adverse outcomes may result from this kind of impairment?
> Injury or death to patient
> Harm to business

What are employee arguments to oppose drug screening?
> Loss of privacy:
>> Disclosure of private information/personal medical information (heart condition, depression, epilepsy, or diabetes)
>> Employer monitoring of off-hour activities (drug ingested on Saturday night may give a positive drug test the following Monday, long after its effects have ceased)
> Damage to reputation:

Assumed guilty and must prove innocence (false positives: Advil for
marijuana, Nyquil for amphetamines, and Vicks Formula 44-M,
Nuprin, Contac, Sudafed, some herbal teas, and poppy seeds for
opiates)

Emotional distress:

Violation of constitutional rights

Embarrassment from being visually supervised while "pissing in a
cup"

Unemployment:

Unfair dismissal from existing job

Unfair not hired for new job

Does the Oath of a Pharmacist speak to the issue of impairment?

Oath of a Pharmacist: "I will maintain the highest principles of moral,
ethical, and legal conduct; I take these vows voluntarily with the full
realization of the responsibility with which I am entrusted by the
public."

How is the issue of confidentiality of research participants linked to impairment?

Federal Certificates of Confidentiality are issued in accordance with the
provision of Section 301(d) of the Public Health Service Act, 42 U.S.C.
Section 241(d). It protects the privacy of research subjects by withholding their identities from all persons not connected with the research. Certificates are available only for research of a sensitive
nature, such as sexual attitudes; use of alcohol, drugs; illegal conduct;
or a situation that could, if released, be reasonably damaging to an
individual's life.

U.S. federal law regulating participant substance abuse treatment links
authorizations for a release of information to the right to consent for
treatment. Thus, only participants may authorize a release of information in states where participants may independently consent to
treatment.

Even with a signed authorization by the participant, U.S. federal law
acknowledges that, without a court order, the final decision concerning release of any information generally rests with the researcher
(Code of Federal Regulations, Title 42, 1995).

Discuss some of the issues surrounding drug testing in the workplace.

Medical surveillance is a proactive stance to meet and concur with the
Drug Free Workplace Act to protect and provide a safe and healthy
environment for all.

The fundamental purpose of surveillance is to detect and eliminate the
underlying causes of any discovered trends; thus, it has a prevention
focus.

Pharmacy's chief professional concern is patient safety.

To keep their jobs, employees may be motivated to alter their urine samples as they are coercively tested to be drug free.

Consequently, the goal of maintaining a safe and healthy working environment is compromised by the drug screening program itself.

Since drug testing only detects prior use of drugs, current work ability is not being tested.

A better method to determine mental fitness is psychomotor testing.

Psychomotor testing has the advantage of being noninvasive, so concerns over constitutional rights (Fourth Amendment, unreasonable search and seizure; Fifth Amendment, right not to self-incriminate) are not violated.

Psychomotor testing determines individual performance and does not penalize recovering addicts or divulge sensitive medical condition compared to drug testing.

## Literature review

To help you get ready to answer certain questions you anticipate being asked during the second part of the case, look in the local medical library and on the World Wide Web for helpful information. Please indicate in the spaces below (1) several helpful articles or books you found, and (2) several helpful Web sites you found.

- **Helpful articles:**
  Bramley, S., Medical records and the law, *BJU Int.*, 86, 286–290, 2000.
  Brody, J.L., Ethical issues in research on the treatment of adolescent substance abuse disorders, *Addict. Behav.*, 25, 217–228, 2000.
  Brown, N.A., Reining in the national drug testing epidemic (case note), *Harvard Civil Rights–Civil Liberties Law Rev.*, 33, 253–272, 1998.
  Carney, P., Current medicolegal and confidentiality issues in large, multicenter research programs, *Am. J. Epidemiol.*, 152, 371–378, 2000.
  Devon, D., Drug testing of health care workers: toward a coherent hospital policy, *Am. J. Law Med.*, 23, 399–448, 1997.
  McBay, A., Legal challenges to testing hair for drugs: a review, *Int. J. Drug Test.*, 1, 34–42, 2000.
  Silverglate, H.A., The right to private pee, *Natl. Law J.*, 22, 22, 2000.
  Simonsmeirer, L.M. and Fink, J.L. III, Legal implications of drug testing in the workplace, *Am. Pharm.*, 28, 30–37, 1988.
  Simonsmeirer, L.M. and Fox, L.A., The law and the impaired pharmacist, *Am. Pharm.*, 25, 63–68, 1985.
  Smith, R.S., Corporations that fail the fair hiring test, *Bus. Soc. Rev.* 88, 29–33, 1994.

- **Helpful Web sites:**
  Defense Environmental Network and Information Exchange:
  www.denix.osd.mil
  American Civil Liberties Union: www.aclu.org
  Department of Health and Human Services: www.health.org
  Drug Policy Foundation: www.soros.org/lindesmith/library/
  Tinelli2.html

## Identify all relevant values that play a role in the case and determine which values, if any, conflict

Nonmaleficence:

Beneficence:

Respect for persons:

Loyalty:

Distributive justice:

## Learning issues for next student-centered problem-based learning session

- List the options open to you. That is, answer the question, "What could you do?"
- Choose the best solution from an ethical point of view, justify it, and respond to possible criticisms. That is, answer the question, "What should you do, and why?"

- What are the different ways of thinking about the problem? Which conflict management techniques can be used in the situation?

## Part two

### Plaintiff's burden on summary judgment under the ADA

Under Section 12112 of the ADA (American with Disabilities Act) and Section 504 of the Rehabilitation Act of 1973 (42 U.S.C. § 794), when plaintiff presents only indirect evidence of discrimination, the court must address a motion of summary judgment within the three-stage, burden-shifting framework first outlined in *McDonnell Douglas Corporation v. Green* [411 U.S. 792, 802–805, 36 L. Ed. 2d 668, 93 S. Ct. 1817 (1973)] and was further explained and refined in *Texas Department of Community Affairs v. Burdine* [450 U.S. 248, 254–255, 67 L. Ed. 2d 207, 101 S. Ct. 1089 (1981)] and *St. Mary's Honor Ctr. v. Hicks* [509 U.S. 502, 506–508, 125 L. Ed. 2d 407, 113 S. Ct. 2742 (1993)]. "This framework allocates burdens of production and orders the presentation of evidence in disparate treatment cases so as to progressively 'sharpen the inquiry into the elusive factual questions of intentional discrimination'" (*Wooster*, 1996 WL 131143 at *8, quoting *Burdine*, 450 U.S. at 255 n.8).

The three stages can be summarized as follows (see *Thomas*, 183 F.3d at 56). First, plaintiff must establish by a preponderance of the evidence a *prima facie* case that she (1) was a member of the protected class (i.e., disabled within the meaning of the ADA and Rehabilitation Act of 1973), (2) was qualified for the job (i.e., she could perform the essential functions of her job with or without reasonable accommodations), and (3) was terminated from her job in whole or in part because of her disability [see *Katz v. City Metal Co.*, 87 F.3d 26, 30 (1st Cir. 1996)].

Once plaintiff establishes her *prima facie* case, at the second stage the burden shifts to the employer–defendant to produce a valid, nondiscriminatory reason for her dismissal (see *Thomas*, 183 F.3d at 56). At this stage, defendant has only a burden of production, and if sustained, the presumption of unlawful discrimination disappears [*Woodman v. Haemonetics Corp.*, 51 F.3d 1087, 1091 (1st Cir. 1995)].

At the third and final stage of the *McDonnell Douglas* framework, the burden shifts back to plaintiff. Now, she has the burden of persuasion to establish by a preponderance of the evidence that the employer's stated reason for her dismissal was a sham, or pretext, and that the real reason was discriminatory (see *Thomas*, 183 F.3d at 56)."At the third stage," the First Circuit Court of Appeals has recently held:

> the ultimate burden is on the plaintiff to persuade the trier of fact that she has been treated differently because of her [disability]. . . . This burden is often broken into two separate tasks. The plaintiff must present sufficient evidence to show both that "the employer's articulated reason for

*[terminating] plaintiff is [1] a pretext" and [2] that "the*
*true reason is discriminatory." . . . For expository conve-*
*nience this court . . . has referred to the First Circuit rule*
*as a "pretext-plus" standard. (Thomas, 183 F.3d at 56).*

## Plaintiff's burden on summary judgment under state law

The courts of this commonwealth follow the same three-stage *McDonnell Douglas* analysis for claims arising under Mass. Gen. Laws ch. 151B [see *Wheelock College v. Massachusetts Comm'n Against Discrimination*, 371 Mass. 130, 134–136, 355 N.E.2d 309 (1976)]. But, plaintiff's burden for avoiding summary judgment is less onerous under ch. 151B because the Supreme Judicial Court identifies Massachusetts as a "pretext only" state [see *Blare v. Husky Injection Molding Systems Boston, Inc.*, 419 Mass. 437, 444–445, 646 N.E.2d 111 (1995)]. In other words, to prevail at the third stage of the burden-shifting regime, plaintiff "must persuade the fact finder by a fair preponderance of the evidence that the defendant's asserted reasons were not the real reasons . . . [for plaintiff's discharge]" [id. at 443, citing *Brunner v. Stone and Webster Engineering Corp.*, 413 Mass. 698, 700, 603 N.E.2d 206 (1992)]. Thus, with respect to summary judgment under ch. 151B, this court must consider "whether there is evidence which generates a genuine dispute of fact on the pretext point" [*Wooster v. Abdow Corp.*, 46 Mass. App. Ct. 665, 669, 709 N.E.2d 71 (1999)(citations omitted)].

## Federal law claims

As stated above, to avoid summary judgment on the claims under the ADA and the Rehabilitation Act, plaintiff must produce enough evidence to raise a triable issue with respect to the three elements of her *prima facie* case. She must provide evidence that (1) she suffers from a "disability," (2) that she was nevertheless qualified for the job, and (3) that Franklin discharged her in whole or in part because of her disability (*Katz*, 87 F.3d at 30). Defendants concede that plaintiff is disabled, and so the court will not analyze the disability issue in this case. However, defendants argue that summary judgment is appropriate because plaintiff cannot make out the "qualification prong" of her *prima facie* case.

### Qualification analysis

It is well settled that, in an ADA case, plaintiff has the burden of showing she is a qualified individual [see *EEOC [Equal Employment Opportunity Commission] v. Amego, Inc.*, 110 F.3d 135, 141 (1st Cir. 1997)]. Under the ADA, the qualification prong of the *prima facie* case is met by showing (1) that the employee satisfied the prerequisites for the position such as experience, education, and other job-related requirements; and (2) that she, with or without reasonable accommodation, can perform the essential functions of such position held or desired [id. at 145 n.7; see 42 U.S.C. § 12111(8); 29 C.F.R.

§ 1630.2(m)]. However, the ADA also says that "the term 'qualification stan-dards' may include a requirement that an individual shall not pose a direct threat to the health and safety of other individuals in the workplace" [42 U.S.C. § 12113(b)]. Therefore, when the essential job functions "necessarily implicate the safety of others, plaintiff must demonstrate that she can per-form those functions in a way that does not endanger others" (*Amego*, 110 F.3d at 144).

Defendants argue that plaintiff is not qualified because she cannot show that she can perform an essential function of the job — overseeing and administering medications — in a way that does not endanger others. They point to the fact that shortly after the hospital lifted her restriction on admin-istering medications, she violated nursing protocols by asking another nurse to administer a narcotic that she prepared, by not obtaining cosignatures for wasted narcotics, by not recording her narcotic administrations in the MAR, and by administering narcotics to a patient for whom all other nurses admin-istered Tylenol. Moreover, defendants argue that these facts are analogous to *EEOC v. Amego, Inc.* [110 F.3d 135 (1st Cir. 1997)], for which the court held that summary judgment was appropriate when the record supported an employer's determination that an employee, who suffered from depression, was unqualified to administer and monitor patients' medication at a resi-dence for severely disabled individuals in light of evidence that the employee made two suicide attempts by medication overdoses (id. at 144–147). As in *Amego*, defendants argue, Franklin's determination that it could not trust Griel to do the medication-related functions of her job was both plausible and supported by undisputed facts; in addition, this court should not sec-ond-guess the hospital's judgment in matters of patient safety (see *Amego*, 110 F.3d at 147).

On this close question, it appears, however, that Griel's situation is distinguishable from plaintiff's situation in *Amego*, and that the record shows sufficient evidence to raise a triable issue as to whether Griel could perform her medication-related job functions without directly threatening others. In determining that plaintiff had failed to prove she was not a "direct threat" to others, the *Amego* court relied on several factors that are absent here. It found, first, that the risk of harm was extremely difficult to guard against because the severely disabled patients were particularly vulnerable to abuse and neglect, and there were no obvious mechanisms to ensure that they were being properly medicated. Here, Franklin had mechanisms that ensured patients were being medicated properly, such as the notations on the medical charts, the sign out and waste procedures governing narcotic administration, the inputting of data in the computer, and the observations of nurses on other shifts. Second, the *Amego* court noted that other measures had not eliminated the risk that the plaintiff had been mishandling medication. For example, plaintiff in *Amego* was obviously not responding to counseling — having attempted suicide — and she failed to complete her therapy sessions despite a modified work schedule. Here, on the other hand, Griel was attending therapy sessions conscientiously, took and passed every drug test that Franklin requested, and attended Alcoholics Anonymous and Nursing Association meetings regularly. Moreover, despite the lapses in protocol, there is no objective evidence that Griel actually compromised the safety of her patients. The evidence of direct threat to patients in this case is so much less than it was in *Amego* that the court cannot rely on it to grant summary judgment.

The weakness of the evidence of record favoring the defendant on this point is further underscored by the strength of the evidence favoring the plaintiff. For example, plaintiff's experts independently reviewed the medical records of the five patients that raised patient safety concerns for defendants. One expert concluded that she "found no deviation from the accepted standards of nursing care on the part of Dolores Griel, R.N. She documented her patients' needs for pain management, intervened appropriately with the proper medication given in the prescribed dose ranges, and she documented the effects of her interventions. The patients appeared to suffer no ill effects after being in her care" (plaintiff's exhibits, Docket No. 45, Exhibit 13 at 22–23). A second expert concluded that "it is my opinion that there were no deviations from accepted standards of nursing care on the part of nurse, Dolores Griel, R.N." (id. Exhibit 14 at 3). Given this body of evidence the court cannot fairly say that no reasonable jury could conclude that plaintiff can perform her job safely, that is, that she is a qualified individual. It therefore follows that plaintiff has cleared the first stage of the [*10] *McDonnell Douglas* analysis and sufficiently established her *prima facie* case.

Before moving to the second portion of the burden-shifting framework, it is worth pausing to address defendant's concern over the status of plaintiff's expert evidence. In their briefs, defendants have moved to strike this evidence. This court disagrees for the following reasons.

Under Fed.R.CIV.P. 56(e), "expert opinion is admissible and may defeat summary judgment only where it appears that the affiant is competent to give an expert opinion" [*Garside v. Osco Drug, Inc.*, 895 F.2d 46, 50 (1st Cir. 1990)]. Here, plaintiff submitted affidavits and two corresponding 26(a)(2)(B) expert reports by Betsy Green, R.N., and Denise Schoen, R.N. Betsy Green is a Massachusetts registered nurse employed as a family nurse practitioner at the Northampton Health Center and the Cooley Dickinson Hospital in Northampton, Massachusetts. She has over 14 years of experience as an acute care nurse, most of which was spent in a critical care unit similar to the one at Franklin. She also holds a master's degree in nursing. Denise Schoen is a Massachusetts registered nurse, employed as an administrative supervisor, and she has over 15 years experience as an acute care nurse in the intensive care/cardiac care/telemetry units at the Cooley Dickinson Hospital in Northampton. Schoen is also a part-time instructor of clinical nursing at Greenfield Community College. Thus, both nurses appear competent to give an expert opinion about whether Griel deviated from accepted standards of nursing care with respect to the five patients at issue in this case.

Moreover, both opinions have a sufficient foundation. "It is fundamental that expert testimony must be predicated on facts legally sufficient to provide a basis for the expert's opinion . . . [thus] an expert should not be permitted to give an opinion that is based on conjecture or speculation from an insufficient evidentiary foundation" [*Damon v. Sun Co.*, 87 F.3d 1467, 1474 (1st Cir. 1996) (internal quotation marks omitted)]. Here, both experts rendered their opinions by reviewing the medical records of the five patients, including the nurses' progress notes. Moreover, both presented detailed and well-reasoned opinions grounded in this data. Thus, this court finds no reason to strike this evidence from this summary judgment proceeding.

### McDonnell Douglas analysis

Since plaintiff can make out her *prima facie* case, the burden now shifts to defendants to articulate a nondiscriminatory reason for terminating Griel. In this case, defendant employer has provided such a reason: Griel's continued employment posed an unacceptable risk to patient safety. This reason is legitimate, nondiscriminatory, and adequately supported by the undisputed evidence. The conclusion that the defendants have indisputably offered a legitimate, nondiscriminatory justification for their termination of Griel is in no way inconsistent with the court's conclusion above, that plaintiff has made out a sufficiently supported *prima facie* case for a least two reasons. First, defendants' burden at this stage is only to articulate a plausible justification; this they have certainly done. Concern about patient safety might well justify an employer's decision to terminate a health care provider. Second, the fact that a jury could conclude that plaintiff was a qualified individual in the sense that she posed no immediate, objective threat to the health and safety of patients in no way rebuts defendants' contention that their concern about patient safety was sincere and well supported. Certainly, the proffered justification is not specious on its face.

Since defendants have provided a legitimate nondiscriminatory reason for their action, the initial presumption of discrimination drops from the case, and the burden now shifts back to plaintiff to prove discrimination (see *Thomas*, 183 F.3d at 61–62; [*11] see also *Hicks*, 509 U.S. at 510–511). Specifically, plaintiff must "produce evidence to create a genuine issue of fact with respect to two points: [1] whether the employer's articulated [nondiscriminatory] reason for its adverse action was a pretext and [2] whether the real reason was [handicap] discrimination" (*Thomas*, 183 F.3d at 62). In other words, plaintiff "must produce evidence to permit a reasonable jury to conclude both that disparate treatment occurred and that the difference in treatment was because of [discrimination]" (id.). Since this court finds that plaintiff has not produced enough evidence to show pretext, the following discussion will analyze only that prong.

The key to showing pretext in a disparate treatment case is comparative evidence; see *McDonnell Douglas*, 411 U.S. at 804 ("Especially relevant to [a showing of pretext] would be evidence that [nonprotected] employees involved in acts against [the employer] of comparable seriousness . . . were nevertheless retained or rehired"); *Thomas v. Eastman Kodak Co.*, 183 F.3d 38, 62 (1st Cir. 1999) ("The [pretext] portion of [plaintiff's] third-stage burden is to produce sufficient evidence to show that she was not evaluated on the same terms as her colleagues, but rather was evaluated more harshly than other nonminority [colleagues]"). Here, "the plaintiff has the burden of showing that she was treated differently from similarly situated [nonhand-icapped] persons" [*Smith v. Stratus Computer, Inc.*, 40 F.3d 11, 17 (1st Cir. 1994)]. She must "identify and relate specific instances where persons simi-larly situated 'in all relevant respects' were treated differently" [*Dartmouth Review v. Dartmouth College*, 889 F.2d 13, 19 (1st Cir. 1989)]. In addition, she must identify these instances "in terms of performance, qualifications and conduct, 'without such differentiating or mitigating circumstances that would distinguish' their situations" [*Stratus Computer*, 40 F.3d at 17 (quoting *Mitchell v. Toledo Hospital*, 964 F.2d 577, 583 (6th Cir. 1992)] [**28] [see *Rod-riguez-Cuervos v. Wal-Mart Stores, Inc.*, 181 F.3d 15, 21 (1st Cir. 1999) (sum-marizing this test for showing pretext)].

Griel proffers the following evidence to show disparate treatment. First, she claims that, while she was placed on a 3-month restriction for her January documentation errors, others were sent to documentation courses or were given verbal or written warnings. Second, while her failure to get signatures for narcotic waste led to her dismissal, it was a ground for merely monitoring others for improvement. In fact, plaintiff noted that discovery revealed over 114 errors in the narcotic administration sheets made by others; defendants have produced no evidence that anyone was disciplined or terminated for these mistakes. Third, while plaintiff concedes that her violation of the rule against administering a drug another nurse drew was very serious and in itself a legitimate ground for termination, Franklin only gave Leete, the other nurse involved in that March incident, a general reprimand.

In response, defendants make two points. First, Griel's mistakes were not evaluated in isolation, one by one, but together as a pattern. Defendants admit that a nurse may make isolated mistakes, such as a failure to obtain a cosignature, and not be disciplined or at least not disciplined severely. But, in Griel's case, she committed three mistakes in March, with two mistakes (failure to obtain a cosignature and failure to document morphine adminis-tration) occurring on the same shift for the same patient. Moreover, these mistakes, according to defendants, continued a pattern of problems that was viewed in the context of the January incidents. Plaintiff cannot identify any other nurse who committed such a series of mistakes, much less committed them within a few weeks after having a narcotics restriction lifted. In other words, defendants claim that no evidence exists of another nurse who was not a former substance abuser who engaged in a similar pattern of mistakes and was not discharged.

Second, according to defendants, even if Franklin terminated Griel based on the incidents in isolation, her violation in March 1997 of the "you draw, you administer" rule was by itself serious enough that Franklin would have fired any nondisabled similarly situated nurse. Defendants explain that Leete was given only a reprimand because she was a new nurse and came forward immediately. Griel, on the other hand, was an experienced nurse, who first denied the accusation and who had just come off restrictions.

Given this pattern of mistakes, defendants are correct that plaintiff proffers insufficient evidence to avoid summary judgment. There is simply no evidence in the record that a nonhandicapped person "similarly situated in all relevant respects" was, or would have been, treated differently (*Dartmouth*, 889 F.2d at 19). In other words, plaintiff provides no evidence that would remotely justify a jury in concluding a nurse who was not a former substance abuser and who committed a similar pattern of similar mistakes was not (or would not have been) terminated.

Moreover, even if Franklin terminated Griel based solely on her violation of the you draw, you administer rule, and not on any pattern of mistakes, she still has not produced sufficient evidence to avoid summary judgment. The evidence is essentially unrebutted that violating this rule is rare and very serious. Although plaintiff's experts rebut the seriousness and the rarity of the documentation and cosignature problems, they are conspicuously silent about Griel's violation of this rule. Griel's only evidence for disparate treatment on this point is that Leete, a neophyte, was treated differently when she participated at Griel's request in violation of this serious rule. But, to use this evidence to raise a genuine issue of material fact, Griel would have to proffer additional evidence to show that she and Leete were similarly situated "in terms of performance, qualifications and conduct, 'without such differentiating or mitigating circumstances that would distinguish' their situations" (*Stratus Computer*, 40 F.3d at 17).

In fact, the evidence is clear that Leete and Griel are not similarly situated. As noted, Leete was new and inexperienced, while Griel had been employed at Franklin since 1992, had been a nurse since 1988, had been recently retrained after returning from her back injury, and had been on restrictions for other mishaps. Leete was forthright in her conduct, while Griel equivocated. Thus, Griel's only evidence of disparate treatment is Franklin's treatment of Leete. Despite plaintiff's counsel's hard work and vigorous argument, this evidence is simply not enough for a reasonable jury to find pretext.

Moreover, there is evidence that, of all the nurses that Franklin terminated in the past 5 years, each committed violations comparable in seriousness to Griel's violations. For example, two were fired for falsifying time cards, and one was caught diverting drugs. Plaintiff argues that these violations are different from hers. But, all that is required for the comparison is that they are of "comparable seriousness," not that they are the identical violation (see *McDonnell Douglas*, 411 U.S. at 804). Since plaintiff offers no evidence that her violation of the you draw, you administer rule was not less serious than the violations used to terminate other nurses, she has not met her burden to show pretext and to avoid summary judgment on her federal claims.

## State law claim

As noted above, Mass. Gen. Laws ch. 151B differs from the federal approach in that, to avoid summary judgment, plaintiff need only show pretext (see *Blare*, 419 Mass. at 444–445). However, with respect to what evidence plaintiff must proffer to demonstrate pretext, the commonwealth has adopted the federal approach requiring the use of comparative evidence [*Matthews v. Ocean Spray Cranberries, Inc.*, 426 Mass. 122, 129–130, 686 N.E.2d 1303 (1997), "adopting the approach taken by" *Dartmouth* and *Smith* whereby plaintiff must identify specific instances when nonhandicapped persons with similar performance, qualifications, and conduct were treated differently].

It is true, as plaintiff points out, that the record contains some evidence of comments by defendants regarding plaintiff's prior drug history. For example, Palmeri noted that it was possible that Griel was diverting drugs, and Moore commented about possibly firing Griel before properly investigating the matter. Under Massachusetts law, however, verbal remarks insufficient to provide direct evidence of discrimination will not, by themselves, demonstrate pretext, but assist in doing so only if linked with comparative evidence demonstrating disparate treatment. See *Tardanico v. Aetna Life and Casualty, Company* [41 Mass. App. Ct. 443, 450, 671 N.E.2d 510 (1996)], granting summary judgment and holding that "isolated or ambiguous remarks, tending to suggest animus . . . are insufficient standing alone, to prove a defendant's discriminatory intent"; *Finney v. Madico, Inc.* (42 Mass. App. Ct. 46, 51, 674 N.E.2d 655 (1997)], reversing summary judgment because plaintiff linked nine remarks sounding of bias against female managers to evidence that defendant laid off only female managers. Here, even if these comments suggest bias, plaintiff has not linked them to evidence of disparate treatment. Therefore, since plaintiff has failed to produce enough evidence to show pretext on her federal claims, summary judgment is appropriate with respect to the ch. 151B claim as well. See *Mullin v. Raytheon Co.*, 164 F.3d 696, 699 (1st Cir. 1999), affirming district court's holding that if "plaintiff makes no showing of pretext, then the state and federal analyses collapse into one another and the summary judgment motion is decided according to familiar standards" [*Mullin v. Raytheon Co.*, 2 F. Supp. 2d 165, 172 (D. Mass. 1998)].

---

*List the options open to you. That is, answer the question, "What could you do?"*

- 
- 
- 
-

*Choose the best solution from an ethical point of view, justify it, and
respond to possible criticisms. That is, answer the question,
"What should you do, and why?"*

- 
- 
- 
- 

*Select one member of your PBL group to role-play as Dolores Griel
and have another member of your PBL group role-play as
William Garrand. How might the two converse about different
ways of thinking and techniques for conflict management?*

- 
- 
- 
- 

*Again, please select one member of your PBL group to role-play as
Dolores Griel and have another member of your PBL group
role-play as William Garrand. How might Dolores Griel use
what is known about stages of change and about motivational
interviewing to solve what you consider the major problem
presented in the case?*

- 
- 
- 
- 

## Part three

Plaintiff provided enough evidence to support a prima facie case for disability discrimination under federal and state law. Defendants, in turn, provided sufficient evidence to rebut plaintiff's prima facie case by providing a legitimate nondiscriminatory reason for her termination, namely, patient safety. To avoid summary judgment, plaintiff had to point to sufficient evidence of record to show that defendants' reason was a sham (i.e., a pretext) by demonstrating that defendants treated other nondisabled, but otherwise similar, nurses differently. As noted, counsel has been vigorous in presenting the record in the light most favorable to plaintiff, but the evidence is just not there. No genuine issue of material fact exists for a jury to resolve. For the forgoing reasons, defendants' motion for summary judgment is allowed on all counts.

## Conclusion

A monitoring system is required to protect the public. As professionals, pharmacists have taken the oath to do no harm. The key is preventing negligence.

# *Index*